DEDICATION

To my son, Christopher Tobias

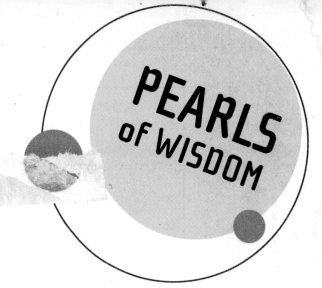

Psychiatry
BOARD REVIEW

Third Edition

Rebecca A. Schmidt, MD
President and Chief Executive
Adult, Child, and Adolescent Psychiatric Associates of Omaha
Assistant Clinical Professor
Department of Psychiatry
Creighton University School of Medicine
Omaha, Nebraska

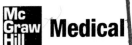 **Medical**

New York   Chicago   San Francisco   Lisbon   London   Madrid   Mexico City   Milan
New Delhi   San Juan   Seoul   Singapore   Sydney   Toronto

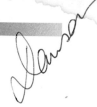
Psychiatry Board Review: Pearls of Wisdom, Third Edition

1 2 3 4 5 6 7 8 9 0   QPDQPD   12 11 10 9

ISBN 978-0-07-154971-4
MHID 0-07-154971-4

Notice

Medicine is an ever-changing science. As new research and clinical experience broaden our knowledge, changes in treatment and drug therapy are required. The author and the publisher of this work have checked with sources believed to be reliable in their efforts to provide information that is complete and generally in accord with the standards accepted at the time of publication. However, in view of the possibility of human error or changes in medical sciences, neither the author nor the publisher nor any other party who has been involved in the preparation or publication of this work warrants that the information contained herein is in every respect accurate or complete, and they disclaim all responsibility for any errors or omissions or for the results obtained from use of the information contained in this work. Readers are encouraged to confirm the information contained herein with other sources. For example, and in particular, readers are advised to check the product information sheet included in the package of each drug they plan to administer to be certain that the information contained in this work is accurate and that changes have not been made in the recommended dose or in the contraindications for administration. This recommendation is of particular importance in connection with new or infrequently used drugs.

This book was set in Adobe Garamond by Aptara®, Inc.
The editors were Kirsten Funk and Peter J. Boyle.
The production supervisor was Sherri Souffrance.
Project management was provided by Deepa Krishnan, Aptara®, Inc.
The cover designer was Handel Low.
The text designer was Eve Siegel.
Quebecor Dubuque was printer and binder.

This book is printed on acid-free paper.

Library of Congress Cataloging-in-Publication Data

Psychiatry board review / [edited by] Rebecca A. Schmidt. – 3rd ed.
    p. ; cm. – (Pearls of wisdom)
  Includes bibliographical references.
  ISBN-13: 978-0-07-154971-4 (pbk. : alk. paper)
  ISBN-10: 0-07-154971-4 (alk. paper)
 1. Psychiatry–Examinations, questions, etc.   I. Schmidt, Rebecca A.
II. Series: Pearls of wisdom.
  [DNLM: 1. Mental Disorders–Examination Questions.   WM 18.2 P97315 2009]
  RC457.P7755 2009
  616.890076–dc22

                                    2009008591

CONTENTS

SECTION I. GENERAL INFORMATION

SECTION II. PSYCHOPATHOLOGY

SECTION III. SPECIAL TOPICS

SECTION IV. SELECT TOPICS IN CHILD PSYCHIATRY

SECTION V. TREATMENT MODALITIES

CONTRIBUTORS

Editor

Rebecca A. Schmidt, MD
President and Chief Executive
Adult, Child, and Adolescent Psychiatric Associates of Omaha
Assistant Clinical Professor
Department of Psychiatry
Creighton University School of Medicine
Omaha, Nebraska

Contributors to This Edition

Judy M. Kisicki, MD
Psychiatrist
Waukesha Memorial Hospital
Waukesha, Wisconsin
ProHealth Care Medical Associates
Oconomowoc Memorial Hospital
Oconomowoc, Wisconsin

William E. Reay, PhD
President and Chief Executive
OMNI Behavioral Health
Omaha, Nebraska
Associate Professor of Psychology
Director, Mental Health Counseling Programs
Northcentral University
Prescott Valley, Arizona

Loreen M. Riedler, MD
Assistant Professor
Department of Psychiatry
Creighton Medical Center
Assistant Professor
Department of Psychiatry
Nebraska Medical Center
Alegent Health Psychiatric Associates
Omaha, Nebraska

Richard Starlin, MD
Infectious Disease and Epidemiology Associates
Clinical Assistant Professor
Department of Internal Medicine
Division of Infectious Diseases
University of Nebraska Medical Center
Omaha, Nebraska

Contributors to Previous Editions

Vimal M. Aga, MD

Anis Ahmed, MD

Ronald C. Albucher, MD

Nicolas Baida-Fragoso, MD

Teresita Awa Bajas, MD*

Denise Barron-Kraus, DO

Ranita Basu, MD

Jennifer Berg, MD

Chad Bradford, MD

Guy E. Brannon, MD

Beverly R. Delaney, MD

John DeQuardo, MD

Karnail S. Dhillon, MD

Theodore B. Feldman, MD

Mary Jo Fitz-Gerald, MD

Kishorchandra Gonsai, MD

Robert J. Gregory, MD

Edward E. Hunter, PhD

Gagan Joshi, MD

Anita S. Kablinger, MD

Helen C. Kales, MD

Gopi Kalla, MBBS*

Jordan Klesmer, MD

Michael Larson, DO

Rajnish Mago, MD

Daniel Maixner, MD

Susan M. Maixner, MD

David M. Marks, MD

Alan M. Mellow, MD, PhD

Merry Miller, MD

K. E. Mitchell, MD

Managalore N. Pai, MD

Melissa Piasecki, MD

Charles J. Rainey, MD, JD

Arthur L. Ramirez, MD

Amaro Reyes, MD

Philip D. Rolland, RPh

Maria Rowdowski, MD

Kemal Sagduyu, MD

Leonard Salazar, MD

Thomas L. Schwartz, MD

Andrew Sewell, MD

Kori Levos Skidmore, PhD

David T. Springer, MD

Oladapo Tomori, MD

Elizabeth Tully, MD

Stacy Volkert, MD

Zia Wahid, MD

William W. Wang, MD, PhD

James A. Wilcox, DO, PhD

Elizabeth Yager, MD

Sidney Zisook, MD

---

*Deceased

INTRODUCTION

Welcome to *Psychiatry Board Review: Pearls of Wisdom.* This text is designed as a study aid to improve performance on the American Board of Psychiatry and Neurology written board examination. Since this book is primarily intended as a study aid, the text is written in a rapid-fire question/answer format. This way, readers receive immediate gratification. Moreover, misleading or confusing foils are not provided. Questions themselves often contain a pearl intended to reinforce the answer. Additional "hooks" may be attached to the answer in various forms, including mnemonics, repetition, and humor. Additional information not requested in the question may be included in the answer. Emphasis has been placed on distilling key facts that are easily overlooked, and quickly forgotten, and, yet, somehow, seem to be needed on board exams.

Many questions have answers without explanations. This enhances ease of reading and rate of learning. Explanations often occur in a later question/answer. Upon reading an answer, the reader may think, "Hmm, why is that?" If this happens to you, go check! Truly assimilating these disparate facts into a framework of knowledge absolutely requires further reading of the surrounding concepts. Information learned in response to seeking an answer to a question is retained better than information that is passively observed. Take advantage of this! Use this book with your preferred source texts handy and open.

This third edition of *Psychiatry Board Review* is separated into five different sections. Section I includes general information related to psychiatry, while Section II addresses specific diagnostic categories. Section III covers special topics associated with psychiatry, and Section IV discusses select psychiatric topics unique to children. Section V concludes the book with a review of psychopharmacology and psychotherapy strategies.

One will find that some information is repeated in various sections, which builds on one's ability to retain the facts necessary to pass board examinations. All efforts have been made to verify information from references with the most accurate information. However, this book does have limitations. Conflicting information can occur between sources and at times within the same source, thereby confounding clarification. Furthermore, new research and practice occasionally deviates from that which likely represents the correct answer for test purposes. As this text is designed to maximize your score on a test, please refer to your mentors and most current sources of information for direction in practice.

Your comments, suggestions, and criticisms are welcome. Please make us aware of any errors you find. As impeccable quality and continuous improvement are the goals of this review text, we would greatly appreciate your input with regard to format, organization, content, presentation, and specific questions. We look forward to hearing from you.

Study hard and good luck!

R.A.S.

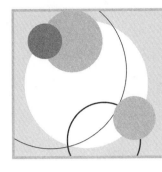

Section I

GENERAL INFORMATION

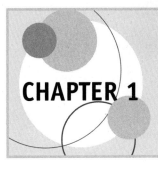

CHAPTER 1
Classification of Mental Disorders

○ **How does the *Diagnostic and Statistical Manual of Mental Disorders, Fourth Edition (DSM-IV)*, compare to the *International Classification of Diseases, 10th Revision (ICD-10)*?**

The *ICD-10*, which is the official system used in Europe, and the *DSM-IV* were developed in a coordinated fashion. The terms in both classification systems and codes correlate and are fully compatible, although the wording may differ. All the *DSM-IV* categories are found in *ICD-10*, but not all *ICD-10* categories are found in *DSM-IV*.

○ **What is the official nomenclature of American psychiatry?**

The *DSM-IV*, published in 1994, is the official nomenclature for psychiatry (as well as other mental health professions) in the United States. The *DSM-IV* is a result of a three-stage revision process, including reviews of scientific literature, data reanalyses, and field trials of diagnostic criteria.

○ **The original *Diagnostic and Statistical Manual of Mental Disorders*, published in 1952 by the American Psychiatric Association, was essentially developed as an adaptation of what publication?**

The Medical 203, a classification system established after World War II by the U.S. Army. Developed by William C. Menniger and others, the Medical 203 was heavily influenced by the theories of Adolph Meyer, who proposed that mental health disorders were a result of one's "reactions" to their environment.

○ **How did the *DSM-II* differ from the *DSM-I*?**

Use of the term "reaction" was discontinued, but use of the term "neurosis" was continued.

○ **Define the difference between "psychosis" and "neurosis."**

According to American Psychiatric Association terminology, the word "psychosis" indicates severe impairment in reality testing and includes delusions and hallucinations, without insight. The *DSM-IV* does not include use of the term "neurosis" in its official nomenclature, but the term is generally accepted to mean a disorder with prominent anxiety and no psychotic features. (The *ICD-10* does include a category of "neurotic" disorders.) On a side note, suggested omission of neurosis from the *DSM-III*, almost caused the APA Board of Trustees to not approve the *DSM-III* for publication in the late 1970s.

○ **How did the *DSM-III*, published in 1980, differ from the *DSM-I* and *DSM-II*?**

The *DSM-III* represented the first widespread use of diagnostic criteria (descriptors) to define mental health disorders in a manner that did not imply etiology. In addition, a multiaxial assessment system was introduced to help "plan treatment and predict outcome."

○ **How many editions of the *DSM* are there?**

Six, soon to be seven: *DSM-I, DSM-II, DSM-III, DSM-III-R, DSM-IV,* and *DSM-IV-TR* (text-revision). The *DSM-V* is due out in 2012.

○ **What disorders are classified on Axis I?**

Major mental health disorders, developmental disorders, and learning disorders. If relational problems (i.e., "V codes" (which include sexual and physical abuse)) are the main reason for treatment, they are also listed on Axis I. If not a focus of treatment, the relational problems are listed on Axis II.

○ **How is Axis II used in the multiaxial evaluation?**

Axis II describes personality disorders as well as mental retardation. Axis II can also be used to describe defense mechanisms characteristic of a certain patient.

○ **What conditions are listed on Axis III?**

Acute and chronic medical conditions.

○ **What is the use of Axis IV?**

Axis IV describes stressors that are part of the patient's presentation. The clinician may consider both positive and negative stressors, as well as the significance of these events on the patient's functioning.

○ **What are general areas to consider for Axis IV?**

Axis IV addresses problems that may occur in the following areas: primary support group, social environment, education, occupation, housing, economics, health care services, and the legal system.

○ **What is the Global Assessment of Functioning (GAF) Scale?**

The GAF is a scale used by clinicians to describe a patient's level of functioning in three areas: social (i.e., marriage, friends), occupational, and psychological. The GAF scale ranges from 100 (highest functioning) to 0. The GAF is recorded on Axis V.

○ **When is the term "provisional" appropriate in evaluating a patient?**

"Provisional" is used when some of the criteria for the diagnosis are present but not all the data are available at the time of presentation. This could be true for the patient who cannot provide a complete history or when exclusionary information (such as laboratory tests to rule out the role of substances) is not available.

○ **How does a health care professional communicate diagnostic uncertainty with a diagnosis?**

Health care professionals have several means of communicating diagnostic uncertainty with a *DSM-IV* diagnosis. They can describe a diagnosis as provisional or atypical, depending on the patient's history and presentation. Health care professionals can also defer the diagnosis or use "NOS type" within a diagnostic category when they are uncertain about the specific subtype of a diagnosis.

○ **How does a health care professional indicate the severity of a patient's clinical presentation?**

DSM-IV guidelines for severity ratings relate to the diagnostic criteria as well as a patient's level of functioning. If a patient's symptoms just meet the level of criteria necessary for the diagnosis and the symptoms lead to mild impairment, the severity is "mild." "Severe" indicates that many more symptoms are present than are necessary to meet diagnostic criteria and that impairment is significant. "Moderate" severity is intermediate.

○ **How does a health care professional describe a mental disorder secondary to a medical condition, such as major depression secondary to hypothyroidism?**

Mental disorders, which are attributable to an underlying medical condition, are listed under Axis I (i.e., mood disorder due to hypothyroidism). The medical condition is also listed on Axis III.

○ **What does "not otherwise specified" (NOS) mean?**

In the *DSM-IV*, NOS is used if the patient's symptoms do not meet criteria for a specific diagnosis—the symptoms are either below the threshold of the criteria or present in mixed or atypical manner. The term NOS is also used when the clinician is uncertain about the etiology of a patient's symptoms (i.e., depression which is primary vs. depression which is secondary to cocaine use).

○ **What is meant by "diagnostic hierarchy"?**

DSM-IV uses a hierarchical scheme to approach diagnoses. This means that certain diagnoses preclude others, such as a substance-induced depression preempting a diagnosis of major depressive disorder. Other hierarchical considerations are when a more pervasive disorder (such as schizophrenia) preempts a less pervasive disorder. Exclusionary criteria are specifically listed as part of the *DSM-IV* criteria and are also reflected in the *DSM-IV* decision trees in the back of the manual.

○ **What is the time criterion for substance-induced disorders?**

For a disorder to be considered directly related to substance use, the *DSM-IV* indicates that the symptoms develop within a month of the substance use. There are times when the symptoms persist beyond 1 month. "Substances" can include medications.

○ **What are the key features of a defined "mental disorder"?**

To be defined as a disorder, the symptoms must be associated with distress and disability or with the risk of "suffering, death, pain, disability, or an important loss of freedom." The symptoms must not be limited to a culturally accepted response to stressors (such as acute bereavement).

○ **Does the *DSM-IV* include any conditions that are not "psychiatric disorders" at this time?**

The *DSM-IV* includes a section on "Other Conditions That May Be a Focus of Clinical Attention." This section includes new or controversial categories under study. Examples of diagnoses in this section include caffeine withdrawal, premenstrual dysphoric disorder, and mixed anxiety-depressive disorder.

○ **When should a health care professional use his or her clinical judgment in using the *DSM-IV*?**

Always! The *DSM-IV* is meant as a *guide* and not as a rigid document. The sequential changes in the *DSM-IV*, with resulting changes in criteria and even the addition or deletion of entire diagnoses, indicate the limitations of the categorical approach and the need for clinical judgment to always be part of a diagnosis.

○ **What is a "V code"?**

A "V code" is a code used to describe a clinical condition that may be important in the overall clinical presentation but not a disorder. Examples of V codes include partner or sibling relational problems, problems related to abuse or neglect, and phase of life problems or bereavement. "No disorder" on Axis I or Axis II is also listed as a V code (V71.09).

○ **What is the use of rating scales in psychiatry?**

Rating scales allow the quantitative measure of a patient's symptoms or functioning. Scales add data to the clinical database and are helpful in measuring treatment effects over time. Rating scales may be clinician rated or patient rated.

○ **What is the Brief Psychiatric Rating Scale (BPRS)?**

The BPRS is a rating scale that assigns number values to 18 different symptoms. The BPRS addresses more severe problems, such as psychosis, and is often used as an outcome measure in clinical trials of antipsychotic medications.

○ **What is the Hamilton Anxiety Scale (HAM-A)?**

The HAM-A is a rating scale that is clinician rated. It assesses a variety of somatic and psychological symptoms of anxiety. The Hamilton Depression Scale (HAM-D) is a clinician-rated depression scale that similarly assesses and assigns a numerical value to the degree of depression found in a patient. Both of these scales are frequently used in the clinical setting as well as in clinical trials of interventions for depression and anxiety.

○ **What is the Beck Depression Inventory (BDI)?**

The BDI is a rating scale that is patient rated. The questions on the BDI target cognitive symptoms and, compared to the HAM-D, has much less emphasis on somatic symptoms. The BDI has wide use both in the clinical setting (where it is easily administered to patients) and in research of depression.

○ **What are some of the advantages to using the *DSM-IV* approach?**

With the *DSM-IV*, the reliability of diagnosis is improved (although never perfect). That is, two observers of the same patient would be likely to agree on the diagnosis. The use of the *DSM-IV* also facilitates history taking because then the clinician is aware of which specific symptoms to target in the interview. In addition, differential diagnosis is facilitated by the *DSM-IV* approach, since the criteria are explicit and overlaps are addressed in the "rule out" part of each diagnostic table.

○ **What are some of the disadvantages of the *DSM-IV* approach?**

The diagnoses, although field tested and based on research, are still relatively arbitrary. In the quest for certainty, clinicians may develop a false sense of security in using the *DSM-IV*. In addition, some of the diagnostic entities change with updated versions of the manual. This makes comparisons difficult for research purposes and leads to confusion for patients and their families.

○ **Do any of the disorders criteria require a "causative" event?**

Posttraumatic stress disorders, acute stress disorders, and adjustment disorders specify in their criteria the presence of an event that then leads to symptoms. One could also conceptualize the substance use disorders and the disorders secondary to a general medical condition as requiring a prior event (drug use) or condition.

○ **On what Axis are learning disorders coded?**

Learning disorders, such as reading disorder and mathematics disorder, are coded on Axis I.

○ **On what Axis are dementias coded?**

The dementias, such as vascular dementia, are coded on Axis I, with the neurological aspects also mentioned on Axis III (i.e., multiple cerebral vascular accidents).

○ **How is the term "remission" used in diagnosis?**

"Remission" indicates that there has been an improvement in the signs and symptoms of the disorder. Partial remission indicates that some of the symptoms remain and full remission indicates that the signs and symptoms have all resolved.

○ **What are "subtypes" and how are they recorded?**

Subtypes are specific subgroupings of a diagnostic entity. An example is the erotomanic subtype of delusional disorder. The *DSM-IV* sometimes uses a five-digit code for the disorders that have subtypes, which allows the clinician to specify the subtype in the diagnostic code.

○ **What are the "specifiers" used in *DSM-IV* diagnoses?**

Specifiers allow the clinician to describe several aspects of the patient's clinical presentation. Severity, presence or absence of psychotic features, chronicity, and certain features of the disorder (such as postpartum onset) are some examples.

○ **What is a differential diagnosis?**

A differential diagnosis is a listing of diagnoses suggested by the patient's clinical presentation. Often, a clinician arrives at a single diagnosis (or possibly more than one diagnosis on Axis I or II but identifies the diagnosis which is the reason for the visit) and lists a differential of other possible diagnoses that he or she would like to keep in mind.

○ **Where does the clinician code medication-induced movement disorders?**

These disorders are coded on Axis I.

○ **What is the "defensive functioning scale"?**

This is a scale that the clinician may use to describe the defense mechanisms or coping style used by a patient. The different defense mechanisms are rated into different levels of adaptation. This scale is under study for possible inclusion into the axes.

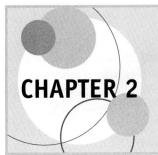

CHAPTER 2   Psychiatric Assessment

○ **What are the three types of clinical psychiatric evaluations according to the American Psychiatric Association (APA)?**

The general psychiatric evaluation, the emergency psychiatric evaluation, and the clinical psychiatric consultation.

○ **What are the goals of a general psychiatric evaluation according to the APA?**

To establish a diagnosis, generate a case formulation, develop a treatment plan, and ascertain if any symptoms (such as suicidal ideation) need emergency treatment. Development of an empathic rapport is also essential to initiating and maintaining treatment compliance.

○ **How do the goals of an emergency psychiatric evaluation differ from the goals of a general psychiatric evaluation?**

Not much, in reality. However, out of necessity, there is a greater emphasis on safety and willingness to participate in treatment during the emergency psychiatric evaluation. In the event that a person is unable to maintain his or her own safety (and/or others), *and* unwilling to participate in an appropriate level of care, involuntary commitment processes are indicated.

○ **What is the essential component of the clinical psychiatric consultation?**

The reason for the evaluation. If you do not answer the question the consulting physician, court, therapist, or caseworker is asking, you will not be consulted again. When the reason for the psychiatric consultation is vague, it is best to ascertain (from the person/institution requesting the evaluation) the exact reason for the evaluation (i.e., psych 2C = call 2U).

○ **True/False: The patient is *not* to be informed of who requested a psychiatric consultation or the reason for the evaluation.**

False. The person/institution requesting the psychiatric evaluation should ideally ask the patient to participate in a psychiatric evaluation and the reason why, while the consultant should clearly state who is requesting the evaluation and the reason thereof. When psychiatric consultations are requested for nonclinical reasons, the limits of confidentiality should be reviewed and agreed to by the patient and/or their guardian before the evaluation begins.

○ **What are the components of a clinical psychiatric examination?**

The components of a clinical psychiatric examination are the reason for evaluation, history of present illness; past psychiatric history; review of collateral sources of information including previous psychiatric records, psychological testing, and rating scales; past medical history; review of pertinent laboratory and radiology studies; review of systems; developmental history; family history; social history; mental status examination; physical examination; risk assessment; multiaxial diagnoses; and treatment recommendations.

○ **What sources of information are utilized during a clinical psychiatric examination?**

The first and foremost source of information for a psychiatric evaluation is the clinical interview with the patient. Additional information can be obtained from structured interview, various questionnaires, and results of psychological testing. With written permission from the patient or their guardian, review of previous records and interviews with appropriate persons involved the patient's life can yield valuable perspectives as to the patient's level of functioning and risk for adverse events.

○ **What factors should be considered when determining the reason for a psychiatric evaluation?**

Who, why, and what services the psychiatrist is expected to render. All these factors will influence the nature and the course of the psychiatric evaluation.

It is important to determine who requested the evaluation, especially if not requested by the patient. Reliability and willingness to be examined can be significantly compromised if the patient did not request the evaluation (such as when the patient is in emergency protective custody or when an examination is requested by the courts), and additional sources of information may need to be pursued more diligently if questions of safety or reliability are present.

Ascertaining the reason for the evaluation is imperative in order to collect sufficient information and make appropriate recommendations. Generally, when a patient requests an evaluation, the reason for assessment is to determine appropriate interventions for distressing symptoms. However, when someone other than a patient requests an evaluation, it is essential to determine the specific reason why the evaluation is needed, again, so that specific and appropriate recommendations can be made.

Finally, determining what services are to be rendered by the psychiatrist will influence what recommendations are made. For instance, if the evaluation is for purposes of disability determination, the psychiatric examination and recommendations will be somewhat different than if the psychiatrist is expected to be the treating physician.

○ **What information should be included in the history of present illness?**

The severity and duration of current symptoms, as well as identifiable stressors. Pertinent negatives as well as statements regarding dangerousness to self and others should also be included.

○ **True/False: A substance abuse history is not a component of the psychiatric evaluation.**

False. A substance abuse history is critical to every psychiatric evaluation, even if it is negative. The use of substances during any psychiatric illness does tend to expand the differential diagnosis and is a major risk factor in dangerousness to self or others.

○ **Past psychiatric history should include what information?**

The past psychiatric history should include information about any inpatient psychiatric hospitalizations, the reason for hospitalization, and diagnoses, if available. Information about index hospitalizations are often very helpful as to the severity of illness and diagnosis, especially if the patient is presenting for treatment in a stable condition. In addition, prior outpatient services by psychiatrists and other mental health providers should be included, as well as a history of previous medication trials and the response thereof.

○ **Why is past medical history an essential component of the psychiatric evaluation?**

Past medical history is essential in ruling out medical causes of psychiatric symptoms, as well as assessing for medication interactions that may be present. In addition, a medical illness may be a major stressor, particularly when that illness is disabling or disfiguring.

○ **What information should be included in a developmental history?**

Information regarding birth history, developmental milestones, relationships, and level of functioning in those relationships are the items that are generally included in a developmental history.

○ **What clinical implications does a family history of psychiatric disorders?**

A positive psychiatric family history may help with establishing risk factors for particular diagnoses, predicting response to various medications, and in developing a greater understanding of the patient's past and current family milieu.

○ **What is one of the best means for evaluating the distribution of mental illness in a family?**

A genogram.

○ **What does the occupational and social history tell the examiner about a patient's level of functioning?**

An occupational and social history gathers information about a person's ability to "work and love." The ability to hold a job for a period of time demonstrates an ability to structure daily activities, meet expectations, relate adequately with peers and supervisors, and take on a certain minimum level of responsibility. The ability to have a long-term relationship indicates an ability to attend to someone else's needs, control impulses, and make a commitment.

○ **List some questions pertaining to a patient's religious background.**

Questions to ask about the role of religion in a person's life could include some of the following: Were there conflicts between the patient's and parent's religious beliefs? How large a role does religion play in the patient's life? How do the parent's religious beliefs impact on the patient's attitude toward emotions, conflict, and psychiatric treatment?

○ **An extensive legal history can lead one to consider which two diagnoses?**

Antisocial personality disorder, and alcohol and/or substance dependence.

○ **Is physical examination included in a psychiatric evaluation?**

Yes. Particularly because some physical findings may be directly related to the patient's psychiatric condition or psychotropic medication side effects.

○ **What conditions can cause increased psychomotor activity?**

Anxiety, akathesia, hyperactivity associated with attention deficit hyperactivity disorder, elevated mood, agitation during psychotic episodes, confusional states due to delirium or dementia, and iatrogenic causes.

○ **What are the components of a mental status examination?**

The components of a mental status examination include general appearance, movements, speech, attitude, thought process, mood, affect, thought content, orientation to time and place, immediate and short-term recall, concentration, fund of knowledge, insight, judgment, and estimate of intelligence.

○ **What aspects of the patient's speech should be assessed?**

Rate and rhythm, quality, volume and tone, grammar and syntax, and vocabulary.

○ **List some possible causes of muteness.**

Aphasia, acute depression, conversion disorder, psychosis, and secondary gain.

○ **What is motor aphasia?**

Motor aphasia is a disturbance of speech in which understanding remains intact but the ability to speak is grossly impaired. Speech is halting, laborious, and inaccurate. Motor aphasia is also known as expressive aphasia, Broca's aphasia, or nonfluent aphasia.

○ **What is echopraxia?**

The pathological imitation of one person's movements by another.

○ **What is alexithymia?**

Alexithymia is the inability or difficulty a person has in describing or even being aware of their emotions or moods.

○ **A patient states, "It's one or my mother, I mean, one or another." Of what psychological phenomenon is this an example?**

Parapraxis or Freudian slip.

○ **What is the difference between a neologism and a word salad?**

Neologisms are new, nonsensical words created by the patient, while word salad is an incoherent mixture of words and phrases.

○ **How is affect characterized?**

Affect is described by its range, lability, appropriateness, intensity, relatedness, and congruence with mood.

○ **How is a patient's mood described in a mental status examination?**

In the patient's own words, usually.

○ **What aspects of thought content are generally included in a psychiatric evaluation?**

The patient's thought content is examined for suicidal or homicidal ideation (and intent): perceptual disturbances such as auditory, visual, tactile, or gustatory hallucinations; delusions, ideas of reference, and ideas of influence.

○ **Name five risk factors for suicide.**

Previous attempts, seriousness of attempts, a history of alcohol or drug usage, lack of social support, and presence of an Axis I disorder.

○ **Does the risk of suicide increase with direct questioning about suicide?**

There is no evidence that it increases risk, and it is likely to increase communication and trust with the patient.

○ **While interviewing a potentially violent patient, what precautions should be taken?**

Do not interview the patient alone. Leave the door to the interview room open, and sit between the patient and the door to allow for unrestricted exit.

○ **What factors are involved in assessing acute dangerousness?**

History of violent behavior, current violent ideation, a realistic and premeditated plan, and intent.

○ **Name three kinds of normal perceptual disturbances?**

Illusions, hypnagogic hallucinations, and hypnopompic hallucinations.

○ **Should a patient's delusions be directly confronted?**

No, the patient will generally become more defensive and even more fixed in their beliefs.

○ **What exactly is a delusion?**

A delusion is a false belief not based on reality.

○ **List five types of delusions?**

Paranoid, somatic, delusions of infidelity, delusions of poverty, and delusions of grandeur are five types of delusions. Other types of delusions include, but are not limited to those of control (thought withdrawal, thought broadcasting, thought insertion, thought control), erotomania, nihilistic delusions, and bizarre delusions. In general, delusions can form about anything or anyone, and may not fit into any particular type of delusion.

○ **How is concentration assessed on a mental status examination?**

By patient report, behavioral observation, serial 7's (or 3's if there are educational or developmental deficits noted), or by spelling the word "world" backward.

○ **In a patient who is disoriented, which sphere is the last to be affected; which is the first?**

Orientation to person; orientation to time.

○ **What is the best way to infer a patient's level of intellectual functioning?**

By considering the patient's vocabulary and ability to interpret proverbs.

○   **What is considered to be a normal digit span?**

The majority of people are able to recall seven digits forward and five to seven digits backward.

○   **What are the essential differences between delirium and dementia?**

Delirium is characterized by an acute state of confusion, disorientation, and varying levels of consciousness, while dementia is a gradual or step-wise decline in intellectual functioning.

○   **What are the characteristic features and course of delirium?**

Delirium is characterized by an acute onset of impaired consciousness, with global impairment of cognitive functions. The course is usually brief and fluctuating, and rapid improvement occurs when the underlying etiology resolves.

○   **How can agitation be distinguished from anxiety in the geriatric population?**

Agitated individuals do not generally complain of a sense of impending doom or dread.

○   **In distinguishing between schizophrenia and bipolar disorder, what single finding on mental status examination would most likely lead to a diagnosis of schizophrenia?**

Flat affect.

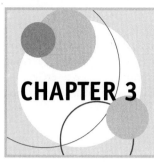

CHAPTER 3   Neuropsychiatry

○ **What percentage of brain tumors will cause psychiatric symptoms?**

Fifty to eighty percent.

In 20%, the psychiatric symptoms are the first indicator that a tumor exists. Of psychiatric patients, between 0.1% and 3% will have a brain tumor.

○ **What is the most common psychiatric presentation of a brain tumor?**

Apathy, depression, irritability, agitation, and an altered level of consciousness—all caused by an increase in intracranial pressure. Often, tumors will cause an exaggeration of previous character traits and coping styles. Delusions caused by tumors are typically less complex than those characteristic of schizophrenia, and hallucinations are more often visual than auditory. Left-sided tumors are associated with depression and akinesia, while right-sided tumors present with euphoria and an underestimation of the seriousness of the illness. Focal neurologic signs are common.

○ **Does the psychiatric presentation depend on the type of tumor?**

Rapidly growing tumors tend to cause severe, acute agitation or psychosis with associated cognitive dysfunction, while slow-growing tumors tend to present with vague personality changes, apathy, and depression, often without cognitive dysfunction. Tumors with multiple foci are associated with a greater frequency of psychiatric symptoms. Gliomas often present with psychiatric symptoms because they are fast growing with multiple foci, as do meningiomas, which are slow growing but often found in the frontal lobes where they interfere with higher-level cognitive functions while producing few focal signs. Supratentorial tumors are twice as likely as infratentorial to produce psychiatric symptoms.

○ **What are the most important factors that predict a psychiatric presentation of brain tumor?**

Important factors include the extent of the tumor, rapidity of growth, and the propensity for increased intracerebral pressure. Also important, but less so, are the patient's past psychiatric history, prior level of functioning, and coping mechanisms. Least important is the location of the lesion.

○   **What are the most common psychiatric presentations of frontal lobe tumors?**

Irresponsibility, childishness, indifference toward others, disinhibition, facetiousness, inappropriate sexual behavior, and witzelsucht—a tendency to make light of everything, albeit with a sarcastic, angry edge to the humor. Previous cognitive skills are preserved and formal intelligence is unaffected, but "executive functioning" can be severely disrupted. Right frontal damage is associated with euphoria; left frontal damage with akinesia, abulia, and flattened affect.

○   **What percentage of frontal lobe tumors present with psychiatric symptoms?**

Ninety percent.

○   **What is the most common psychiatric presentation of temporal lobe tumors?**

Cancer in the temporal lobes often presents with a schizophrenia-like illness, but can also cause depressed mood, apathy, irritability, euphoria and hypomania (because of interference in the connections between the temporal and frontal lobes/limbic system), lability and intensification of premorbid personality traits, anxiety, and panic attacks.

○   **How can temporal lobe tumors be distinguished from schizophrenia?**

Temporal lobe tumors will often be associated with visual, olfactory, and tactile hallucinations as well as auditory hallucinations, while affect is typically spared. The psychosis will usually present as repeated "spells," staring behavior or dreamlike episodes, and there can also be episodic mood swings. Tumors in the dominant lobe are associated with receptive aphasia or deficits in the ability to learn and remember verbal information; those in the nondominant lobe with disruption in the discrimination of nonspeech sounds.

○   **What is the psychiatric presentation of parietal lobe tumors?**

Symptoms of parietal lobe tumors are often more cognitive than behavioral. There is often a marked lack of awareness of deficits or even frank denial on the part of the patient (anosognosia or "neglect syndrome"), and the often-bizarre neurologic presentation can lead to incorrect diagnoses of conversion or somatization disorders.

○   **How about occipital tumors?**

Also fairly silent psychiatrically, fewer than 20% of occipital tumors have an initial behavioral presentation. The characteristic visual hallucinations tend to be simple and unformed, often little more than flashes of light, but can be associated with agitation, irritability, fatigue, suspiciousness, and prosopagnosia (an inability to recognize familiar faces). Homonymous hemianopsia is common.

○   **What is the psychiatric presentation of diencephalic tumors?**

Tumors of the thalamus, hypothalamus and the area surrounding the third ventricle often interrupt the cortical–striatal–pallidal–thalamic–cortical loop, affecting many frontal functions and presenting as a frontal lobe syndrome. Hypothalamic tumors can cause hyperphagia, daytime somnolence, or anorexia nervosa. Diencephalic tumors often cause a subcortical dementia affecting memory and causing slowing of thought processes, apathy, abulia, depression, and inability to manipulate acquired knowledge. Interruption of CSF flow by tumor growth can cause hydrocephalus and consequent generalized cognitive dysfunction.

○ **What are the five signs that should lead one to suspect a brain tumor in a psychiatric patient?**

Seizures, especially if focal or new onset (this is the initial manifestation of 50% of brain tumors), headaches (especially if dull, new onset, poorly localized, nocturnal or positional, present on awakening, and worsening with time), nausea and vomiting, sensory changes (especially visual changes, vertigo, or unilateral hearing loss), and focal neurological signs (such as weakness, ataxia, or localized sensory loss).

○ **What procedures may aid the diagnosis of a brain tumor?**

CT scans are good for identifying small soft-tissue mass lesions and concomitant calcifications, obstructive hydrocephalus, and midline shift. They may not reveal very small tumors, however, and can miss isodense tumors and carcinomatosis (diffuse meningeal involvement). MRIs have better resolution and are thus better at revealing very small tumors; the drawbacks are cost, the inability to detect calcifications, and the restriction of subjects to those without metal in their heads. Cisternography, in which dye is injected into the ventricles, can aid in the differential diagnosis of intraventricular tumors and tumor-associated hydrocephalus. Skull x-rays can diagnose craniopharyngiomas, pituitary tumors, and "empty sella" syndrome, but bone scans are better at detecting bony metastases. Chest x-rays are useful for detecting primary neoplasms of the lung, the most frequent source of brain metastases. A lumbar puncture is useful only for diagnosing meningeal carcinomatosis or leukemia if other tests are unrevealing, and requires a preliminary CT scan or MRI if there is any suspicion of increased intracerebral pressure. EEGs are frequently normal, but sometimes there are diffuse or focal spikes or slow waves, either continuous or paroxysmal. Angiography is useful for establishing the vascular supply of a tumor prior to surgery. Neuropsychiatric testing, formerly used to localize the lesion before the advent of modern imaging, now is useful to establish the extent of the dysfunction, provide a baseline measurement of cognitive function, and help to optimize rehabilitation posttreatment. The advantages of SPECT, PET, BEAM, and MEG scans over the above diagnostic tests are as yet unclear.

○ **How should therapy be altered if a patient with preexisting psychiatric disease presents with a brain tumor?**

Clinicians should be especially aware of drug–drug interactions, drugs that cause delirium, and those that cause seizures, because patients with cranial neoplasms become more sensitive to all three. Drug dosages should be decreased (use 1–5 mg of haloperidol, for example, instead of 10–20 mg) and serum levels should be monitored. To decrease the risk of delirium, it is better to substitute haloperidol, carbamazepine, valproate, or benzodiazepines for lithium. Likewise, SSRIs, MAOIs, or secondary amines are better tolerated than TCAs, high-potency neuroleptics are safer than low-potency, and the antiparkinsonian agents amantadine or diphenhydramine much less likely to cause anticholinergic delirium than benztropine, trihexyphenidyl, or orphenadrine. Attention should also be paid to the seizure-causing potential of antipsychotics—haloperidol, molindone, and fluphenazine are somewhat safer than chlorpromazine or clozapine for the control of psychotic symptoms; and lithium, bupropion, and maprotiline are best avoided for mood control for the same reason. Methylphenidate does not lower the seizure threshold and offers the advantage of rapid onset of action. Psychotherapy should be concrete and reality based, involving the family and focusing on education and issues of loss and death. Denial is a useful defense mechanism early in the course of the illness but becomes maladaptive later on. ECT is contraindicated if there is any evidence of increased intracranial pressure, but a tumor per se is no longer an absolute contraindication.

○ **How should one modify one's pharmacologic treatment of anxiety disorder in someone with a cranial mass?**

Short-acting, low-dose benzodiazepines are much less likely to cause a paradoxical reaction of increased arousal and agitation than longer-acting agents, which also have an increased propensity to cause delirium, especially in older people. Benzodiazepines also raise the seizure threshold. Buspirone does not cause paradoxical reactions or delirium; its only disadvantage being delayed onset and weak effects. Panic attacks from temporal lobe tumors may respond to carbamazepine, valproic acid, and primidone as well as more conventional antidepressants and anxiolytics.

○ **What are the characteristics of a seizure?**

Impairment of consciousness (if complex), involuntary movement, behavioral changes, or altered perceptual experiences.

○ **What is temporal lobe epilepsy?**

Although the term no longer officially exists, it is still used clinically to describe seizures that are associated with sensory hallucinations (particularly olfactory), flashbacks, *déjà vu* or *jamais vu*, complex verbalizations, automatisms, and autonomic symptoms such as piloerection and nausea. Rarely, TLE can present with cataplexy or catatonia.

○ **How can TLE be differentiated from complex partial or petit mal seizures?**

TLE may be either complex or simple. The term "complex partial seizure" is restricted to patients with focal firing combined with an altered level of consciousness; automatisms alone do not make a complex partial seizure. Petit mal or absence seizures tend to be shorter in length without automatisms or postictal features, unlike TLE.

○ **What characteristics can help confirm the diagnosis of temporal lobe epilepsy?**

Subjective alterations, postictal confusion, impaired memory of event, postictal depression, other episodes of nearly identical behavior, and observer confirmation of characteristic automatisms.

○ **Is there any relation between TLE and psychiatric pathology?**

The incidence of psychiatric problems is four to seven times greater in those with TLE than in those without.

○ **What psychiatric issues confront patients with epilepsy?**

Epileptic patients daily confront the fear of performing normal social activities (such as dating, during adolescence), because their interpersonal relations typically suffer if a seizure is witnessed. American culture stigmatizes epileptics as an inferior minority group, with consequent negative effect on the self-esteem of those affected by it. Restrictions on activity (operating machinery, driving, swimming, etc.) can be burdensome, and epileptics suffer guilt and possible legal consequences when they ignore these restrictions. As a result of this, family relationships can evolve into abnormal patterns of isolation or dependency.

○ **What patterns of psychopathology are common in those with a seizure disorder?**

There are three patterns of psychopathology associated with seizure disorders, but they are poorly characterized and overlap. The first pattern is characterized by perceptual changes, alterations in consciousness, and poor memory of events. The second is more chronic, associated with paranoia, simple auditory hallucinations, and perceptual changes. The third is characterized by persistent depersonalization and/or visual distortions.

○ **How can a seizure be distinguished from a pseudoseizure?**

The distinction can sometimes be tricky, as patients often have both.

Seizure	Pseudoseizure
Related to sleep deprivation	No relation to sleep
Marked by incontinence	No incontinence
Patient sustains injuries (tongue biting, head trauma, broken bones)	Injuries unusual
Abrupt onset and termination	Gradual onset and termination Triggered by interpersonal stress
No "epileptic personality" exists	Positive findings on MMPI
Elevated serum prolactin levels	Prolactin levels normal at 15–30 min postseizure Bizarre, purposeful movements—pelvic thrusts side-to-side movements
Reflexes impaired	Intact reflexes Seizure exacerbated by restraint
Loss of consciousness	Consciousness preserved during seizure No autonomic instability No postictal changes (such as lethargy) No amnesia for seizure Extremity movements are out of phase

○ **What are some other terms for "pseudoseizure"?**

Conversion reaction, hysteroepilepsy, and nonepileptic seizure (the preferred term).

○ **How can a seizure disorder be distinguished from schizophrenia?**

Altered mentation from a seizure tends to be ego-dystonic, and the patient can talk about the symptoms in a detached manner. There is generally no evidence of interictal changes on the mental status examination, and the premorbid social histories are generally good. The seizure disorder is characterized with abrupt rather than gradual alterations in personality, mood, and ability to function that are unresponsive to psychiatric or psychological intervention. The patient generally does not quite meet *DSM-IV* criteria for schizophrenia.

○ **How can a seizure disorder be distinguished from a panic disorder?**

Often a difficult distinction, because both conditions have overlapping symptoms—depersonalization, fear, *déjà vu* and *jamais vu*, dizziness, illusions, paresthesias, chills, and flushes, which are in part mediated by a similar underlying limbic dysfunction (the temporal lobe modulates fear, for example) and amenable to similar pharmacologic intervention, i.e., benzodiazepines. However, in panic disorders, consciousness is preserved, an EEG will be normal, there are seldom olfactory hallucinations, family history is usually positive, there are no automatisms, and a positive response is found not to anticonvulsants but to antidepressants (which would typically worsen complex partial symptoms). In addition, panic attacks usually last longer than seizures, and agoraphobia is a prominent symptom in panic but not seizure.

○   **Is there a particular personality type associated with seizure disorder?**

Of the qualities traditionally associated with the "epileptic personality type"—dependency, humorlessness, hypergraphia, hyposexuality, religiosity, viscosity, paranoia, and a preoccupation with philosophical or moral concerns—evidence exists only for hyposexuality, as a reflection of a secondary endocrine abnormality evoked by seizures.

○   **Are seizures associated with aggression?**

Aggression during a seizure is very unusual, and when it does occur is typically disordered, uncoordinated, undirected, and associated with restraint or postictal paranoid psychosis.

○   **What strategies can be used in treating psychiatric symptoms associated with a seizure disorder?**

Strategies that can be used to treat the neuropsychiatric aspects of seizure disorders include assessment of the social factors that aggravate the seizure disorder; adjustment of the anticonvulsant as necessary to minimize seizures, using monotherapy if possible; use of psychotropic medications to target specific psychiatric symptoms, anticipating interactions, using low initial dosages, and waiting for a response plateau before changing the dose again; targeting psychotherapeutic approaches to specific behaviors or stressors; and finally collaboration with all caregivers.

○   **What are the symptoms of Parkinson's disease?**

Parkinson's is a progressive, nongenetic disorder that presents with both motor and cognitive symptoms. The motor symptoms typically have an asymmetric onset, and consist of bradykinesia and muscular rigidity, flexion at trunk and neck leading to postural instability, difficulty initiating movements, lack of facial expression, and a 4 to 6 Hz resting tremor. Ninety-three percent of those with Parkinson's suffer cognitive deficits—reduced verbal fluency and naming difficulties, deficits in visual analysis and constructional praxis, and executive dysfunction similar to frontal lobe syndrome—difficulties in selective attention and set maintenance. Recognition memory is usually unimpaired, but procedural memory shows deficits.

○   **What is the etiology of Parkinson's disease?**

The etiology is unknown, although some hypothesize that it is related to exposure to environmental toxins. The bradykinesia and rigidity can be related to progressive loss of neurons in the substantia nigra. There is reduced dopamine uptake in the putamen. In addition to dopamine, neurotransmitter abnormalities are found in the somatostatin and CRF systems. There is an increase in the number of muscarinic cholinergic receptors (unlike in Alzheimer's) but a decrease in nicotinic. Pathology shows Lewy bodies in the locus ceruleus, substantia nigra, and hypothalamus (in contrast to Lewy body dementia, in which Lewy bodies are found in the cortex also).

○   **What are the neuropsychiatric symptoms in Parkinson's disease?**

Depression occurs in 40% to 60%, often before the onset of motor symptoms, and is unrelated to either the duration or severity of the disease or the response to medications, but is associated with dementia. Parkinson's depression is characterized more by dysphoria, sadness, irritability, pessimism, and suicidal ideation, less by guilt and self-blame. Actual suicide is rare, unlike in Huntington's chorea. Psychotic symptoms are common (occurring in up to 50% of patients at some point of the disease) usually as a side effect of anticholinergic medications, but can also occur as a result of mood disturbance, other medications, sleep deprivation, or the dementia associated with Parkinson's disease. The psychotic symptoms can range in severity from hallucinations that cause no distress to delusional states with agitation and terrifying hallucinations of all types.

○ **What tests can help diagnose Parkinson's?**

PET scans show decreased uptake in the striatum, while CT scan and MRI show decreased volume in the substantia nigra of advanced cases. EEG shows nonspecific slowing.

○ **What percentage of patients with Parkinson's disease manifest dementia?**

From 10% to 40%, the risk rising with age. Other risk factors for dementia in Parkinson's disease are family history, depression, and motor disability.

○ **What are some treatments for Parkinson's and its associated neuropsychiatric symptoms?**

L-Dopa is a dopamine agonist that can help compensate for the bradykinesia and rigidity, as do anticholinergics, but there is no treatment for the postural instability except for physical and occupational therapy. Antidepressants work normally on Parkinson's patients, but this population is very sensitive to the anticholinergic, sedating, and orthostatic effects of these drugs. ECT is effective for both the affective and motor symptoms. If antipsychotics must be used, atypicals with minimal extrapyramidal side effects will have the least effect on motor symptoms. Quetiapine and clozapine have been shown to be the most effective in controlling psychotic symptoms in Parkinson's-related psychosis, while aripiprazole is minimally effective and can exacerbate motor function. Risperdal is generally poorly tolerated in these patients and should be avoided. Whenever the use of atypicals is indicated in patients with Parkinson's disease, monitoring for neuroleptic malignant syndrome–like symptoms is essential, and can be very difficult to distinguish from baseline symptoms. Again, the use of typical neuroleptics such as haloperidol is generally contraindicated, although may be necessary when agitation becomes a safety issue.

○ **What symptoms can occur as a side effect of treating a patient with Parkinson's disease?**

Anticholinergic drugs, while being the most effective in suppressing the parkinsonian tremor, are also the most prone to induce psychosis. Delusions are usually dose related, frequently persecutory, and preceded by vivid dreams or visual hallucinations. Risk factors for delusions are age and concurrent dementia. Thirty percent of treated Parkinson's patients will hallucinate fully formed animal or human figures, typically at night and with the hallucinations associated with sleep disturbance. These differ from typical anticholinergic hallucinations in that they are less threatening, more fully formed, not combined with tactile or auditory stimuli, and not associated with delirium. Delirium occurs in 5% to 25% of patients as a medication side effect, with bromocriptine and pergolide particularly implicated. L-Dopa can cause anxiety.

○ **What is delirium?**

Delirium is a pattern of diffuse, reversible cognitive deficits with acute onset, and a waxing and waning course. The deficits can include delusions (20%–70%), perceptual disturbances, mood alterations, language (50%–90%) and thought disorders (95%), sleep/wake disturbance (50%–95%), hallucinations (30%), and psychomotor alterations. Disorientation is common, to time (80%), place (70%), and person (20%). Twenty percent of hospital patients will become delirious, and if elderly, the 1-year mortality will be 40%. Some clinicians distinguish between *acute confusional state*, a disorder of attention associated with frontostriatal dysfunction, and *acute agitated delirium*, a disorder of emotion associated with middle temporal gyrus dysfunction, but many patients present with a mixed picture.

○ **What is the etiology of delirium?**

The anticholinergic hypothesis of delirium holds that it is a result of decreased levels of acetylcholine. Medications or medical conditions causing decreased oxidative metabolism of glucose in the brain decrease the levels of acetyl CoA and thus acetylcholine, causing mental status changes. However, cholinergic medications can cause delirium also. Both decreased glucose and hypoxia can increase dopamine activity, while GABA levels are decreased in delirium tremens. Other neurotransmitters have also been implicated. Delirium is a final common pathway that can result from intoxication, withdrawal, metabolic dysfunction, infection, concussion or cerebral contusion, epilepsy (ictal, postictal, or interictal), neoplasm, cerebral vascular disease, hematologic processes, hypersensitivity reactions, or exposure to excessive radiation or electricity. Small thalamic lesions can also cause delirium. Delirium is sometimes divided into *hyperactive* or *hypoactive* delirium on the basis of psychomotor symptoms, but the difference is not standardized and the two cannot be distinguished on the basis of cognitive impairment or EEG findings, although hyperactive delirium is associated with a somewhat better prognosis.

○ **What are the risk factors for delirium?**

Risk factors for delirium include polypharmacy, multiple medical problems, alcohol and sedative/hypnotic dependence, severe burns, status postsurgery (particularly hip replacement and cardiotomy), HIV/AIDS, hypoxemia, organ insufficiency, preexisting brain disease, and increased age.

○ **What are risk factors for delirium in the elderly?**

In addition to the ones already listed, additional risk factors for delirium in the elderly include dementia, low albumin levels, few social interactions, age above 80 years, infection (especially UTI), visual impairment, fractures, fever/hypothermia, and thiamine deficiency.

○ **What laboratory tests can help diagnose delirium?**

An EEG will show slowing for both hypo- and hyperactive delirium, but this can precede or lag behind clinical changes. Alpha activity is decreased, and delta and theta activity is increased, with slowing of both peak and mean activity. TBI delirium and hepatic encephalopathy shows decreased blood flow globally on SPECT, particularly to the frontal lobes. Delirium tremens, in contrast, shows low-voltage *fast* activity on EEG, and is associated with *increased* cerebral blood flow. Evoked potentials will be abnormal in delirium.

○ **How is delirium best treated?**

First, find and eliminate the underlying etiology. Manipulation of the environment can be helpful—reorientation, visible and prominent calendars, night-lights, and natural lighting. Neuroleptics are the standard pharmacologic treatment, with benzodiazepines for ethanol withdrawal. For anticholinergic delirium, physostigmine can be effective (though it has a short half-life and can cause seizures). Tacrine or donepezil can reverse a central anticholinergic delirium. Psychostimulants worsen delirium and should be avoided. Haloperidol usually causes improvement within hours by decreasing glucose uptake in the limbic cortex, caudate, frontal lobes, and anterior cingulate. Haloperidol will cause fewer extrapyramidal side effects if given intravenously, because hepatic first-pass metabolism is avoided. Patients with HIV and Lewy body dementia remain unusually susceptible, however. One risk of haloperidol is torsades de pointes, but this is idiopathic and unrelated to dose, cardiovascular disease, or QTc prolongation. Droperidol may also be used for increased sedation and faster onset of action.

○ **What is dementia?**

Dementia is a global cognitive impairment including memory loss combined with aphasia, apraxia, agnosia, or an executive deficit severe enough to interfere with functioning. Memory loss alone is referred to as amnesia.

○ **How is dementia distinguished from delirium?**

In dementia, arousal is intact, attention is preserved, and the intellectual deficits are persistent, while in delirium, level of arousal fluctuates and deficits should remit once the underlying cause of the delirium is treated.

○ **What is the prevalence of dementia of the Alzheimer's type in the United States?**

It is age related. The prevalence of Alzheimer's in the 2000 census (Hebert et al. 2003) in persons 65 to 74 years old was 5%, while 20% of persons of age 75 to 84 years were affected and 50% of persons older than 84 years were affected. Over half of the dementias are of the Alzheimer's type, followed by vascular dementia, and the rest are attributable to other causes such as Huntington's, Parkinson's, Pick's, or Lewy body dementia. One in six cases of dementia is at least partly reversible—caused by infection, metabolic diseases, toxins, or deficiency states.

○ **What is the epidemiology of Alzheimer's disease?**

Alzheimer's affects two and a half to four million citizens of the United States. With the aging of the baby boomer generation, this number is expected to significantly increase over the next 30 years. The biggest risk factor is age (with prevalence doubling with every 5 year increase), others being sex (women are slightly more prone), family history, Down's syndrome, history of head injury, and alleles for the E4 apolipoprotein. (No alleles means a 15% chance of late-onset Alzheimer's disease; one copy means a 50% chance and both copies a 90% chance of expressing the disease by age 80 years, with risk increased for women.)

○ **How is Alzheimer's diagnosed?**

A diagnosis of Alzheimer's dementia is warranted if the patient exhibits memory impairment and cognitive deficits (aphasia, apraxia, agnosia, or disturbances in executive functioning) that occur in a gradual and progressive manner, and causes significant impairment in functioning. Other factors that could cause a decline in functioning should be ruled out. Up to 90% of clinically diagnosed Alzheimer's disease will be confirmed on subsequent pathology. A definite diagnosis requires an autopsy or brain biopsy showing amyloid plaques and neurofibrillary tangles. Neuropsychological testing can be useful in determining extent of dysfunction, while use of the Mini-Mental Status Examination is a good screening tool for the presence of deficits, and severity/progression thereof.

○ **What are the usual causes of death in Alzheimer's disease?**

Aspiration pneumonia, sepsis from an infected decubitus ulcer, or death from concurrent cardiovascular disease or cancer.

○ **What neuropsychiatric symptoms occur in Alzheimer's?**

Personality alterations include passivity and disengagement, loss of enthusiasm and energy, and decreased affection. Patients become emotionally coarse, labile, insensitive, excitable, and unreasonable, and often self-centered, resistive, and disinhibited. Delusions occur in 30% to 50%, usually in the middle of the illness, typically with themes of theft, infidelity of spouse, or abandonment. "Phantom boarder" and the Capgras syndrome are common. Patients with delusions do not necessarily have more severe illness, but they do tend to be more behaviorally disturbed and difficult to manage, and manifest a more rapid intellectual decline. Hallucinations are not common, found in only 10% of Alzheimer's sufferers, and mostly visual, consisting of people from the past, intruders, animals, objects, or scenes. Hallucinations are more likely to be secondary to concurrent delirium, or alternately, Lewy body dementia. Auditory hallucinations are usually persecutory and occur in the context of delusions. Mood changes are common, with tearfulness, feelings of worthlessness and thoughts of being a burden characteristic. Suicide is nevertheless rare. Elation occurs in one in five, angry outbursts in half. Forty percent manifest anxiety, usually in the form of excessive anticipatory concern surrounding upcoming events. Psychomotor symptoms include wandering and pacing (in the middle and late stages of the disease), assaultiveness (one in five), and most commonly, apathy, agitation, and anxiety. There are also frequent interruptions in sleep, decreased interest in food with anosmia, and decreased sexual activity.

○   **What laboratory tests can help diagnose Alzheimer's?**

Laboratory studies are useful in excluding other causes of dementia. Serum tests in patients with Alzheimer's disease should be normal. CT scan and MRI show striking cortical atrophy, particularly in the medial temporal lobes. EEG may show theta and delta wave slowing, with maximal abnormality in the parietal lobes. PET scans show early abnormalities, in particular hypometabolism in the parietal lobes, later extending to the frontal lobes, with subcortical structures spared. SPECT scans are similar. Although measurement of more specific markers associated with Alzheimer's is being developed, multiple studies have shown that a clinical diagnosis of dementia may be more sensitive and specific than these tests.

○   **What is the etiology of Alzheimer's disease?**

Genetic contributions to Alzheimer's disease include mutations on chromosomes 14 and 21, the latter of which contains the gene for the β-amyloid precursor protein. Alleles for the apo-E4 protein (chromosome 19) facilitate deposition of amyloid, leading to amyloid plaques, neurofibrillary tangles, and neuronal death through a mechanism that is not entirely clear. The presence of Alzheimer's-like dementia symptoms in many individuals with Down's syndrome over the age of 40 years supports the role of β-amyloid precursor protein in disease development, as these individuals have an extra 21st chromosome. Findings of increased aluminum in the senile plaques and neurofibrillary tangles have raised questions about the role of the metal in the etiology of the disease, but it does not appear related to dietary intake. Head injuries predispose patients to the later development of Alzheimer's, and there are probably other, as yet unidentified, environmental factors. The indifference manifested by those with the disease is likely secondary to the temporal and parietal lobe damage, which also accounts for disorientation and lack of visuospatial skills; frontal lobe damage causes the disinhibition and lability. Delusions may be the result of temporoparietal alterations combined with an acetylcholine deficit.

○   **What is the treatment for Alzheimer's disease?**

There is no cure, but several acetylcholinesterase inhibitors (e.g., donepezil, galantamine, and rivastigmine) may allay some symptoms of Alzheimer's, but not delay progression. The NMDA receptor antagonist, memantine, is also available and can be used in lieu of or in combination with the existing acetylcholinesterase inhibitors. Again, the improvement seen with these medications is symptomatic only and the progression of the disease does not seem to be altered. It has been estimated that a treatment that could delay onset of Alzheimer's disease by 5 years would halve the nursing home population in the United States.

○   **What are the symptoms of Pick's disease?**

Personality changes include apathy or disinhibition—patients become boisterous, irritable or overly familiar, show social and occupational withdrawal, and show decreased motivation and engagement. There can be some early, transient depression. One-third of patients will manifest elation, one-quarter will have delusions, and some may even show symptoms of the Klüver-Bucy syndrome with its consequent weight gain. Patients may be restless and roam incessantly, and engage in complex repetitive acts and compulsive rituals. Memory, visuospatial, and mathematical skills are relatively spared, consistent with the pattern of cortical atrophy. The biggest deficits are in executive functioning (set shifting tasks, word-list generation, and response initiation) and language function. Pick's patients usually have naming deficits, echolalia, impaired auditory comprehension, and poverty of speech, sometimes to the point of mutism.

○ **What is the etiology of Pick's disease?**

Pick's disease is one of a class of disorders known as *frontotemporal dementias*. The cause is unknown; some are genetic, but most sporadic. At autopsy, Pick cells are found in all cortical layers, albeit with a regional and laminar distribution pattern, the neurons lacking dendritic spines and containing intracytoplasmic argyrophilic "Pick bodies" consisting of straight filaments. Enlarged "ballooned cells" containing a uniform argyrophilic cytoplasm are also found. (In other dementias, atrophy is usually confined to the outer layers (layers I–III) and there are no Pick bodies or ballooned cells in the cortex.) Cortical acetylcholine, glutamate, and dopamine systems are unaffected, but there is a decrease of serotonin and in the basal ganglia, dopamine, GABA, and substance P levels are decreased. Most of the degeneration is confined to the frontal lobes, with some temporal involvement.

○ **What is the epidemiology of Pick's disease?**

It is an autosomal dominant trait, affecting males and females equally.

○ **What laboratory tests help diagnose Pick's disease?**

CT scan or MRI often shows focal atrophy in the frontal or temporal lobes, but PET and SPECT are better methods of diagnosis. PET will show decreased glucose utilization, particularly in the midfrontal convexity, and SPECT will show hypoperfusion in the frontal convexity or orbitofrontal cortex. Some frontotemporal dementias (not Pick's) are due to amyotrophic lateral sclerosis, so motor neuron disease should be ruled out. A patient with ALS will have decreased numbers of spinal motor neurons, and they will contain nonstaining inclusions.

○ **How can one distinguish a frontotemporal dementia such as Pick's disease from Alzheimer's?**

Frontotemporal dementia	Alzheimer's
Early loss of social skills	Social skills preserved until late
Memory loss late in disease	Memory loss often presenting symptom
Early loss of executive function	Late loss of executive function
Stereotyped speech with terminal mutism	Fluent aphasia
Semantic anomia	Lexical anomia
Visuospatial deficits late in disease	Visuospatial deficits characteristic
Frontotemporal hypoperfusion/hypometabolism	Parietal and posterior temporal abnormalities
No specific neuron type affected	Cholinergic neurons targeted
Initial presentation of personality change	Personality change is late

○   **What is Lewy body dementia?**

Also known as Lewy body disease, Lewy body variant of Alzheimer's disease, diffuse Lewy body disease, diffuse cortical Lewy body disease, senile dementia of the Lewy body type (SDLBT), Lewy body dementia presents with parkinsonism, progressive dementia, mental status fluctuations, and paranoid ideation. It is notable for a delirium-like presentation with periods of mental coherence, making diagnosis difficult, and also visual hallucinations that are much more prevalent than in Alzheimer's disease, typically of brightly colored animals or people, vivid and often frightening. The classic triad of Lewy body dementia is visual hallucinations, fluctuation of consciousness, and spontaneous parkinsonism. Patients with Lewy body dementia are unusually sensitive to neuroleptics, and therefore, must be started at very low doses.

○   **What characteristics distinguish vascular dementia from other dementias?**

Vascular dementias, which make up almost a third of all dementias depending on the population, present with focal neurological signs, stepwise deterioration, patchy intellectual deficits, abrupt onset and a history of cardiovascular disease, hypertension, or transient ischemic attacks. Common onset of over the age of 50 years, with males affected more than females, and death usually occurs in 6 to 8 years from cardiovascular disease or stroke.

○   **How can one diagnose vascular dementia?**

A definite diagnosis requires pathology, but a probable diagnosis can be made by noting the correlation between the dementia and corresponding cerebrovascular disease already diagnosed through imaging studies or the presence of focal neurological signs or stroke. The onset of the dementia should be within 3 months of the stroke. The profile of deficits varies depending on the location of the infarcts, slowness of cognition and impaired executive function are typical, as are decreased cognitive, memory, and visuospatial abilities. Language function is usually preserved. Laboratory tests are normal, but if the patient is young or lacks risk factors for stroke, an ANA, antiphospholipid antibody and lupus anticoagulant should be checked to rule out a treatable inflammatory vasculitis. CT scan can show cortical infarctions or evidence of periventricular ischemic changes, and an MRI, the technique of choice, will reveal small subcortical infarcts and white-matter changes. SPECT and PET scans should show multiple small areas of hypometabolism. History and physical is key, i.e., stepwise decline, abrupt onset, and focal signs.

○   **What causes vascular dementia?**

There are a number of different etiologies. *Multi-infarct dementia*, a term often used to refer to vascular dementia, is a result of many small-vessel infarcts affecting different areas of the brain. A *strategic single infarct* affecting the left angular gyrus or medial thalamic nuclei will cause dementia, as will *hypoperfusion* from a hemorrhage or cardiac arrest, which causes border-zone ischemia. *Binswanger's disease* is caused by white-matter changes, usually secondary to fibrinoid necrosis of the small vessels from hypertension. *Hemorrhages*, such as chronic subdurals, a ruptured cerebral aneurysm or subarachnoid hemorrhage, can also cause dementia.

○   **How does one treat vascular dementia?**

Control hypertension (or any other causes) and give aspirin, ticlopidine, or clopidogrel to decrease platelet aggregation. Baclofen is effective for poststroke spasticity, and nortriptyline for pseudobulbar affect. Mood disorders and psychosis can be treated in the usual manner. Patients also benefit from gait retraining and speech therapy if warranted.

○ **What is the relationship between stroke and depression?**

Thirty to fifty percent of stroke sufferers will become depressed, with 20% meeting criteria for major depression. The average duration of the depression is 1 year. There is an inverse relationship between the severity of the depression and the distance of the anterior border of a left-hemisphere lesion from the left frontal pole. Risk factors include preexisting subcortical atrophy, a family history of depression, lack of a meaningful life, and overprotection by a caregiver. Lesions of the left dorsolateral frontal cortex, left basal ganglia, or cerebellum/brainstem produce a transient depression rarely lasting more than 6 months. The test of growth hormone response to desipramine is 100% sensitive and 75% specific for poststroke depression, although this has yet to be recognized as a valid marker.

○ **What is the relationship between stroke and mania?**

Mania can occur with right basitemporal lesions, presumably reflecting the region's close connection with the limbic system. Risk factors are subcortical atrophy and family history of bipolar disorder.

○ **What are the symptoms of progressive supranuclear palsy?**

There are several, both motor and cognitive. Patients will show profound bradykinesia, axial rigidity (neck and trunk more than limbs), and a pseudobulbar palsy (dysphagia, sialorrhea, and dysarthria). There are restrictions in gaze, vertical gaze more than horizontal (often leading to falls). Cognitive difficulties include deficits in verbal memory, calculating ability, and synthesis of complex information, with slowed central processing. There should be no agnosia, apraxia, or aphasia. Personality changes are consistent with impaired frontal function—apathy, emotional indifference, depression, irritability, forced inappropriate laughing or crying, outbursts of rage (often responsive to trazodone), or OCD-like symptoms.

○ **What laboratory tests can help in the diagnosis of progressive supranuclear palsy?**

Serum test results are normal. An EEG will be normal or show nonspecific findings, i.e., generalized background slowing or diffuse theta activity. CT scan and MRI will show diminished midbrain size with frontotemporal atrophy later on in the disease, PET scan reveals frontal hypometabolism, and SPECT shows a bilateral frontal hypoperfusion.

○ **What is the etiology of progressive supranuclear palsy?**

The exact etiology is unknown. There is decreased striatal dopamine formation and storage, and in the cortex, numbers of nicotinic acetylcholine receptors are decreased. Dopamine D_2 receptors are diminished cortically and subcortically. Neurofibrillary tangles are formed of straight rather than as twisted filaments (as in Alzheimer's disease), and are concentrated at the mesencephalic–diencephalic junction. The cortex, thalamus, and hypothalamus are typically spared.

○ **What is Wilson's disease?**

Also known as *hepatolenticular degeneration*, Wilson's disease affects males and females equally and has both motor and psychiatric symptoms. Motor symptoms usually present first—tremor, rigidity, dystonia, poor coordination, abnormal gait and posture, dysarthria, dysphagia, and hypophonia. Psychiatric symptoms will be the initial presentation in 20% of cases, however, and consist of mild memory and executive disturbances usually in parallel with the extrapyramidal signs. Twenty to thirty percent of patients will have depression, but mania or hypomania can be present also. Personality changes can consist of impulsivity, irritability, and lability. Wilson's should always be suspected in young psychiatric patients who have movement disorders.

○   **What is the etiology of Wilson's disease?**

Wilson's disease is an autosomal recessive disease present in 1 in 40,000, caused by a gene defect on chromosome 13 coding for a protein used in copper metabolism. Copper accumulates to toxic levels in the liver, cornea, and basal ganglia, causing symptoms by the age of 20 to 30 years, the psychiatric symptoms correlating with signs of neurological dysfunction rather than hepatic disease. The copper causes a cavitary necrosis of the putamen, and atrophy of the brainstem and dentate nucleus. *Opalski cells* (large oval cells with a finely granular cytoplasm) will be found on pathology, as well as *Alzheimer's II astrocytes*, large watery astrocytes.

○   **What laboratory tests can help diagnose Wilson's disease?**

Low levels of ceruloplasmin (the serum copper-carrying protein), increased 24-hour urine copper, and increased copper on hepatic biopsy. Patients will have chronic hepatitis and hemolytic anemia. The classic finding is Kayser–Fleischer rings, green copper deposits in the cornea, but in practice these are usually visible only on slit-lamp examination. Because Wilson's disease is entirely treatable, a high index of suspicion should be maintained.

○   **How is Wilson's disease treated?**

With penicillamine. If this is not tolerated, because of neutropenia or proteinuria, then triethylenetetramine may be suggested. Liver transplantation becomes an option in end stage disease.

○   **What is Fahr's disease?**

An idiopathic calcification of the basal ganglia that causes abnormal involuntary movements and neuropsychiatric disturbances. The etiology is unknown. Motor symptoms include parkinsonism, choreoathetosis, dystonia, and ataxia. Dementia is common, with deficits in concentration, memory, and abstraction, although language is preserved. Mood disorders are common, and a schizophrenia-like psychosis may in fact predate both the dementia and the neurological symptoms. A CT scan or MRI will show mineral deposits in the basal ganglia, periventricular white matter, and dentate nuclei. There is no treatment, although psychiatric symptoms can be controlled with the appropriate medications.

○   **What is corticobasal degeneration?**

This dementia is caused by a focal cortical degeneration in the frontal and parietal lobes as well as neuronal loss and inclusion bodies in the substantia nigra. Patients usually present with a primary movement disorder, such as complex tremor, asymmetric rigidity, or supranuclear gaze palsy, with secondary cognitive changes, such as aphasia, apraxia, visuospatial deficits, and personality changes consistent with the areas of the brain affected. One notable psychiatric symptom is the "alien hand" syndrome, in which the hand of the patient, while retaining full sensation, takes on a mind of it's own.

○   **How does hydrocephalus present?**

There are two types: *noncommunicating hydrocephalus*, caused by an acute obstruction to CSF flow, which presents with the usual symptoms of increased intracranial pressure, headache, confusion, and ophthalmoplegia; and *communicating hydrocephalus* or *normal-pressure hydrocephalus*, caused by a deficiency in the resorption of CSF and responsible for 2% to 5% of all dementias. Normal-pressure hydrocephalus causes a characteristic triad of dementia, gait disturbance, and (later) incontinence. The dementia is frontal–subcortical in nature, characterized by deficits in attention, visuospatial skills, abstraction, judgment, and new learning. The gait slows, strides become shorter, and step height decreases, producing a characteristic "magnetic gait." Incontinence is more likely to be urinary than fecal.

○ **What causes hydrocephalus?**

Subarachnoid hemorrhage, head trauma, encephalitis, meningitis, carcinomatous disease, and partial aqueductal obstruction, among others.

○ **How can normal-pressure hydrocephalus be diagnosed?**

A CT scan will show increased ventricular size, particularly anteriorly, with periventricular lucencies. A lumbar puncture will show no elevation of pressure and will be otherwise normal. Cisternography will show reflux into the ventricles, and no flow into the superior sagittal sinus where CSF is normally resorbed.

○ **What is the treatment for normal-pressure hydrocephalus?**

Shunting, either ventricle to peritoneum or lumbar subarachnoid to peritoneum. Not all patients improve, unfortunately. Good prognostic signs include a short duration of symptoms, a known etiology, gait disturbance presenting before dementia, visible periventricular changes on imaging, and a temporary improvement following the removal of 50 mL of CSF on lumbar puncture.

○ **What percentage of patients with Huntington's disease present first with psychiatric symptoms and what are those symptoms?**

Fifty percent of Huntington's patients will present first with emotional or cognitive symptoms such as depression, irritability, apathy, or hallucinations.

○ **What is the epidemiology of Huntington's disease?**

It is an autosomal dominant trait with complete penetrance, caused by an expanded and unstable CAG trinucleotide repeat in chromosome 4, which affects 5–7 out of 100,000 people, depending on the population studied. The principal causes of death, which typically occurs around 14 years after diagnosis, are pneumonia, trauma, and suicide. Family members of Huntington's patients show increased psychopathology, but this is uncorrelated with the length of the trinucleotide repeat in asymptomatic carriers.

○ **What is the etiology of Huntington's disease?**

Degeneration begins in the medial caudate nucleus (the degree of degeneration correlating with the degree of cognitive dysfunction) and proceeds laterally to the putamen and occasionally to the pallidum. Somatostatin levels are increased, and GABA and acetylcholine levels in the striatum are decreased. There are also smaller decreases in dopamine and neurokinin. Because the major sources of input to the caudate are the limbic system and motor cortex, emotional and motor symptoms tend to be intertwined.

○ **What are the signs and symptoms of Huntington's disease?**

Initial motor symptoms are mild rigidity, restlessness, and tic-like jerks, exacerbated by emotional stress, mental concentration, and sleep deprivation, combined with slower writhing movements such as flexion and extension of the fingers ("piano playing"). There is an ulnar deviation of the hands on walking. Later symptoms include grimacing, nodding, head bobbing and rolling, a "dancing" gait; later still, akinesia, and dystonia. Abnormalities of articulation, coordination of limb movements and saccadic motions of the eyes are strongly correlated with intellectual and functional impairment. Cognitive deficiencies occur in visuospatial skills and memory, and skill acquisition is also impaired. Language skills are preserved except for fluency and prosody, with resulting impairment in interpersonal communication—patients will answer in single words or in short, infrequent phrases lacking emotional valence.

○   **How do the cognitive deficits of Huntington's disease differ from those in other dementias?**

Huntington's patients will show greater impairment in symbol manipulation, such as serial 7's, than in memory. Object naming is preserved, unlike in Alzheimer's, and the language functions are relatively spared until late in the course of the disease. Patients will have difficulties in sustained concentration, and also in discriminating facial affect and identity. Because memory retrieval is more impaired than encoding, Huntington's patients are far more able to recognize than to recall information. Also unlike Alzheimer's, in which memory loss follows a clear temporal gradient, Huntington's patients will have both recent and remote amnesia. There is also evidence of frontal dysfunction, i.e., decreased mental flexibility and difficulties in planning and organizing, that appear early, but are less severe than in Alzheimer's disease or Korsakoff's syndrome.

○   **What are the psychiatric complications of Huntington's disease?**

Two-thirds of patients will present with a psychiatric complaint before the onset of cognitive or motor symptoms. Typically, personality changes occur, such as apathy, lability, egocentrism, impulsivity, and decreased self-control (manifested through promiscuity or substance abuse). One-third will meet criteria for major depression or dysthymia, this often predating the dementia by several years, and 1 in 10 will have mania or hypomania. Huntington's patients, unlike those with Alzheimer's, Parkinson's, or stroke, are unusually prone to suicide, with one quarter making an attempt and 6% succeeding. Six to twenty-five percent of patients will become psychotic, usually with persecutory delusions and auditory hallucinations, and occasionally with fixed, specific delusions. Intermittent explosive disorder is found in one-third of patients. Substance abuse is no more common than in the general population. Thirty percent will have altered sexual behavior, either increased aggression or promiscuity, exhibitionism, voyeurism, or pedophilia.

○   **What laboratory tests aid in the diagnosis of Huntington's disease?**

Serum lab tests should be normal. CT scan/MRI will show atrophy of the caudate or putamen, manifested by enlarged frontal horns of the lateral ventricles. PET scan will show glucose hypometabolism in the striatum. An EEG will be low voltage, with poor or absent alpha waves. There is also a genetic test for the Huntington's gene, that is considered positive if more than 38 to 40 of the trinucleotide repeats are present.

○   **How should one treat Huntington's disease?**

There is no treatment. Antipsychotics will work on some patients to reduce psychosis, but the lowest dose possible should be used because neuroleptics will exacerbate the cognitive dysfunction, and they should generally be withheld until the involuntary movements become disabling. Fluphenazine is less apt to cause dysphoria than haloperidol, but not always. Antidepressants are effective against concomitant depression, as is ECT, and Huntington's-associated mania responds better to carbamazepine than lithium. There is no reliable treatment for the irritability and aggression, though a reduction in environmental complexity and establishment of unchanging routines is helpful. Unlike in Korsakoff's, memory retrieval is a problem rather than encoding, so increased rehearsals are generally not effective. However, patients are able to make use of verbal mediators to aid recall.

○   **What is the epidemiology of traumatic brain injury (TBI)?**

Of the two million a year in the United States, 300,000 require hospitalization and 80,000 have chronic sequelae. TBI accounts for 26% of injury deaths and 2% of all deaths, and is the most common neurological disease other than headache. Half are from motor vehicle crashes. Alcohol is involved in 50% of TBIs.

○ **What are the three basic patterns of traumatic brain injury?**

Contusions, diffuse axonal injury, and subdural hematomas are the three basic patterns of TBIs. Contusions, which usually affect the basal and polar areas of the temporal lobes, are typically the result of low-velocity injuries, such as falls. *Contrecoup* injuries result from abrupt pressure changes on the opposite side of the brain from the injury. Diffuse axonal injury is usually caused by acceleration or deceleration, and results in stretched axons and disrupted axonal transport, that causes axonal swelling and detachment and wallerian degeneration of the distal stump of the axon. The most vulnerable regions of the brain susceptible to axonal injury include the reticular formation, the superior cerebellar peduncles, the basal ganglia, hypothalamus, limbic fornices, and corpus callosum. Subdural hematomas, which have effects specific to location as well as more generalized effects on affect, arousal, and cognition, occur when an injury precipitates intracranial venous bleeding between the dura and the underlying cortex.

○ **What are the effects of TBI on brain chemistry?**

Initially, norepinephrine levels are elevated, with the degree of elevation correlating both with worse injuries and poorer outcome. The effect of TBI on other neurotransmitters is uncertain. Following the initial injury is secondary neurotoxicity from calcium influx, exotoxin release, phospholipase activation, and lipid peroxidation that further damages axons and neuronal systems. Free radicals and the neurotransmitter glutamate have both been implicated in causing further neuronal damages, and levels of both remain elevated for days postinjury.

○ **What laboratory tests can help in the diagnosis of TBI?**

CT scans may not show visible lesions until months after the injury. MRI is sensitive for frontal and temporal lesions that are often not visualized on CT scan, and can show diffuse axonal injury that do not show on CT scan. SPECT will show abnormalities that correlate with the degree of trauma. EEG can show abnormal foci or areas of seizure activity, particularly if measured under conditions of sleep deprivation, photic stimulation, or hyperventilation, or with anterotemporal or nasopharyngeal leads.

○ **What are the sequelae of traumatic brain injury?**

Sequelae of TBIs include slowed cognitive processing, deficits in attention and arousal, concentration, executive function, memory, personality changes (typically childishness, emotional lability, restlessness, decreased social contact, poverty of interests, and loss of spontaneity), anxiety, psychosis, and epilepsy.

○ **What are the prognostic indicators for recovery from TBI?**

Good prognostic indicators are high premorbid intelligence and preserved olfaction. Poor prognostic indicators are long posttraumatic amnesia, intoxication, chronic substance abuse, increased age, psychiatric history, learning disability, and a history of preexisting behavioral problems.

○ **What is the definition of a mild traumatic brain injury?**

Mild traumatic brain injury occurs when trauma to the head is characterized by a loss of consciousness less than 30 minutes, antero- or retrograde amnesia that lasts less than 24 hours, an altered mental status (dazedness, disorientation, or confusion) with a Glasgow Coma Score above 13, or focal neurological deficits.

○ **Describe three "frontal lobe syndromes."**

The orbitofrontal syndrome is characterized by impulsivity, disinhibition, hyperactivity, distractibility, and lability, while the dorsolateral syndrome is characterized by slowness, apathy, perseveration (negative symptoms), and is also known as *akinetic mutism*. The inferior orbital/anterior temporal syndrome is characterized by sudden outbursts of rage, withdrawal, fearfulness, and loss of inhibitions.

○ **What are the long-term neuropsychiatric sequelae of TBI?**

TBI causes increased deposition of β-amyloid protein, raising the risk of Alzheimer's disease 10-fold in those who already have one copy of the apo-E gene. The incidence of postinjury depression is difficult to assess methodologically because of confounding with posttraumatic apathy and unknown premorbid states, but it seems to be from 10% to 40%. In the first year after injury, 10% will have suicidal ideation and 2% will attempt suicide (15% in the 5 years postinjury). More common is a sadness, described as "mourning" for the lost self. The risk of depression is related to a premorbid psychiatric history and the degree of neuropsychiatric impairment, but not to loss of consciousness, amnesia, or presence of skull fractures. Poor premorbid social adjustment predicts poor recovery of ADLs and social function postinjury. Left frontodorsolateral and left basal ganglia lesions are associated with a transient depression. Mania, by contrast, is correlated with lesions at the base of the right temporal lobe or in the right orbitofrontal cortex, has an incidence of 3% in the 10 years postinjury, and is associated with a positive family history of bipolar disorder. Up to 15% of TBI sufferers will develop symptoms indistinguishable from schizophrenia, especially those with left temporal lesions. One study of a 100 homeless schizophrenics found that 55 of them had a history of TBI. The risk of epilepsy is 1% with mild, 2% with moderate, and 12% with severe TBI. Factors that increase this risk include skull fractures, penetrating wounds (50% risk of epilepsy), chronic alcoholism, intracranial hemorrhage, and increased severity of injury. Often this epilepsy does not develop until many years later (as with Phineas Gage). Ten to thirty percent develop an anxiety disorder, but PTSD is rare thanks to posttraumatic amnesia.

○ **What is postconcussion syndrome?**

Even mild injury or brief loss of consciousness can lead to attentional and information-processing impairment. Somatic symptoms include headache (50%), dizziness, insomnia, and fatigue (25%). Cognitive symptoms include memory impairment and decreased concentration. Perceptual symptoms include tinnitus and sensitivity to sound and light. Emotional symptoms include anxiety, depression, and irritability.

○ **How does one treat postconcussion syndrome?**

Early treatment includes education of the patient and family regarding predictors of symptoms and their resolution, validation of the patient's cognitive and emotional difficulties, and acknowledgment that the symptoms have an emotional component.

○ **How can one distinguish postconcussion syndrome from PTSD?**

Postconcussion syndrome generally remits within 3 months.

○ **What are the characteristics of the aggressive outbursts sometimes displayed by TBI patients?**

Aggression associated with TBI is usually triggered by very trivial stimuli, lacks planning or premeditation, occurs suddenly rather than building slowly over time, is brief and punctuated by interepisodic calm, serves no long-term goals, and is ego-dystonic, in that patients will be upset and embarrassed by their violence rather than attempt to justify it or blame others.

○ **What are some considerations regarding the pharmacologic treatment of those with TBI?**

The damaged brain is very sensitive to side effects of medication, so doses should be raised and lowered in small increments over long periods of time. An adequate therapeutic trial should be given at the highest dose before a medication is abandoned. Continuous reassessment is warranted given the continually changing status of the patient. The most disabling side effects tend to be anticholinergic (impairment of memory, concentration, and attention), so SSRIs are the best medications to use for depression and emotional lability. Seizure risk can be minimized if the medications are introduced gradually and the patient is on an anticonvulsant. Lithium decreases the seizure threshold and aggravates confusion, so carbamazepine or valproate is better tolerated. Dextroamphetamine or methylphenidate, which block the norepinephrine receptor, can increase concentration and arousal while decreasing fatigue, but the response might not be sustained. Bromocriptine increases alertness, concentration, memory, and speech while decreasing fatigue, hypersomnia and apathy in those at least a year postinjury. Amantadine improves anergia, abulia, mutism, anhedonia, impulsivity, and lability. Benzodiazepines increase GABA and glutamate toxicity (in animals) and should be avoided. Antipsychotics can be used to treat psychosis, but at low doses, because of the increased incidence of extrapyramidal side effects (EPS). Haloperidol, fluphenazine, and molindone lower the seizure threshold least, but haloperidol has been shown to delay recovery and the long-term effect of the others is uncertain.

○ **What is the best treatment for aggression following head injury?**

There is no medication approved by the FDA. Aggression can be controlled acutely through the use of sedating medications, i.e., neuroleptics or benzodiazepines, although the latter can produce disinhibition and paradoxical worsening of symptoms. Neuroleptics are a poor choice for chronic control, as tolerance to the sedation develops, while EPS and akathisia can increase agitation. Risperidone has been used effectively in low doses, however. Propanolol can also be effective in controlling aggression, and pindolol may be used if bradycardia develops. Anticonvulsants and antidepressants are sometimes effective. Behavior modification is effective in 75% of patients, in that teaching new cognitive strategies helps compensate for lost functions.

○ **What are three common reactions to brain injury?**

Three common reactions to brain injury are catastrophic reactions, indifference, and pseudobulbar affect. Catastrophic reactions, frequent with left-sized lesions, are characterized by anger, frustration, depression, tearfulness, shouting, swearing, and aggression, caused by the patient's inability to cope when faced with defective physical and cognitive functioning. Indifference, frequent with right-sided lesions and associated with hemineglect, is characterized by the lack of interest in family and friends, minimization of physical disabilities, and enjoyment of foolish jokes. Finally, pseudobulbar affect is characterized by pathological laughing or crying unrelated to one's inner emotional state (also known as pathological emotionalism or emotional lability).

○ **What is the epidemiology of HIV dementia?**

HIV dementia, also known as AIDS dementia complex, AIDS encephalopathy, subacute encephalitis, HIV encephalopathy, and HIV-1-associated minor cognitive/motor disorder (HAMCMD), will affect 30% persons infected by HIV. The median survival time postdiagnosis is 6 months.

○ **What is the etiology of AIDS dementia?**

It is caused by direct infection of the brain by HIV, which targets temporolimbic structures, the thalamus, and the basal ganglia, causing extensive atrophy (manifested through increased ventricular size rather than widened sulci). Neurons are not direct targets, but they are susceptible to associated neurotoxicity. The gp120 protein in the viral capsid binds irreversibly to calcium channels, increasing intracellular free calcium and increasing neurotoxin production. In addition, macrophages, once they have incorporated the viral genome into their own, are induced in the presence of cytokines and infectious byproducts to produce high levels of free radicals, quinolinic acid, TNF-α, IL-1β, interferon-γ, and arachidonic acid, which in turn increase intracellular calcium and nitric oxide. Neuronal apoptosis is also triggered by TNF-α and the viral *tat* protein.

○ **What is the differential diagnosis for mental status changes in AIDS patients?**

The differential diagnosis for mental status changes in AIDS patients is extensive. *Toxoplasmosis*, the most prevalent AIDS-related CNS infection, presents as focal or diffuse cognitive or affective disturbance, with ring-enhancing lesions on imaging. It is diagnosed by biopsy. *Cryptococcus neoformans*, presents as meningitis with headache, altered mental status, nuchal rigidity, nausea, and vomiting. An LP and CSF analysis is diagnostic. *Cytomegalovirus* can cause encephalitis, retinitis, peripheral neuropathy, and demyelination, and is treated with intravenous foscarnet or ganciclovir. *Herpes simplex* causes temporal lobe encephalitis or encephalomyelitis; severity is correlated with the severity of immune dysfunction, and it is treated with intravenous acyclovir. *Varicella zoster* causes peripheral and cranial nerve inflammation, encephalitis, and vascular inflammation, also treated with intravenous acyclovir. *Non-Hodgkin's lymphoma*, the primary CNS tumor in AIDS patients, causes altered mental status, hemiparesis, aphasia, seizures, and focal signs. Other CNS pathogens include *syphilis, TB, adenovirus type II, papovavirus, MAC, metastatic Kaposi's sarcoma, Candida, Aspergillus, Coccidioides, Rhizopus, Acremonium, Listeria, Nocardia, vasculitis, thrombotic emboli*, and *vasculotoxicity from AIDS medications*.

○ **What diagnostic tests can aid in determining the etiology of mental status changes in AIDS patients?**

CT scan and MRI are both good for showing ring-enhancing lesions, with MRI particularly suited as it shows high-signal intensities in subcortical white and gray matter. PET imaging will show increased glucose metabolism in basal ganglia and thalamus early in the disease, with hypometabolism late, and can be used to assess response to treatment. SPECT has an uncertain role. A lumbar puncture and CSF analysis can show toxoplasmosis, cryptococcus, HSV, VZV, CMV, and HIV, the signs of which include virions, increased IgG, HIV-specific antibody, neopterin, increased numbers of mononuclear cells, β_2-microglobulin (which is correlated with the severity of the dementia), and oligoclonal bands. EEG will show abnormal frontotemporal theta slowing in 25% of otherwise asymptomatic HIV-positive patients, and is thus very sensitive for early signs of the disease. Of those with AIDS, 65% will show intermittent or continuous theta or delta slowing. Evoked potentials are also abnormal even in the asymptomatic, and manifest delayed latency in the brainstem auditory and somatosensory evoked potentials. Polysomnography shows gross disturbances in sleep architecture.

○ **What are the symptoms of AIDS dementia?**

Impaired attention and concentration, mental slowing, impaired memory, slowed movements, incoordination, personality changes (irritability and lability) and, as the disease worsens, severe cognitive deficits, psychomotor slowing, seizures, muteness, catatonia, psychosis, mania, ataxia, spasticity, hyperreflexia, and bladder and bowel incontinence occur.

○ **What psychiatric conditions are associated with AIDS dementia?**

The incidence of depression is uncertain given the confounding substance abuse histories of many AIDS sufferers, but appears to be about 30%, with a risk factor being a past history of depression. Suicidal ideation has been measured at 55% in the HIV-positive population. Mania, when it appears, can be from a right frontal tumor or infection, or as a side effect of zidovudine. Anxiety can be triggered by knowledge of the diagnosis, PCP prophylaxis, CNS infections, or pulmonary insufficiency, and can often result from the zidovudine or steroids used in treatment. Delirium is also common and difficult to reverse.

○ **What are some treatments for AIDS dementia?**

The prerequisite for effective treatment is a high index of suspicion, because subtle cognitive deficits are often overlooked. Zidovudine, which penetrates the blood–brain barrier more effectively than ddI, ddC, 3TC, or d4T, is associated with increased cognitive function when administered in doses above 2 grams a day. Nimodipine (a calcium channel blocker) helps to block calcium channel–mediated neurotoxicity, although verapamil and diltiazem are not similarly effective. Methylphenidate increases verbal rote memory, rate of cognitive tracking, and mental set shifting by increasing dopaminergic function and will often return patients back to the normal range on neuropsychiatric testing. Vitamin B_6 will increase the production of serotonin at the expense of quinolinic acid and acts as a cofactor in the transformation of tryptophan to serotonin; administration of B_6 along with B_{12} can correct subclinical deficiencies in both. Vitamin E and *N*-acetylcysteine can both act as antioxidants. Behavioral plans include the keeping of notebooks, cueing signs and timers, labeling cabinets with contents rather than relying on memory, and keeping daily activity checklists. For delirium, molindone, which has little D_1 or D_2 affinity, is well tolerated in those with a history of EPS or neuroleptic malignant syndrome. For depression, anticholinergic medications are best avoided. The psychostimulants are as effective as the TCAs and have a faster onset of action. ECT is effective but may increase confusion in the encephalopathic patient. Lithium, carefully administered, or valproate is effective for mania. Neuroleptics can treat overwhelming panic, but EPS effects are common. Benzodiazepines are also effective for anxiety, although they occasionally have a disinhibiting effect, and trazodone helps with sleep. β-Blockers are unwise, because they can cause hypotensive episodes in those with undiagnosed HIV-related dysautonomia. Buspirone is excellent if immediate control of anxiety is not necessary, and is useful in treating substance abusers; however, dyskinesias with buspirone are more easily elicited in the neurologically impaired.

○ **What kinds of neuropsychiatric disturbances are associated with systemic lupus erythematosus?**

Seventy-five percent of lupus patients will have some sort of neuropsychiatric disturbance, which can be cognitive, psychiatric, or neither. Cognitive impairment is present in 20% to 30% and tends to fall into two general patterns of either failure of recognition memory associated with past or present brain involvement, or impaired immediate memory and concentration associated with systemic disease activity. Psychiatric symptoms include depression, anxiety, ethanol abuse, and psychosis; suicidality is increased in those with active disease and is associated with diffusely slow EEG measurements, but can also be from psychosocial causes. Cognitive and psychiatric symptoms tend to fluctuate concurrently and are not permanent once the disease is treated.

○ **What is the etiology of the neuropsychiatric manifestations of lupus?**

There are several. Small-vessel vasculopathy results when antiphospholipid antibodies cause endothelial injury; the resulting connective tissue proliferation causes an occlusive vasculopathy, which after repeated brief attacks, leads to a chronic noninflammatory vasculopathy. Large-vessel vasculitis occurs when intravascular complement activation and deposition of immune complexes in vessel walls attracts inflammatory cells. Finally, the direct effect of antinuclear antibodies (ANA) against brain constituents may play a role, although evidence for this is mixed. Other brain injuries occur in the form of emboli, infections, or TTP associated with lupus.

○ **How is lupus cerebritis best diagnosed?**

Unfortunately, the standard lupus antibody tests are not correlated with CNS disease activity (except possibly ribosomal P protein antibody). Serum and CNS ANA titers are equivocal and antiphospholipid antibodies–although correlated with stroke, chorea, and seizures—are likewise equivocal for cognitive and psychiatric symptoms. EEG is insensitive and nonspecific. MRI can show cerebral atrophy or T_2 hypointensity in subcortical regions (as opposed to multiple sclerosis, which tends to be more periventricular and also less enhanced by gadolinium), but these are not well correlated with symptoms. Flow to frontal lobes on SPECT is well correlated with psychosis, but the role of SPECT in diagnosing lupus is unclear. CSF from lumbar punctures can show pleocytosis, elevated IgG levels, and oligoclonal bands, but the sensitivity is low.

○   **How is lupus best treated?**

The treatment of lupus includes the use of high dose steroids, which ironically worsen psychiatric symptoms, anticoagulation for symptoms related to antiphospholipid antibodies, and IV pulse cyclophosphamide for severe cases. Psychiatric disease can be treated symptomatically in the usual fashion.

Note: This chapter is intended as an adjunct to preparation for the neurology section of ABPN boards. Multiple references are available for study, including the *Neurology: Pearls of Wisdom* review book.

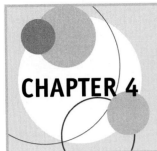

CHAPTER 4 Psychological Sciences

○ **Name three kinds of learning (conditioning).**

Classical, operant, and observational (or modeling).

○ **According to classical conditioning, in order to achieve a conditioned response, what must be paired with the neutral object?**

An unconditioned stimulus.

○ **Classical conditioning is generally thought to be most relevant to which form(s) of psychopathology?**

Anxiety disorders (or specific forms such as panic, phobia, and obsessive–compulsive disorder).

○ **Which psychiatric disorder might be thought of as an example of "one trial learning"?**

Posttraumatic stress disorder (or acute stress disorder).

○ **What do we call that which we place after a behavior that increases the likelihood that a behavior will occur again or more frequently?**

A reinforcer (or reward). Negative or positive

○ **If you reward (or reinforce) someone for successive approximations toward some goal, what is this called?**

Shaping.

○ **Punishment stops behaviors from occurring, but it has undesirable consequences. Name three.**

1. Emotional reactivity (sometimes including aggression) that may interfere with learning.

2. Avoidance of the punishment in ways that are unanticipated and negative.

3. It does not teach alternative desired behaviors, it only stops what is not desired.

○ **If you wish for a behavior to be maintained, even after reinforcements (or rewards) no longer follow the behavior, the behavior will be more likely to last longer under which initial reinforcement schedule: continuous or partial?**

Partial.

○ **If a behavior is maintained by a reinforcer that is not inherently desirable, but which has become associated with an inherently desirable reinforcer, what is that reinforcer called?**

A secondary reinforcer.

○ **What is the "Premack principle"?**

The Premack principle is a theory that states that a frequently occurring behavior (for instance, something that a person likes to do) can be used as a reinforcement (or reward) for a less frequently occurring behavior (by making the opportunity to engage in the desired behavior contingent upon the less frequently occurring behavior). Or in other words, a naturally occurring high-frequency response reinforces a lower frequency target response.

○ **Exposure and response prevention (a behavioral approach to the treatment of obsessive–compulsive disorder) is an example of which classical conditioning principle?**

Extinction (or possibly habituation) or systematic desensitization.

○ **If you recommended to a patient with agoraphobia to take several steps outside the door to the home for a few minutes each day, this would be an example of which classical conditioning principle?**

Extinction (or possibly habituation) or systematic desensitization.

○ **Anticipatory anxiety is an example of which form of conditioning?**

Classical.

○ **Albert Bandura focused a major portion of his research on demonstrating that observational learning or modeling was an important factor in the development of which behavior problem?**

Aggression (or violence).

○ **Martin Seligman exposed dogs to painful electrical shocks and the dogs tried to find a safe place in their cage. Eventually, the dogs gave up and did not learn that one side of the cage had become shock free. What did Seligman call this phenomenon?**

Learned helplessness.

○ **Learned helplessness is considered by Seligman to be a model for which form of psychopathology?**

Depression.

○ **What did Seligman do to get his dogs to learn that they could escape the shock?**

The dogs had to be repeatedly taken over to the shock-free area of the cage.

○ **Name the other animal model for depression.**

The forced swim test (or Porsolt test) induces a state of depression in mice by forcing them to swim in an enclosed container (I wonder if this is not more a state of desperation and therefore a less than satisfactory model, although it does seem like we're often drowning in own sorrows). Apparently, the mouse tends to "give up" after a certain period of time and takes on a characteristic "immobile posture." Administration of antidepressants apparently decreases the amount of time that the mouse is immobile (Porsolt et al. 1997).

○ **What is the name given to treatment for social deficiencies in people with schizophrenia that is most heavily based on observational learning?**

Social skills training.

○ **Which experimental design was popularized by the behaviorists, and which can be readily employed in the clinical setting?**

Single subject design or multiple baseline single subject design, commonly known as $N = 1$ designs.

○ **Which behavioral approach has the best likelihood of success for treating obsessive–compulsive disorder—systematic desensitization, in vivo exposure, or reverse conditioning?**

In vivo exposure.

○ **If a parent intentionally ignores a child's misbehavior, this is an example of which operant conditioning principle?**

Extinction.

○ **Define negative reinforcement.**

Negative reinforcement, by definition, is the application of an event that increases the probability of a target behavior occurring in the future. For example, when a fire truck comes by with the loud siren, one puts their fingers in their ears to eliminate the loud noise. Placing one's fingers in the ears is negatively reinforced by the reduction of a painful noise. A teacher expelling a youth from a classroom when the child says a curse word is negatively reinforced by the elimination of the noxious stimulus (youth). It is also positively reinforced in the youth if he or she wants to escape the classroom.

○ **How many "bits" of information can be stored in immediate memory for the average human?**

Seven. This phenomenon is actually called the "seven plus or minus two phenomena." That is why phone numbers and zip codes are about five to nine characters.

○ **To enhance the amount of retention, several pieces of information can be associated together to form a single "bit" in immediate memory. What is this process called?**

Chunking.

○ **To enhance memory, various investigators have demonstrated that pieces of information can be associated together with one another according to various mental pictorial schemes or other cognitive techniques. What are such techniques called?**

Mnemonic devices.

○ **Jean Piaget developed four stages of cognitive development. What are these stages?**

(1) Sensorimotor, (2) preoperational, (3) concrete operations, and (4) formal operations.

○ **What did Piaget call the process in which an experience is integrated into existing cognitive structures?**

Assimilation.

○   **What did Piaget call the process whereby cognitive structures change, based on new information that cannot be assimilated into existing structures (scheme)?**

Accommodation.

○   **According to Piaget, before the individual progresses to the preoperational stage, what must be achieved, and at about what age does this happen?**

Object permanence, which occurs between 18 and 24 months of age.

○   **Name the six stages of moral development, as formulated by Lawrence Kohlberg.**

(1) External reward and punishment stage, (2) bargaining or marketplace stage, (3) conformist stage, (4) law and order stage, (5) social contract stage, and (6) universal ethical principles stage.

○   **What are the most common individually administered intelligence tests?**

The Wechsler scales (specifically, the Wechsler Adult Intelligence Scale III, the Wechsler Intelligence Scale for Children, and the Wechsler Preschool and Primary Intelligence Scale-Revised).

○   **What are the means and standard deviations of all of the Wechsler scales?**

The means are 100 and the standard deviations are 15.

○   **What are the levels of mental retardation, based on IQ scores?**

Mild: 50/55 to 70
Moderate: 35/40 to 50/55
Severe: 20/25 to 35/40
Profound: less than 20/25

Note: because of the standard error of measurement, a given IQ test score should not be taken as absolute, and allowance is made in diagnosis for the test score to vary approximately five points in either direction. That is, a person may have an IQ of 65 on a given test, but be judged appropriately by a clinician to NOT be mentally retarded.

○   **Why did Alfred Binet originally develop an IQ test?**

To have an objective means of assessing mental retardation.

○   **What are the two most commonly used projective personality tests for adults?**

The Rorschach (inkblot test) and the thematic apperception test (TAT).

○   **What is the difference between an objective and a projective personality test?**

Objective tests have a limited set of responses (such as true/false or multiple choice), facilitating reliability and ease of scoring. Projective tests have a potentially unlimited number of possible responses to items or stimuli, such that considerable time and training is required for scoring.

○ **What does the term reliability mean, as it relates to a psychological test?**

There are several kinds of reliability, such as test-retest reliability, interrater reliability, alternate forms reliability, and split halves reliability. In general, reliability refers to the dependability of scores obtained from a psychological assessment or from a psychological test. A reliable psychological test will yield highly dependable or highly consistent results if administered to the same person or persons under similar circumstances.

○ **What is validity as it refers to a psychological test?**

There are many forms of validity, such as predictive validity, construct validity, face validity, concurrent validity, content validity, convergent validity, discriminant validity, consequential validity, and criterion validity. In general, validity describes the extent to which a psychological instrument measures what it is supposed to measure.

○ **If you want to evaluate personality, what tests should you order?**

Most clinical psychologists prefer to select their own tests, based on the referral question, so you do not need to order specific tests. If you want the results of a specific test, you can request that it be included in the battery that the psychologist will use.

○ **What areas of assessment are included in a full neuropsychological test battery?**

While there are no absolute rules, and while the clinical psychologist or neuropsychologist in general will select tests based on your referral question and personal preferences, the areas evaluated tend to include the following: psychomotor and sensory–perceptual functioning, general intelligence, language functioning, memory and immediate problem solving, attention and concentrational functions, practice functions (complex organized executive/motoric activities), visuospatial and constructional functions, abstracting/higher order conceptualization capacities, and emotional/behavioral functioning. The most common and widely used neuropsychological batteries include the Luria–Nebraska neuropsychological battery and the Halstead–Reitan Battery.

○ **Which classic psychological test was developed on the basis of the statistical difference between the way people with psychiatric disorders and normal controls respond to test items?**

The Minnesota Multiphasic Personality Inventory (MMPI).

○ **What are the factors of the five-factor theory of personality, and why is this theory considered important?**

Neuroticism, extraversion, openness to experience, conscientiousness, and agreeableness. This theory is considered important because these factors have arisen consistently in many factor-analytic studies of personality traits, because the factors have been replicated across many cultures, and because the factors emerge even if the people rating others have almost no contact with the people they are rating, i.e., the factors seem to be intrinsic to all humans, forming an "implicit personality theory."

○ **What is the most important factor in determining behavior, the situation or one's personality traits?**

While on the average, situations exert more influence on behavior than personality traits, the combination of the personality traits and the situation under consideration is the most predictive model, based on empirical investigation.

○ **What are the three qualities of the psychotherapist considered by Carl Rogers to be the most important for the outcome of the psychotherapy?**

Empathy, warmth, and genuineness.

○ **For which of the following disorders would psychotherapy alone most likely be an *in*appropriate treatment: major depression, posttraumatic stress disorder, or panic disorder?**

Major depression.

○ **What factor is in general most influential in the development of friendship relationships?**

Proximity.

○ **What is the next most influential factor in the development of friendship relationships with others?**

Personal similarity.

○ **Leon Festinger demonstrated that people tend to be consistent in the way they conduct themselves. When people's inconsistencies are pointed out, it produces distress. In general, people will try to reduce perceived inconsistency in some way. What is the name of the theory associated with these findings?**

The theory of cognitive dissonance.

○ **Stanley Milgram conducted a now famous set of experiments in which he demonstrated that people under certain circumstances were willing to deliver (what they believed to be) painful electrical shocks to others. What phenomenon was Milgram studying in this set of experiments?**

Obedience to authority. Note: these studies caused such a stir with the APA that IRBs were created. Milgram was interested in general compliance related to Nazi Germany.

○ **What activity did Muzafer Sherif demonstrate to be most effective in reducing destructive intergroup rivalry or competition?**

Focusing attention on to a common enemy, which resulted in the groups joining together in cooperation.

○ **Philip Zimbardo tried to conduct studies of the behavior of prisoners and guards by having ordinary people role play prisoners or guards interacting with one another. Why did he have to halt his now famous Prison–Guard experiment?**

The guards started abusing the prisoners. Note: important related to Labeling Theory.

○ **Name two intrinsic psychological motivational systems.**

Appetitive (or approach) and aversive (or avoidance).

○ **Paul Ekman demonstrated that several emotional expressions seem to be biologically based or at least intrinsic to all humans, i.e., they are universally understood by humans studied across many cultures. Name six such emotional expressions.**

Anger, fear, sadness, joy, disgust, and surprise.

○ **What are the two factors in Stanley Schacter's two-factor theory of emotion?**

(1) Arousal or activation and (2) cognitive interpretation or attribution.

○ **Albert Bandura demonstrated that a person's belief that he or she could accomplish a specific activity was, in general, highly predictive of whether the person could, in fact, accomplish that activity. What is the name of the theory derived from this area of research?**

Self-efficacy theory.

○ **Which theory of perception is most aligned with the view that "the whole is more than the sum of the parts"?**

Gestalt theory.

○ **Which early school of psychology had as its goal an analysis of the contents of consciousness?**

Structuralism.

○ **Which early schools of psychology emphasize a biological model of human behavior?**

- Functionalism.
- Mechanistics, described by Ernst Brucke (1819–1892), a physiologist, was the first academic advisor of Freud. Ernst worked for Franz Brentano (1838–1917), an "act psychologist."
- Classical ethology, developed by Konrad Lorenz. Konrad joined the Nazi party in 1938 and was affiliated with its Race Policy Department. After a long history in POW camps after the war, Lorenz received the Nobel Prize in medicine in 1973.
- Psychoanalysis, although Sigmund Freud was, of course, a medical doctor and not an academically trained psychologist.

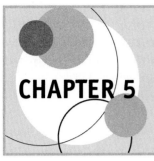

CHAPTER 5

Quantitative and Experimental Methods

○ **What is a direct interview?**

An important source of information about a subject is the direct interview, which is a person-to-person interaction.

○ **What are indirect surveys?**

Indirect surveys are structured self-report forms that may be used for gathering research data. However, they lack the clinical judgment of an experienced practitioner that is necessary in some instances.

○ **What is reliability?**

Reliability refers to whether or not the findings of the assessment instrument or diagnostic procedure are reproducible (i.e., whether or not the quality of the data is trustworthy or dependable). In psychometrics, reliability is a measure of the internal consistency and stability with which a measuring instrument performs its function. Generally, reliability roughly corresponds to the everyday concept of accuracy.

○ **What is interrater reliability?**

Interrater reliability means the results of the survey can be replicated when the instrument is used by different examiners. A measure of the consistency of rating, interrater reliability is equal to the correlation between the ratings given by different raters of the same people or stimulus.

○ **What is test-retest reliability?**

Test-retest reliability means the results of the survey can be replicated when the instrument is used on different occasions. A measure of a test's reliability, or more specifically its stability, test-retest reliability is based on the correlation between scores of a group of respondents on two separate occasions.

○ **What is validity?**

Validity refers to whether the test measures what it is supposed to measure, or in other words, the soundness or adequacy of something or the extent to which it satisfies certain standards or conditions. In psychometrics, validity is the extent to which a test measures what it purports to measure, or the extent to which specified inference from the test's sores are justified or meaningful.

○ **What are the subcategories of validity?**

There are many. They include criterion validity, face validity (a priori validity), content validity, concurrent validity, internal validity, external validity, ecological validity, congruent validity, consensual validity, construct validity, content validity, convergent validity, incremental validity, intrinsic validity, predictive validity, and trait validity.

○ **What is bias?**

There are different types of biases. The first is construct bias, which occurs when what the construct measures is not identical across groups. Method bias refers to all sources of assessment problems emanating from an instrument or its administration, such as the influence of the person or the tester on the best outcome. Finally, item bias (or differential item functioning) refers to anomalies at the item level, such as a poor translation of words.

○ **What does the double-blind design method help with?**

The double-blind design is helpful in controlling experimenter effects and the influence of demand characteristics. Neither the experimenter nor the research participants or subjects know, until after the data have been collected, what participants received during the experiment. The double-blind method is often used with a placebo to avoid contamination of the results from biases and preconceptions on the part of the experimenter.

○ **What is randomization?**

Randomization of a sample is a method in which each member of the total group studied has an equal chance of being selected. It also helps eliminate bias.

○ **What is sensitivity?**

Sensitivity is the ability of an assessment instrument to detect the item/quality being measured.

○ **What is specificity?**

Specificity refers to the ability of an assessment instrument to assess *only* the variable chosen for study.

○ **What is predictive value?**

Assessment instruments should also have a good predictive value, which is the proportion of true-positive to true-negative results. In psychometrics, predictive value is a form of criterion validity in which the predictor scores are obtained in advance of the criterion scores, as when a test of scholastic aptitude is validated against scores on tests of school performance obtained months or years later. Note: most tests have poor predictive utility.

○ **What is analysis of variance (ANOVA)?**

ANOVA is a set of statistical procedures designed to compare three or more groups of observations and determines whether the differences between groups are due to experimental influence or chance alone. Note: a two-group test is called the *t*-test, or to be more specific the Student's *t*-test.

○ **What is factor analysis?**

Factor analysis is a statistical technique for analyzing the correlations between a large number of variables in order to reduce them to a smaller number of underlying dimensions, called factors, in a manner analogous to the way in which all spectral colors can be reduced to combinations of just three primary colors.

○ **What is multivariate statistics?**

Multivariate statistics is a branch of statistics devoted to investigating the influence of one or more independent variables acting on more than one dependent variable.

○ **What is a coefficient of correlation?**

A coefficient of correlation shows the relationship between two sets of paired measurements. In statistics, a coefficient of correlation measures the degree of linear relationship between two variables such that high scores on one tend to go with high scores on the other and low scores on one with low scores on the other (positive correlation), or such that high scores on one tend to go with low scores on the other (negative correlation). The most commonly used index of correlation, the "product-moment" correlation coefficient, symbolized by r, ranges from 1.00 (for perfect) to 0 (no relationship).

○ **What is a Chi square?**

A Chi square is a nonparametric statistic used to evaluate the relative frequency or proportion of events in a population that falls into well-defined categories.

○ **Name four multivariate methods.**

Multiple regression, discriminant analysis, canonical correlation, and factor analysis are multivariate methods.

○ **What is the null hypothesis?**

The null hypothesis is the assumption that there is no significant difference between two random samples of a population. When it is rejected, observed differences between groups are deemed to be improbable by chance alone. In inferential statistics, the null hypothesis is the provisional hypothesis that there is no difference or no relationship between random samples and that the observed experimental results can therefore be attributed to chance alone.

○ **What does the "p value" mean?**

In inferential statistics, the "p value" is the probability of obtaining a result as extreme as the one observed, in either direction from the expected value, if the null hypothesis is true. A "p value" of 0.05 means that the result will occur 5 times out of every 100 times by chance alone.

○ **What is a t test?**

A statistical procedure designed to compare two sets of observations is the t test.

○ **What is a type I error?**

The false claim of a true difference because the observed difference is due entirely to chance is a type I error. In statistics, a type I error occurs by rejecting the null hypothesis when the null is true. The significance level determined from a statistical test is the probability of a type I error.

○ **What is a type II error?**

The false acceptance of the null hypothesis when, in fact, there is a true difference but the difference is so small that it falls within the acceptance region of the null hypothesis is a type II error. In statistics, a type II error occurs by failing to reject the null hypothesis when it is false.

Note: type III error is a term used to refer to an error arising from a misinterpretation of the nature of the scores being compared in a significance test.

○   **What are independent variables?**

Independent variables are those qualities that the experimenter systematically varies (e.g., time, age, sex, type of drug).

○   **What are dependent variables?**

Dependent variables are those qualities that measure the influence of the independent variable or the outcome of the experiment (e.g., the measurement of a person's specific physiological reactions to a drug).

○   **What is the sensitivity of a test?**

Sensitivity is the proportion of patients with the condition in question that the test is able to detect.

○   **What is the specificity of a test?**

Specificity is the proportion of patients who do not have the condition that the test calls negative.

○   **What is the sensitivity in the following test?**

	Disease	No Disease
Test +	90	20
Test −	10	80
Total	100	100

$$\text{Sensitivity} = \frac{\text{True Positive}}{\text{True Positive} + \text{False Negative}}$$

    In the table shown in the question, it is clear that **90** people who were tested have the disease, which means they are **true positive**. **Twenty** people tested positive but have no disease so they are **false positive**. **Eighty** people tested negative and have no disease so they are **true negative**. **Ten** people have the disease but tested negative (hence, they are **false negative**). Know the formulas and fill in the numbers to get correct answers in % values.

○   **What is the specificity in the above test?**

$$\text{Sensitivity} = \frac{\text{True Nagative}}{\text{True Negative} + \text{False Positive}}$$

○   **What is the positive predictive value in the above test?**

$$\text{Positive predictive value} = \frac{\text{True Positive}}{\text{True Positive} + \text{False Positive}}$$

○ **What is the negative predictive value in the above test?**

$$\text{Negative predictive value} = \frac{\text{True Negative}}{\text{True Negative} + \text{False Negative}}$$

○ **A college student had the following scores in the simulated examination he tried at home: 11, 9, 7, 6, 6, 4, and 6. What is the mode in this case?**

The mode is the number 6. The most important precaution is to ARRANGE the given numbers in an ascending pattern; otherwise answers will be wrong. Once arranged, find the middle number; and that is the median. Since there is a total of seven numbers, the middle number is 6 in the series 4, 6, 6, 6, 7, 9, 11. Had there been 8 numbers (4, 6, 6, 6, 7, 8, 9, 11) we would have had to take average of the two middle numbers (6, 7) to get the median, which would then be 6.5. The mode is the number that occurs MOST frequently. (Remember: Mode and Most start with MO and the number 6 is the number occurring most frequently in the above series.)

○ **What is the median in the above case?**

Six.

○ **The average duration of dementia is 4.5 years and its incidence is 3 per 1,000 each year. What is the prevalence of dementia?**

$$\text{Prevalence} = \text{incidence} \times \text{duration of a disease}.$$

Since incidence = 3 and duration of dementia = 4.5 years (in the given population), prevalence can be calculated by multiplying 4.5 by 3. The answer is 13.5.

○ **What is the definition of the standard deviation?**

The standard deviation is the square root of the variance, which gives an estimate of the average deviation from the mean.

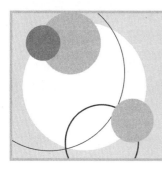

Section II

PSYCHOPATHOLOGY

CHAPTER 6

Schizophrenia

○ **Who first coined the term "dementia praecox" referring to patients with schizophrenia?**

Emil Kraepelin delineated the difference between manic-depression and schizophrenia with his observations that patients with schizophrenia had a premature and long-term deterioration in functioning versus the more cyclic and nonprogressive course of manic-depression.

○ **What were the "Four A" symptoms Eugen Bleuler used to describe the primary symptoms of schizophrenia in the early 1900s?**

The "Four A" symptoms include abnormal (loose) associations, autistic behavior and thinking, abnormal (flat) affect, and ambivalence. Note: Bleuler was the one to coin the term "schizophrenia" in 1908.

○ **What are schneiderian or first-rank symptoms?**

Kurt Schneider characterized psychotic symptoms of schizophrenia as those of thought control, thought insertion, thought withdrawal, thought broadcasting, and auditory hallucinations composed of a running commentary about one's actions or voices conversing with each other. Many of these symptoms are present in the current *DSM-IV* criteria.

○ **What are the risk factors for schizophrenia?**

Risk factors for schizophrenia include the presence of an affected first-degree relative (3%–7%), perinatal insults (low birth weight, prematurity, preeclampsia, prolonged labor, fetal distress, hypoxia—1%), and a winter birth.

○ **In monozygotic twins, what is the concordance rate for schizophrenia?**

The concordance rate for schizophrenia in monozygotic twins is 40% to 50%, suggesting a strong genetic contribution to the development of schizophrenia; environmental causal factors are suspected of being involved as well.

○ **What are the risks to family members of developing schizophrenia?**

Siblings of patients with schizophrenia have approximately a 10% lifetime risk of developing schizophrenia. In a family with one parent diagnosed with schizophrenia, children have a 12% risk of schizophrenia. When two or more family members have schizophrenia, the risks increase dramatically. Children in families with two parents diagnosed with schizophrenia have a 40% lifetime risk of schizophrenia, while a monozygotic twin is diagnosed with schizophrenia has a 47% risk of developing schizophrenia during his/her lifetime. A clinical observation has been noted in which siblings of affected patients will often be high achievers.

○ **What are the lifetime prevalence rates and incidence rates for schizophrenia?**

The lifetime prevalence rate for schizophrenia is estimated to be between 0.5% and 1%, while incidence rates are approximately 1 per 10,000.

○ **What gender-specific factors have been noted in schizophrenia?**

Women show a peak age of onset in the late 20s compared to the early 20s in men. Women also tend to have more prominent mood symptoms and a better overall prognosis. The male-female ratio is 1:1. Women tend to respond better to antipsychotic medication, but are at higher risk for developing tardive dyskinesia.

○ **What season of birth is associated with a disproportionate number of patients with schizophrenia?**

Winter birth is associated with a higher occurrence of schizophrenia. Theories attempting to explain "why" include potential environmental stressors such as temperature, nutritional deficiencies, and exposure to infectious agents.

○ **What is the relationship between symptoms of schizophrenia and employability?**

Unemployment rates in patients with schizophrenia are as high as 70%. However, there is a relatively low correlation between psychopathology and the ability to hold a job, the level of negative symptoms being a more important predictor of work performance than positive symptoms.

○ **How does the life expectancy of individuals with schizophrenia compare to the general population?**

The life expectancy of persons with schizophrenia is estimated to be about 10 years less than in the general population. This is accounted for in part by a high suicide rate (10%) and a relatively higher prevalence of general medical illness with lesser tendency to receive treatment. They may be at special risk for illnesses associated with poor self-care and exposure to pathogens, e.g., tuberculosis, and substance abuse-related illnesses such as emphysema and HIV-related disorders.

○ **What evidence supports the dopamine hypothesis of schizophrenia?**

The dopamine hypothesis is supported by observations that drugs with increased dopaminergic activity, such as amphetamines and levodopa, can cause psychosis, while drugs with postsynaptic dopamine blockade activity improve psychotic symptoms. Also, plasma levels of homovanillic acid (a dopamine metabolite) have been noted to increase during acute psychosis and fall with symptomatic improvement in some patients. PET studies have shown increased dopamine receptors in the caudate nucleus in drug-free patients.

○ **What are the most consistently replicated postmortem structural abnormalities in schizophrenia?**

The basal ganglia, limbic system, and cerebral cortex have all been implicated in structural studies of schizophrenia. But the most consistent findings in these studies appear to be reduced volume and cytoarchitectural abnormalities in the hippocampus of patients with schizophrenia.

○ **Why is glutamate, an excitatory amino acid neurotransmitter, of interest in schizophrenia research?**

The NMDA glutamate receptor subtype is blocked by phencyclidine (PCP or angel dust) and produces a clinical syndrome similar to schizophrenia, including positive and negative symptoms, and a formal thought disorder. Glutamate may also be relevant to schizophrenia because it is the primary neurotransmitter of descending projections from cortical and hippocampal regions. Abnormalities in subcortical areas may be involved in altered neuronal information processing in schizophrenia.

○ **Are immunological abnormalities associated with schizophrenia?**

Disturbances in cellular immunity, such as morphologically atypical lymphocytes, deficient natural killer cell production, abnormal helper–suppressor cell ratios, and increased CD5+ beta-lymphocytes, have been described in patients with schizophrenia. Investigators have also reported increased endogenous CNS immunoglobulin and interferon levels as well as the possibility of CNS antibodies. If these findings are verified by future studies, an autoimmune reaction or infectious agent may be implicated in the development of schizophrenia.

○ **What are the psychiatric indications for neuroimaging studies (CT scan, MRI)?**

First-episode psychosis, confusion or dementia of unknown cause, prolonged catatonia, movement disorder of unknown etiology, and first episode of personality change or mood disorder after the age of 50 years.

○ **What structural neuroimaging findings are characteristic of schizophrenia?**

No structural findings are pathognomonic of schizophrenia, the diagnosis of which remains a clinical one at this time. A number of nonspecific markers, however, have been identified. Enlargement of cortical sulci, ventriculomegaly in lateral and third ventricles, reduction in temporal lobe gray matter and whole brain volume, decrease in size of temporal lobe structures, cerebellar atrophy, and alterations in corpus callosum shape and size have been identified in samples of patients. An increased ventricle to brain ratio (VBR) is the best-replicated neurobiological finding in schizophrenia.

○ **What are the clinical correlates of increased ventricular size in schizophrenia?**

Ventricular enlargement in schizophrenia is associated with a greater degree of negative symptoms, cognitive impairment, poor premorbid social adjustment, and decreased antipsychotic response with increased incidence of extra pyramidal side effects. Overall, the prognosis is poorer. Ventriculomegaly, however, is a nonspecific finding, reflecting diminution of brain tissue and is seen in a variety of neuropsychiatric conditions.

○ **What is the most consistent functional neuroimaging study finding in schizophrenia?**

Hypofrontality, especially evident during neuropsychological tests such as the Wisconsin card sort test (which places demands on the dorsolateral prefrontal cortex) is the most consistent finding.

○ **List substances of abuse and medications that can be a cause of psychosis?**

Substances of abuse such as hallucinogens, phencyclidine, amphetamines, cocaine, and alcohol may be associated with psychotic symptoms. One must also rule out exposure to commonly prescribed medications, including anticholinergics, corticosteroids, and levodopa that have been associated with psychosis. Finally, use of cannabis may be associated with precipitation of psychotic episodes.

○ **Abnormal smooth pursuit eye movements are found in what percent of first-degree relatives of schizophrenic patients?**

Forty percent (50%–80% in patients with schizophrenia).

○ **What single symptom satisfies Criterion A (active phase) in the *DSM-IV* diagnosis of schizophrenia?**

Delusions judged to be bizarre OR auditory hallucinations experienced as two or more voices conversing with one another or keeping a running commentary on one's thoughts or behavior can each alone satisfy Criterion A.

○   **What are the three symptom domains of schizophrenia?**

(1) Hallucinations, delusions, and paranoia; (2) thought disorder and bizarre behavior; and (3) Anhedonia, thought poverty, and social withdrawal.

○   **What is the triad of cognitive deficits present in schizophrenia?**

Memory, executive functions, and motor performance.

○   **What is the strongest predictor of treatment outcome in first-episode schizophrenia?**

Duration of presenting symptoms before treatment. Patients with a shorter duration of psychotic symptoms have more rapid and higher rates of remission. First-episode patients also have a greater therapeutic response at lower doses of antipsychotic medication and are more sensitive to side effects, most notably extrapyramidal symptoms.

○   **What subtype of schizophrenia is associated with better short- and long-term outcomes?**

The paranoid subtype is associated with fewer negative symptoms and less deterioration resulting in better overall treatment outcome.

○   **How does the long-term outcome of schizophrenia in developing countries compare with that in industrialized nations?**

Individuals in developing countries tend to have a more acute course and better outcome than those in industrialized nations. Psychosocial factors are felt to affect the course to a greater degree than causal factors of the illness. The more sociocentric culture of developing countries appears to produce a more favorable outcome than in industrialized nations that are egocentric.

○   **Describe the concept of "schizophrenia spectrum disorders."**

Schizophrenia spectrum disorders are the Cluster A personality disorders (schizoid, schizotypal, and paranoid personality disorders) that are characterized by odd and eccentric behavior, unusual ideas, mild formal thought disorder, and social withdrawal. Higher rates of these disorders have been noted in the families of patients with schizophrenia than in those of normal subjects.

○   **List the *DSM-IV* criteria for schizophrenia.**

The *DSM-IV* criteria for schizophrenia require that two or more characteristic symptoms (delusions, hallucinations, disorganized speech or behavior, and negative symptoms) are present for at least 1 month. The symptoms must cause significant decline in functioning, and cannot be primarily due to a mood disorder, substance use, medical condition, or pervasive developmental disorder.

○   **How is schizophrenia subtyped in the *DSM-IV*?**

Schizophrenia is subtyped on the basis of the most predominant symptoms at the time of the most recent evaluation and therefore may change over time. Five subtypes have been identified: paranoid, disorganized, undifferentiated, catatonic, and residual. The paranoid and disorganized subtypes have the best and worst outcomes, respectively.

Describe the three general stages of schizophrenia and its course.

The first stage is the onset of the illness that can either be insidious or acute. The majority of individuals display some form of prodromal phase manifested by gradual development of signs and symptoms (e.g., social withdrawal, unusual behavior, loss of interest in work or school). The second stage follows with either years of chronic psychotic symptoms (varying in severity) or years of episodic psychotic symptoms with relatively complete recovery. The final stage (residual phase) typically encompasses a lessening in the severity of psychotic symptoms, but patients often continue to exhibit chronic symptoms of their illness.

Describe the onset of schizophrenia.

Schizophrenia typically becomes manifest in adolescence or early adulthood and has a rather heterogeneous natural history. About half of cases present with the insidious onset of subtle progressive impairment of function in personal, social, school, or work areas lasting weeks to years, prior to the onset of psychosis. However, a rapid onset of psychosis may also be seen in persons with no prior disturbance of personal or social functioning.

What are the differences in diagnostic criteria for schizophrenia in children versus adults?

Essentially, features are the same in both age groups and a single *DSM-IV* criteria set is utilized in both populations. Delusions and hallucinations may be less elaborate in children, whereas visual hallucinations may be more common. Diagnostic confusion, however, can arise between pervasive developmental disorder, autism, communication disorders, and schizophrenia in children.

In the differential diagnosis of schizophrenia, what other major psychiatric diagnoses should one consider?

Schizophreniform disorder, schizoaffective disorder, mood disorders, delusional disorder, personality disorders (especially schizotypal, schizoid, paranoid, and borderline), brief psychotic disorder, psychotic disorder NOS, obsessive–compulsive disorder, malingering, factitious disorder, autism, substance-induced psychosis, and psychosis secondary to a general medical/neurological condition.

What feature delineates schizophrenia from delusional disorder?

Delusions in delusional disorder are by definition nonbizarre, and do not occur in the presence of other psychotic symptoms such as hallucinations or aberrant thought processes.

Describe the features of late-onset schizophrenia.

Typically, late-onset schizophrenia is defined as onset of illness after 45 years of age. It occurs more frequently in women, and is often characterized by paranoid delusions and lesser degrees of disorganization and negative symptoms. Patients with late-onset schizophrenia have better occupational histories and are more likely to have been married than early-onset patients. It is important to exclude psychosis due to a general medical condition or a brain lesion.

Differentiate schizophrenia from schizophreniform disorder.

The distinction is primarily based on the symptom duration. A diagnosis of schizophrenia requires the presence of psychotic symptoms for at least 1 month, with a history of prodromal symptoms for 6 months, while the symptoms of schizophreniform disorder (prodromal, acute, and residual) must be present for at least 1 month, but less than 6 months. Also, no decline in functioning is required for the diagnosis of schizophreniform disorder, although this is often evident.

○ **Describe the clinical course and outcome of schizophreniform disorder.**

It is estimated that one-third of individuals with the diagnosis of schizophreniform disorder recover within 6 months, with a final diagnosis of schizophreniform disorder. Two-thirds will ultimately be diagnosed with schizoaffective disorder, schizophrenia, or a psychotic mood disorder.

○ **Describe Capgras syndrome.**

Capgras syndrome describes delusions of impostures. Affected individuals are convinced that doubles of important persons, significant others, or oneself exist. This may be seen in a variety of psychiatric conditions; however, 60% of cases are associated with schizophrenia.

○ **What is the prevalence of substance use disorders in schizophrenia?**

Thirty-five to fifty percent of patients with schizophrenia have a substance use disorder; not including nicotine dependence. This rate compares with 27% in the general population, 56% in bipolar disorder, and 84% in antisocial personality disorder. Many patients with schizophrenia meet criteria for abuse of multiple substances.

○ **What percentage of schizophrenic patients develop severe depressive symptoms?**

Up to 60% of patients with schizophrenia develop depression at some point during the illness, but the diagnosis of depression is complicated by phenomenological overlap with negative symptoms and extrapyramidal side effects of antipsychotic medications.

○ **Describe factors associated with suicide in schizophrenia.**

Approximately 10% of patients with schizophrenia commit suicide, primarily in the first 10 years of the illness. Risk factors include male gender, age under 30 years, college education, paranoid subtype, comorbid substance use, depressive symptoms, unemployment, frequent exacerbations of the disease, prior suicide attempts, living alone, and recent hospital discharge.

○ **A patient with schizophrenia presents with persistent hyponatremia and low urine specific gravity. Discuss diagnostic considerations and management approach.**

It is important to consider psychosis-induced polydipsia causing water intoxication and hyponatremia. Of course, diabetes insipidus, diabetes mellitus, chronic renal failure, and other potential medical problems should be ruled out. SIADH also causes hyponatremia, and medical or medication-induced etiologies should be considered in the differential diagnosis. In psychosis-induced polydipsia, the goal is to control psychosis and water intake. Water restriction and sodium replacement may be necessary. Lithium, phenytoin, and clozapine have been reported to show benefit.

○ **What is the current thinking regarding schizophrenia and violence?**

The data related to this issue are conflicting secondary to methodological problems. Certain observations have, however, been noted. Well-planned, directed violence may be associated with paranoid delusions. Violence in more disorganized psychotic states is poorly focused and generally nondirected. ECA data reported that 12.7% of individuals with schizophrenia reported violent behavior in the previous year compared with 25% of those with alcoholism. Generally, individuals with schizophrenia are at higher risk to be victims of violent crimes rather than to be perpetrators.

○ **What is metabolic syndrome?**

Metabolic syndrome is a constellation of symptoms associated with increased risk for diabetes mellitus type 2 and cardiovascular disease. Symptoms include elevated fasting glucose levels (>110 mg/dL), hypertension (BP > 140/90), abdominal obesity (BMI > 27 kg/m²), elevated triglycerides (>250 mg/dL), and decreased high-density lipoproteins (HDL, 25 mg/dL). Metabolic syndrome is essentially an epidemic in the United States, with some studies estimating the prevalence rate to be at 25% (American Diabetes Association parameters).

○ **What classes of medications are associated with increased risk for metabolic syndrome?**

Atypical antipsychotics, protease inhibitors, β-blockers, thiazide diuretics, and corticosteroids to name a few.

○ **Are people who have a diagnosis of schizophrenia (and bipolar disorder) at increased risk for diabetes mellitus type 2, regardless of what type of medications they are prescribed?**

Yes. There is a two to three times higher prevalence rate of diabetes mellitus type 2 in individuals affected by schizophrenia (16–21%) than the general population (7.3% as of 2000). Several hypotheses have been proposed for this increased prevalence, including increased genetic predisposition, sedentary lifestyle, and poor dietary habits, in both the mental health and general population, but individuals with a diagnosis of schizophrenia or bipolar disorder are at greater risk due to lower socioeconomic standing and negative symptoms of their disease.

○ **What mechanisms of action have been proposed for the increased risk of metabolic syndrome associated with atypical antipsychotic treatment?**

Insulin resistance (due to increased weight gain, i.e. adipose tissue) and inhibition of pancreatic β-cell 5-HT$_{1A}$ receptors (resulting in decreased insulin secretion).

○ **What two atypical antipsychotics are most often associated with metabolic syndrome?**

Clozapine and olanzapine, but all atypicals are associated with increased risk for metabolic syndrome.

○ **Which three atypical antipsychotics are most often associated with elevated triglyceride levels and reduced HDL levels?**

Clozapine, olanzapine, and quetiapine.

○ **What are the recommendations from the 2004 Consensus Development Conference between the American Diabetes Association and American Psychiatric Association for monitoring the metabolic syndrome in patients prescribed atypical antipsychotics?**

Baseline: family history, BMI, blood pressure, fasting glucose, and lipid profile. Upon initiation of treatment with an atypical antipsychotic, check BMI every 4 weeks for 12 weeks and then quarterly thereafter; and check blood pressure, fasting glucose, and lipid profile quarterly for 1 year and then annually (actually, every 5 years thereafter for the lipid profile).

○ **What is the recommended treatment for metabolic syndrome?**

Reduction of weight gain through increased physical activity (30 minutes of walking a day) and dietary change, specifically a diet lower in total calories and low in saturated fats and complex carbohydrates (starches and sugars). Easier said than done in America.

○ **What medications may be useful in treating symptoms of metabolic syndrome?**

Appetite suppressants, fibrates, nicotinic acid, statins, ACE inhibitors, angiotensin receptor blockers, metformin, and thiazolidinediones can be used to treat the symptoms of metabolic syndrome, but ultimately, physical exercise and dietary change provide the best results.

○ **How are the atypical antipsychotics different from traditional antipsychotics in receptor affinities?**

Atypical antipsychotics are relatively selective in binding to mesolimbic dopamine sites compared to nigrostriatal dopamine receptor blockade that produces extrapyramidal side effects. They also bind more extensively to serotonin receptors to a greater degree than dopamine receptors, hence the term serotonin–dopamine antagonists.

○ **What are the indications for ECT in schizophrenia?**

Catatonia, patients with prominent mood symptoms, and medication refractory symptoms are the most common indications. An acute, severe episode of psychosis that is life threatening and refractory to usual therapeutic modalities is also an indication for ECT. Positive symptoms are more responsive to ECT, whereas negative symptoms typically do not improve.

○ **Name currently available forms of depot antipsychotics in the United States and their indications.**

Fluphenazine decanoate, fluphenazine enanthate, haloperidol decanoate, and Risperdal Consta®. Common indications are nonadherence to oral agents and patient preference.

○ **A 25-year-old man with schizophrenia previously in remission on fluphenazine decanoate 12.5 mg IM q 2 weeks presents with rapidly progressing psychotic symptoms. What would be the most appropriate medication intervention?**

Consider the addition of oral fluphenazine during the crisis, which would be more beneficial in the short term than adjusting the depot dosage *alone*. Depot dosage changes may not be reflected in steady state blood levels for several weeks. There may also be a role for the short-term use of benzodiazepines.

○ **What is the current thinking regarding an adequate trial of antipsychotic medications?**

Most experts consider a medication trial at a minimum daily dosage of 300 to 1,000 mg chlorpromazine equivalents for a period of 4 to 6 weeks as adequate.

○ **What antipsychotic medication is associated with pigmentary retinopathy?**

Thioridazine (Mellaril) at doses above 800 mg.

○ **A 21-year-old male presents with agitation, hallucinations, and paranoid delusions of 6-month duration. Describe the dosage of haloperidol that is likely to be effective in treating the acute psychosis.**

Studies indicate that there is no significant advantage in using a dosage above the 10 to 20 mg a day range. Doses above 20 mg may be associated with substantial side effects potentially leading to increased rates of noncompliance.

○ **What atypical antipsychotic is currently the only medication shown to be effective in the treatment of refractory schizophrenia?**

Clozapine (Clozaril).

○ **Briefly, describe the prominent receptor interactions of clozapine and some significant side effects.**

Clozapine has relatively weak D_2 blockade, strong D_4, 5HT-2, alpha-1, cholinergic, and histaminergic blockade. Side effects include weight gain, sedation, hypotension, constipation, sialorrhea, dose-dependent seizures (5%–10% at dosages over 600 mg daily), and agranulocytosis (1%–2%, with most episodes of bone marrow toxicity occurring in the first 3–6 months of treatment).

○ **When monitoring blood counts during treatment with clozapine, when should clozapine be discontinued?**

Clozapine should be discontinued when the WBC drops to 2,000 to 3,000/mm^3 or the absolute neutrophil count (ANC) is <1,500/mm^3. The WBC with differential should then be checked daily, and the patient should be closely monitored for signs of infection. If the WBC and/or the ANC drop even farther, bone marrow aspiration and protective isolation should be considered.

○ **What are the current recommendations for monitoring of blood counts during treatment with clozapine?**

During treatment with clozapine, blood counts should be monitored at baseline and weekly for 6 months during the initial treatment phase, then twice a week for 6 months, and then monthly. Generally, if the WBC remains above 3,500/mm^3 and the ANC is >1,500/mm^3, clozapine treatment can continue.

○ **What are some choices for augmenting somatic treatments in patients with schizophrenia?**

Lithium, valproic acid, carbamazepine, benzodiazepines, and ECT have all been used for refractory symptoms. Comorbid disorders such as depression must be assessed and are often treated with combinations of antipsychotic and antidepressant medications. Augmentation choices are typically driven by target symptoms such as mood symptoms or severe behavioral disturbances.

○ **Describe prognostic factors often associated with good long-term outcome of schizophrenia.**

Good prognostic factors include female gender, family history of affective disorder, absent family history of schizophrenia, good premorbid functioning, higher IQ, acute onset, and being married. Other important factors are minimal comorbidity, paranoid subtype, and absence of significant disorganization or negative symptoms.

○ **Describe neurological phenomena identified in some patients with schizophrenia.**

Ten to twenty-five percent of patients with schizophrenia have motor findings unrelated to antipsychotic medication use. Spontaneous dyskinesias, abnormal gait, stereotypy, grimacing, abnormal motor tone, and motor apraxia may be seen. Abnormal ocular signs, such as frequent blinking, have also been noted. Abnormal smooth pursuit eye movements have been reported in 50% to 80% of patients with schizophrenia. Other nonlocalizing neurological signs seen more frequently than in controls include dysdiadochokinesia, poor right–left discrimination, and abnormal performance on sequenced repetitive tasks involving the frontal lobe.

○ **Describe the neuroendocrine side effects of neuroleptics.**

Neuroleptic medications block dopamine receptors, thereby causing prolactinemia. This in turn causes a variety of potential side effects including gynecomastia (in men) and amenorrhea and galactorrhea (in women). Amantadine or bromocriptine can be used to lower prolactin levels and thus decrease these neuroendocrine side effects.

○ **List the four types of extrapyramidal side effects of antipsychotic medications.**

Akathisia, parkinsonism, dystonia, and neuroleptic malignant syndrome.

○ **What are the treatment strategies for neuroleptic-induced akathisia?**

Akathisia is often associated with high potency neuroleptic medications and switching to a lower potency medication or lowering the dose, if possible, may be helpful. Akathisia is generally nonresponsive to anticholinergic medications, but benzodiazepines and β-blocking medications have been found to be useful. Switching to an atypical antipsychotic is another treatment strategy.

○ **What extrapyramidal side effect of antipsychotic medications is difficult to distinguish from the negative symptoms of schizophrenia?**

Medication-induced parkinsonism, which affects 20% of patients treated with typical neuroleptics, generally occurs within the initial treatment phase. Characterized by bradykinesia, cogwheel rigidity, tremor, and akinesia, it can be difficult to distinguish from the avolition, alogia, and flat affect (negative symptoms of schizophrenia). Catatonia and depression (akinetic depression) may also be a result of medication-induced parkinsonism. Treatment generally consists of the use of anticholinergic agents such as benztropine.

○ **How common is antipsychotic-induced acute dystonia? Mention associated risk factors.**

It is estimated that about 10% of newly exposed patients experience acute dystonic reactions, most often within the first 3 days of treatment initiation. Risk factors include male gender, African American ethnicity, young age, use of high-potency agents, high doses, and intramuscular administration.

○ **Discuss the management of acute dystonic reactions.**

Parenteral administration of anticholinergic medications or benzodiazepines produces dramatic responses. Maintaining or assuring the patient's airway is imperative, and reassurance and support is essential. Oral anticholinergic maintenance is often necessary.

○ **What is neuroleptic malignant syndrome (NMS)?**

The syndrome consists of the development of severe muscle rigidity and elevated temperature with exposure to neuroleptic medications at any time during the course of treatment. Autonomic and metabolic instability can lead to tachycardia, hypertension, hypotension, leucocytosis, and elevated creatine phosphokinase associated with muscle breakdown. Other symptoms of this potentially lethal condition include diaphoresis, dysphagia, tremor, incontinence, delirium, mutism, and coma.

○ **Neuroleptic malignant syndrome occurs how frequently?**

Approximately 0.5% to 1% of patients taking neuroleptics develop NMS.

○ **Describe the treatment of NMS.**

Antipsychotic medications should be withdrawn immediately. Supportive and symptomatic treatment consists of correcting fluid and electrolyte imbalances, treating fevers, and managing blood pressure instability. Studies have indicated that the treatment with dantrolene, bromocriptine, or amantadine may be helpful. In a number of cases, ECT has been shown to effectively treat NMS.

○ **Describe risk factors for tardive dyskinesia.**

Tardive dyskinesia occurs in about 20% of patients receiving traditional antipsychotics for long periods of time and in up to 50% of high-risk patients such as the elderly. Atypical antipsychotics, while less prone to causing tardive dyskinesia, still do, and require constant vigilance for symptoms thereof. Other risk factors include total duration of exposure to antipsychotics, female gender, history of extra pyramidal side effects, and a mood disorder diagnosis. Spontaneous dyskinesias are seen in 1% to 2% of antipsychotic naive patients.

○ **What patient characteristics are associated with medication noncompliance?**

Severe anxiety, paranoia, grandiosity, depression, hostility, personality disorder traits, disorganization in thought, sensitivity to medication side effects, and substance abuse are each associated with decreased compliance with medications. Important psychological considerations include denial about having an illness, attempts at gaining control of one's life by oppositional behaviors, expression of anger toward one's therapist or family by noncompliance, and the painful recognition that one is severely ill when symptoms are treated and the psychosis lifts.

○ **What cognitive problems may be seen in individuals with schizophrenia?**

Deficits in the processing of complex information, in maintaining a steady focus of attention, in working memory, in distinguishing between relevant and irrelevant stimuli, and in abstract thinking have all been identified in samples of patients with schizophrenia.

○ **What limitations have been identified in social skills training of persons with schizophrenia?**

Studies have shown that individuals with schizophrenia can learn to improve targeted behaviors in structured environments but have difficulty with generalizing to real-life settings.

○ **What qualities help the psychiatrist build a psychotherapeutic relationship in working with patients with schizophrenia?**

A straightforward and direct manner assists in building rapport with patients, whereas being aloof and authoritative hinders the relationship. An active and assertive posture coupled with patience, can assist the clinician to provide structure in the therapeutic situation. This aids the physician in tolerating intense affects periodically exhibited by patients diagnosed with schizophrenia.

○ **What are some generalizations regarding group therapy for patients with schizophrenia?**

Group therapy is not well tolerated during an acute psychotic episode due to overstimulation. However, patients in the subacute or chronic phase benefit from interaction-oriented, behavioral, and social skills training groups. Only highly functioning and stable schizophrenic persons can tolerate insight-oriented groups.

○ **What are the major themes in family therapy when a family member has schizophrenia?**

Families learn to set realistic expectations based on a thorough education of the disorder and its treatment, with a focus placed on teaching families that they are not to blame for their relative's disorder. Constructive ways of dealing with negative feelings that occur when facing frustrating aspects of the disorder are explored and information regarding community support groups such as the National Alliance for the Mentally Ill (NAMI), which provides practical advice, experience, and advocacy, is given.

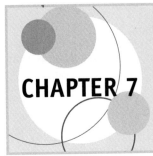

CHAPTER 7

Other Psychotic Disorders

○ **What is psychotic disorder not otherwise specified (psychosis NOS)?**

This diagnosis is used if there are psychotic symptoms that do not meet the full criteria for a specific disorder, or if there are psychotic symptoms without enough information to make a specific diagnosis.

○ **What are some examples of psychosis NOS?**

Postpartum psychosis that does not meet criteria for other disorders, psychotic symptoms that have lasted less than 1 month, but have not yet resolved, auditory hallucinations occurring in the absence of other symptoms, and nonbizarre delusions with overlapping mood symptoms that are persisting for long periods of time.

○ **What diagnoses other than schizophrenia include psychotic symptoms in their criteria?**

Schizophreniform disorder, schizoaffective disorder, delusional disorder, shared psychotic disorder, and brief psychotic disorder. One must also consider substance-induced psychotic disorder, psychotic disorder due to a general medical condition, and an affective disorder with psychotic features.

○ **What are the diagnostic criteria for postpartum psychosis?**

There are no specific diagnostic criteria in *DSM-IV*. Diagnosis is made when psychosis occurs in close temporal association with childbirth.

○ **What symptoms characterize postpartum psychosis?**

Symptoms of postpartum psychosis, which can present dramatically within 48 to 72 hours postpartum, include depression, delusions, thoughts by the mother of harming the infant or herself, cognitive deficits, mood abnormalities, and occasional hallucinations. Psychotic symptoms usually occur after symptoms such as insomnia, restlessness, agitation, lability of mood, and mild cognitive defects. Good premorbid adjustment and a supportive family are good prognostic indicators. The course of the illness is similar to a mood disorder.

○ **What is the significance of postpartum psychosis?**

Postpartum psychosis is a psychiatric emergency as reality testing becomes so impaired that both the lives of the mother and the infant may be in jeopardy. The rate of infanticide, however, is rare, occurring in less than 1 of 50,000 births, while the rate of suicide by the mother can approach 4%.

○ **What is the incidence of postpartum psychosis?**

It occurs in one to two women per 1,000 childbirths (0.1%–0.2% postpartum women), and 50% to 60% of the women who have just had their first child.

○ **What are the risk factors for developing postpartum psychosis?**

Risk factors for postpartum psychosis include a prior history of depression (25%), a history of depression during the prenatal period (75%), prior episodes of postpartum depression (50%–80%), a family history of depression, a complicated pregnancy, shorter inter-pregnancy period, low birth weight, stressful life events, a complicated relationship with the infant's father, and a history of bipolar disorder (50%).

○ **What somatic treatments are recommended for postpartum psychosis?**

Antipsychotics and mood stabilizers are generally used initially to treat psychotic symptoms. In situations where psychotic symptoms or suicidal/homicidal ideation persists, or when the psychotic/bipolar symptoms occur during pregnancy, ECT can be quite effective and poses little risk to the fetus. Once psychotic symptoms are stabilized, ongoing medication management and social support of the mother and the child is indicated, especially in situations where there is limited psychosocial support.

○ **How do you differentiate delusional disorder from schizophrenia?**

In contrast to schizophrenia, the delusions of delusional disorder are nonbizarre in that they involve situations that could occur in real life. Also, there is not the deterioration in functioning that usually occurs in schizophrenia. Patients with delusional disorder do not have negative symptoms or loose associations, but olfactory and tactile hallucinations may occur in delusional disorder in the context of the delusion.

○ **What is the duration requirement for delusional disorder?**

The delusions must be present for at least a month.

○ **Is functioning impaired in delusional disorder?**

In general, social and marital functioning is more likely to be impaired than intellectual and occupational functioning.

○ **What factors can predispose an individual to delusional disorder?**

Hearing deficiency, severe psychosocial stressors, immigration status, and low socioeconomic status.

○ **What is the prevalence of delusional disorder?**

Delusional disorder is uncommon in clinical settings—accounting for only 1% to 2% of admissions to mental health facilities.

○ **What is the usual course of delusional disorder?**

Onset is generally in middle or late adult life, but may occur at a younger age. The persecutory type is the most common subtype and may be chronic, with a waxing and waning course.

○ **What subtypes of delusional disorder exist?**

The seven types of delusional disorder are the erotomanic type, the grandiose type, the jealous type, the persecutory type, the somatic type, the mixed type (no one theme predominates), and the unspecified type.

○ **What is the erotomanic type of delusional disorder?**

Delusions that someone, usually of higher stature, is in love with the patient.

○ **Define grandiose type of delusional disorder?**

Delusions of extraordinary talents, abilities, worth, or having a special relationship to someone who is famous.

○ **What is the jealous type of delusional disorder?**

Delusions that one's sexual partner is unfaithful.

○ **What is the somatic type of delusional disorder?**

Delusions that the patient has a physical defect or illness.

○ **Define delusional disorder of persecutory type?**

Delusions that oneself, or a close relative, is being harmed or mistreated in some way.

○ **What defense mechanisms are common in delusional disorder?**

Reaction formation, projection, and denial.

○ **What is the treatment for delusional disorder?**

The treatment is usually antipsychotic medication. Pimozide (Orap®) may be a specific treatment for the somatic type of delusional disorder.

○ **Which neuroanatomical structures are usually associated with delusions?**

Lesions of the basal ganglia and limbic system are the structures that are associated with delusions.

○ **What is Capgras's syndrome?**

Capgras's syndrome is the delusion that imposters have replaced familiar people.

○ **What is Fregoli's syndrome?**

Fregoli's syndrome is the delusion that a persecutor is taking on a variety of faces like an actor.

○ **What is lycanthropy?**

Lycanthropy is the delusion of being a werewolf.

○ **What is heutoscopy?**

Heutoscopy is the false belief that one has a double.

○ **What is Cotard's syndrome?**

Cotard's syndrome is the delusional belief that the individual has lost everything, including one's bodily organs.

○ **What is another name for erotomania?**

De Clerambault syndrome.

○   **What is another term that refers to grandiose type of delusional disorder?**

Another term is megalomania.

○   **What are other terms for the jealous type of delusional disorder?**

Conjugal paranoia and Othello syndrome.

○   **What factors are associated with a good prognosis in delusional disorder?**

Good prognostic factors include female gender, onset before the age of 30 years, higher levels of social and occupational functioning, sudden onset, short duration, and the presence of precipitating factors.

○   **What is brief psychotic disorder?**

Brief psychotic disorder is an episode of psychosis characterized by the presence of at least one psychotic symptom (delusions, hallucinations, disorganized speech, disorganized, or catatonic behavior) that lasts for at least 1 day, but less than a month, with full recovery of functioning. The disorder does not meet the criteria for another disorder.

○   **What qualifiers are there for brief psychotic disorder?**

Practitioners should specify if the psychotic episode occurs "with marker stressor" (the psychotic symptoms occur in response to a stressor that most people in the culture of origin would consider stressful), "without marked stressor," or "with postpartum onset" (the psychotic episode occurs within 4 weeks postpartum).

○   **What is the prognosis for brief psychotic disorder?**

While some patients may develop schizophrenia, European studies show that 50% to 80% of affected individuals have no recurrence of symptoms.

○   **What drugs are useful in treating brief psychotic disorder?**

The only drugs, which have been reported in long-term studies to be effective, are low-dose, high-potency antipsychotics and benzodiazepines. Medications are only used for short term, and one should reexamine the diagnosis if it appears that a longer duration of treatment is necessary.

○   **What are the diagnostic criteria for schizoaffective disorder?**

An uninterrupted period of illness during which, at some time, there is either a major depressive episode, a manic episode, or a mixed episode concurrent with the psychotic symptoms characteristic of schizophrenia, and, during the same period of illness, there have been delusions or hallucinations for at least 2 weeks in the absence of prominent mood symptoms.

○   **What is the minimum duration of time for a schizoaffective episode?**

One month. The minimum duration of time for a manic episode is 1 week, 2 weeks for a depressed episode, and 1 month for an episode of schizophrenia.

○   **What associated features may occur with schizoaffective disorder?**

There may be poor occupational functioning, a restricted range of social contact, difficulties with self-care, and increased risk of suicide.

○ **What associated disorders may occur with schizoaffective disorder?**

Individuals with schizoaffective disorder may be at increased risk for later developing episodes of pure mood disorders, schizophrenia, or schizophreniform disorder.

○ **Are there any gender differences?**

Schizoaffective disorder affects more women than men when compared to schizophrenia. Women are more likely to have a later onset, more prominent symptoms, and a better prognosis.

○ **What are the two types of schizoaffective disorder?**

Schizoaffective disorder, bipolar type, and schizoaffective disorder, depressive type.

○ **What is the typical onset of schizoaffective disorder?**

Typically, the onset is in early adulthood.

○ **What is the prognosis for schizoaffective disorder?**

The prognosis for patients with schizoaffective disorder is better than schizophrenia but considerably worse than the prognosis for mood disorders. The bipolar type has a better prognosis than that of the depressive type.

○ **What medications are used in the pharmacological management of schizoaffective disorder?**

In addition to antipsychotics, carbamazepine, lithium, and valproate are used for the bipolar type. Antipsychotics plus antidepressants are used for the depressive type. Electroconvulsive therapy and clozapine are alternative therapies.

○ **What is another name for shared psychotic disorder?**

Folie à deux.

○ **What is shared psychotic disorder?**

A person, in close relationship with another person, who has psychotic symptoms develops a shared delusion with that person.

○ **What is the treatment for shared psychotic disorder?**

The initial treatment is to separate the two individuals. The source of the delusion is usually from a dominant partner. If the delusion does not abate in the submissive partner after 1 to 2 weeks, medication may be necessary.

CHAPTER 8 Mood Disorders

○ **What is the lifetime prevalence in the United States for major depressive episode (MDE)?**

Results from the National Comorbidity Survey Replication (Kessler et al. 2003) indicate that the lifetime prevalence of major depression is 16.2%, with 6.6% of the population having experienced an episode of depression within the last year. The point prevalence of major depression in the primary care physician's office is between 5% and 10%, roughly the same as hypertension, and it is even higher, ranging from 10% to 20%, among medical–surgical admissions and in the institutionalized elderly.

○ **How did the 1990 World Health Organization/World Bank Study (Murray and Lopez) rank major depression as a cause of morbidity?**

Fourth. By 2020, it is estimated that major depression will be the second leading cause of morbidity.

○ **What is the ratio of females to males among people with major depressive disorder?**

Virtually all countries and all cultures demonstrate approximately a 2:1 ratio of females to males. It is unclear why this is the case; hormonal factors, childbirth, greater expressivity, role dissatisfaction and other sociological factors, and cognitive–behavioral models (such as learned helplessness) have been suggested to play a role in this gender difference.

○ **Have different prevalence rates of major depressive disorder been demonstrated for different ethnic groups?**

The prevalence rate of all or most mood disorders is believed to be equal among different racial or ethnic groups. It has been suggested that clinicians may underdiagnose mood disorders (and overdiagnose schizophrenia) in patients of different ethnicity.

○ **What findings from twin studies suggest a genetic susceptibility to major depression?**

The difference in concordance rates for major depression between monozygotic twins, about 50%, versus 10% to 25% in dizygotic twins, suggests that a genetic predisposition for depressive disorders exists.

○ **Briefly describe the biochemical synthesis pathway for serotonin.**

Tryptophan $\xrightarrow{A}$ 5-Hydroxy - tryptophan $\xrightarrow{B}$ 5-Hydroxytryptamine (serotonin)

A = tryptophan hydroxylase*   B = amino acid decarboxyla

*TPH has at least two isoforms, 1 and 2, with TPH2 being the brain-specific form. Some evidence exists that mutations of the TPH2 gene are associated with a higher risk for depression (Zhang et al. 2004).

○　**Briefly describe the biochemical synthesis pathway for norepinephrine.**

Tyrosine $\xrightarrow{A}$ DOPA $\xrightarrow{B}$ Dopamine $\xrightarrow{C}$ Norepinephrine

A = tyrosine hydroxylase　　B = DOPA decarboxylase　　C = dopamine β-hydroxylase

○　**The "monoamine hypothesis" postulated what mechanism of action for antidepressants?**

The monoamine hypothesis postulated that antidepressants increased the amount of norepinephrine and serotonin in the brain, primarily by increasing the concentration of these neurotransmitters in the synapse and by downregulation of their postsynaptic receptors. The various ways that increased concentration of these neurotransmitters can be achieved include increased cellular production, increased release, or decreased removal.

○　**What phenomena tend to indicate that the monoamine hypothesis of depression is not sufficient to account for the mood improvement associated with use of antidepressants?**

The lag time between initial administration of antidepressants and relief of depressive symptoms (at least 2–3 weeks) and the finding that monamine depletion in healthy individuals does not correspond to an onset of depressive symptoms (Goodwin et al. 1972) tend to refute the monoamine hypothesis of depression.

○　**What additional mechanisms of actions are postulated for antidepressants?**

An increasing amount of research suggests that antidepressant efficacy may be accounted for by its restorative properties. Stress (the most common precipitant of depressive episodes) has been demonstrated to cause significant reductions in neurotrophins such as brain-derived neurotrophic factor (BDNF) and neuroprotective proteins such as B-cell lymphoma protein-2 (Bcl-2). The use of antidepressants in mice has been demonstrated to increase levels of BDNF and Bcl-2d, suggesting that antidepressants may improve not only norepinephrine and serotonin levels, but also the overall health of neurons. Other mechanisms that may contribute to antidepressant action at the molecular level include activation of the cAMP response element binding protein (CREB), which in turn activates BDNF and tyrosine kinase receptor type B (trkB). Allelic variation in the structure of the serotonin transporter gene may also predispose individuals to depression (the shorter form of the serotonin transporter promoter is associated with a higher susceptibility to depression as well as reduced response rate to SSRIs). All in all, the next motto for the APA may be "The Decade of Gene."

○　**What does the hippocampus have to do with above?**

The hippocampus appears to be especially sensitive to the neurotoxic properties of cortisol, which is elevated during times of stress. In fact, hippocampal volume (if ones does not include amygdala volume) may be correlated with depressive episodes. Interestingly, infusion of BDNF into the hippocampus (again, in mice; Shirayama et al. 2002) produces an antidepressant effect.

○　**PET and SPECT studies of depressed patients have demonstrated what findings?**

Hypointensity in frontal lobe areas (compared to scans of controls), representing decreased metabolic activity of these regions. Although this finding has been replicated in multiple studies, other studies have failed to demonstrate this hypointensity.

○　**Who described depression as anger turned inward?**

Sigmund Freud. Freud's classic 1917 paper *Mourning and Melancholia* described depression and its distinction from grief. He described depression as introjected rage over object loss, and differentiated depression from grief by postulating that depression (melancholia) invoked self-reproach and guilt, whereas mourning did not.

○   **What are the consequences of untreated depression?**

Lack of adequate treatment not only prolongs personal suffering, but can destroy families and has great societal costs. Depression, as much as any other chronic medical condition, leads to disability, role dysfunction, psychosocial deterioration, days in bed (and out of the work force), and even complaints of physical pain. When untreated, its course tends to be chronic and chronically recurrent with an increased frequency of episodes over time. Of most importance, mortality rates are higher in individuals with major depression than in individuals who are depression free.

○   **What are the risk factors for an MDE?**

The single greatest risk factor for an MDE is a past history (a previous episode). Other important risk factors include a family history of depression, female gender, youth, being single/widowed/divorced, and poor general medical health. In addition, individuals with underlying dysthymia (i.e., clinical low-grade depression) and with subthreshold depressive symptoms (especially problems with sleep) are at risk.

○   **What life event is most often associated with development of depression later in life?**

The loss of a parent before the age of 11.

○   **What life event is commonly associated with the onset of a depressive episode?**

Loss of a spouse.

○   **What stressor(s) is(are) associated with the onset of mania?**

None, unless one considers a substance-induced (illegal, legal, or prescribed) mania as a stressor.

○   **What general medical conditions have been associated with high rates of depression, as well as a high relative mortality risk when associated with depression?**

Myocardial infarction, cerebrovascular accident, hip fracture, and many others, including cancer and dementia.

○   **What did findings of the SADHART trial (Shapiro et al. 1999) indicate?**

An unexpected observation from the SADHART trail indicated that the use of Zoloft for depression occurring after a myocardial infarction was safe and may actually improve cardiovascular functioning.

○   **What percentage of people who experience an MDE will go on to experience a second episode?**

Approximately 50%. Of those who experience two episodes, approximately 70% will go on to experience a third episode, and 90% of those experiencing three or more will experience another. These statistics should be taken into account when deciding how long to treat patients with antidepressants after resolution of an episode.

○   **What symptom(s) must be present for a diagnosis of MDE?**

Either a depressed mood *or* anhedonia must be present a good deal of the time for at least two consecutive weeks.

○ **What other symptoms contribute to a diagnosis of MDE?**

Change in appetite or weight (increase or decrease), insomnia or hypersomnia, observable psychomotor agitation or retardation, fatigue or decrease in energy, feelings of worthlessness or inappropriate guilt, impaired concentration or indecisiveness, and recurrent thoughts of death or suicidal ideation or behavior. To meet criteria for major depressive disorder, five out of the nine criteria (including at least one of the two from the last question) must be present for a duration of 2 weeks. In addition, the syndrome is not considered an MDE if it can be accounted for on the basis of a known medical condition that can cause depression (e.g., hypothyroidism), a medication that can cause depression (e.g., corticosteroids) or a substance of abuse.

○ **What other diagnoses should be considered in the differential of a patient with symptoms suggestive of MDE?**

- Substance-induced mood disorder (if symptoms begin within 1 month of substance intoxication or withdrawal, or during medication use).
- Mood disorder due to a general medical condition (depressive symptoms believed to be directly due to physiological effects of medical illness).
- Bereavement (if symptoms are relatively mild, do not include feelings of worthlessness, psychomotor retardation, suicidal ideation, and begin and end within 2 months of the death of a loved one).
- Adjustment disorder with depressed mood, full criteria for an MDE are not met.
- Dysthymic disorders where patients have chronic, low-grade depressive symptoms for at least 2 years but do not meet criteria for MDE.
- The bipolar disorders. Recurrent depressive episodes refractory to treatment or partially responsive to treatment are especially suspected.

○ **What percentage of persons diagnosed with major depression will have at least one other psychiatric condition?**

Seventy-five percent of individuals diagnosed with major depression will have a comorbid psychiatric diagnosis (Kessler et al. 2003). The most common comorbid conditions are anxiety disorders (59%), impulse control disorders (30%), and substance abuse disorders (24%).

○ **What is the difference between an adjustment disorder with depressed mood and an MDE?**

If criteria are met for an MDE, this diagnosis should be applied, whether or not the symptoms are chronologically/etiologically related to a stressor. Adjustment disorder with depressed mood should be diagnosed if depressive symptoms occur but either is not sufficient to meet criteria for major depression (less than five criteria), or do not last for 2 weeks. Adjustment disorders do not represent normal bereavement and occur within 3 months of an identifiable stressor. Of note is that symptom disturbance in adjustment disorders does not persist for more than 6 months after the termination of the stressor. Acute and chronic modifiers are used to denote the duration of the stressor, not the symptoms.

○ **According to *DSM-IV*, when is it appropriate to diagnose major depressive disorder in a person recently bereaved?**

If symptoms consistent with MDE develop or persist beyond 2 months past the death of a loved one, a diagnosis of normal bereavement gives way to major depressive disorder. It must be understood that there is extensive variation between individuals and cultural groups in what is considered "normal" bereavement. Nonetheless, even in the first few months of bereavement, certain features have been described that fall outside the usual realm of bereavement, and these demand clinical attention. Some of these features include hallucinations other than hearing the voice of the deceased or briefly seeing the image of the deceased, marked psychomotor retardation, inappropriate and excessive guilt, suicidal rumination, persistent feelings of worthlessness, and persistent functional impairment.

○   **How is an MDE differentiated from dysthymic disorder?**

Dysthymic disorder is differentiated from an MDE primarily by duration and number of symptoms. In dysthymic disorder, a depressed mood must be present most of the time for a period of more than 2 years (1 year in children and adolescents), which is obviously much longer than the 2-week period minimum required for the diagnosis of an MDE. At least two symptoms of the following must be present to make a diagnosis of dysthymic disorder: changes in sleep, changes in appetite, reduced energy, reduced concentration, reduced self-esteem, and hopelessness. In contrast, a diagnosis of MDE requires at least four of these symptoms. The presence of suicidal ideation or actions practically rules out dysthymic disorder as a diagnosis in most cases.

○   **What is meant by "double depression"?**

Dysthymia with superimposed MDE.

○   **What percentage of individuals diagnosed with dysthymic disorder will eventually experience an episode of major depression?**

Seventy to eighty percent. Many patients with a history of dysthymic disorder will present for treatment initially during an episode of major depression.

○   **What medical conditions tend to mimic or produce depressive symptoms?**

The list is rather exhaustive. More common conditions include *endocrine* disorders (hypothyroidism or more rarely hyperthyroidism, adrenal dysfunction including Addison's disease), *neurological* disorders (Parkinson's disease, dementias), *cancer* (particularly gastrointestinal—pancreatic carcinoma classically presents with depression), viral or other *infections* (e.g., hepatitis, mononucleosis, HIV), and *metabolic* disorders (B_{12} deficiency). These and other medical conditions should be considered and possibly ruled out in patients presenting with depressive symptoms.

○   **What medications tend to produce depressive symptoms?**

Major medications that have been reported to evoke depressive symptoms include alpha-methyldopa, reserpine, propanolol, guanethidine, clonidine, thiazide diuretics, digitalis, oral contraceptives, L-dopa, adrenocorticotropic hormone (ACTH) and corticosteroids, anabolic steroids, benzodiazepines, cimetidine, ranitidine, cyclosporin, neuroleptics, nonsteroidal anti-inflammatory agents, ethambutol, cycloserine, disulfiram, sulfonamides, baclofen, metoclopramide, cocaine, and amphetamines (compiled from Cassem 1987, Fava et al. 1988, Hall 1980, Pascually and Veith 1989).

○   **When can the specifier "with melancholic features" be applied to an MDE?**

When either anhedonia or lack of reactivity to usually pleasurable stimuli is present, and when three of the following are present: distinct quality of depressed mood such that it is different from typical grief situations, diurnal variation with mood worse in the morning, early morning awakening (terminal insomnia), marked psychomotor agitation or retardation, anorexia or weight loss, and excessive or inappropriate guilt.

○   **When can the specifier "with atypical features" be applied to an MDE?**

When mood reactivity is present and when two of the following are present: weight gain or increase in appetite, hypersomnia, leaden paralysis, and long-standing hypersensitivity to rejection. Atypical depression tends to be common in patients with bipolar disorder, seasonable mood disorders, and possibly in individuals with comorbid Axis II pathology.

○ **When is the specifier "with postpartum onset" applied to an MDE?**

When the symptoms appear within 4 weeks of childbirth. Many clinicians, however, believe the period following childbirth during which the new mother is at increased risk of affective illness is much longer than 4 weeks. This specifier can apply to a manic, hypomanic, or mixed episode as well.

○ **What is the incidence of MDE among postpartum women?**

Approximately 10% to 15%. This condition should be differentiated from "maternity blues," which is a mild dysphoria occurring in up to 50% of postpartum women. A postpartum depression, especially when relatively severe, is a risk factor for bipolar disorder.

○ **What longitudinal diagnoses should be considered in patients presenting with MDE?**

Major depressive disorder, single episode is used to describe a presentation of MDE when no prior episodes of major depression, mania, or hypomania have occurred. When a history of prior episode(s) of major depression is present, major depressive disorder, recurrent should be diagnosed. Also, MDE can occur in the context of bipolar disorder. If a patient has had one or more previous episodes of mania or hypomania, the diagnosis of bipolar disorder should be made.

○ **What are the lifetime prevalences of bipolar I and bipolar II disorders, respectively?**

For bipolar I disorder, 0.4% to 1.6% and for bipolar II disorder, 0.5%.

○ **Is there an increased risk for bipolar I disorder in various ethnic or racial groups?**

No. However, bipolar disorder tends to be underdiagnosed in some ethnic groups and in young persons.

○ **What percentage of individuals diagnosed with bipolar I disorder complete suicide?**

Ten to fifteen percent.

○ **What is the ratio of females to males among those diagnosed with bipolar I disorder?**

In contrast to unipolar depression, the prevalence of bipolar disorder shows a 1:1 gender ratio.

○ **How does the presentation of bipolar I disorder differ between males and females?**

Generally, males will present with a manic episode first, while females will more often present with an episode of depression. However, the presence of recurrent depressive episodes in any gender should alert the clinician to the possibility of a bipolar diagnosis, rather than recurrent depression, especially when the depressive episodes respond poorly to treatment with antidepressants.

○ **What is unique about the postpartum period in women diagnosed (or eventually diagnosed) with bipolar I disorder?**

The postpartum period can be the first time a woman presents with symptoms of mania or depression. Women who do have a history of bipolar I disorder are particularly at risk for postpartum psychosis.

○ **What percentage of teenagers diagnosed with recurrent major depression eventually become diagnosed with bipolar I disorder?**

Ten to fifteen percent, again underscoring the fact that recurrent depressive episodes are a risk for bipolar I disorder.

○ **What percentage of individuals with a history of one manic episode will have another manic episode?**

Ninety percent. At times, manic episodes can be associated with changes in time zones (jet lag) and sleep deprivation (studying for finals).

○ **When is complete interepisode recovery less likely in individuals diagnosed with bipolar I disorder?**

When mood-incongruent psychotic symptoms are present in the last episode of mania or depression.

○ **What symptom must be present for a diagnosis of manic or hypomanic episode?**

A distinct period of elevated, expansive, or irritable mood. In a manic episode, this period of abnormal mood must last 1 week unless hospitalization is necessary, and it must be severe enough to interfere with functioning. In a hypomanic episode, this abnormal mood must last 4 days and is less severe and disruptive.

○ **What other symptoms characterize a manic or hypomanic episode?**

If the mood is elevated or expansive (see previous question), three other symptoms must be present. If the mood is irritable, four other symptoms must be present. Other symptoms include inflated self-esteem or grandiosity, decreased need for sleep, pressured speech, racing thoughts or flight of ideas, distractibility, increase in goal-directed activity, and excessive involvement in pleasure-seeking activities with potential for negative consequences.

○ **What medical conditions tend to mimic or produce manic symptoms?**

The list is exhaustive. Some of the more common causes are *endocrine disorders* (including hyperthyroidism and Cushing's syndrome), *neurological conditions* (including multiple sclerosis, Huntington's disease, viral encephalitis, and cerebral tumors), and *systemic disorders* (including uremia, pellagra, vitamin B_{12} deficiency, and carcinoid syndrome).

○ **What medications and recreational drugs tend to produce manic symptoms?**

Medications include stimulants such as methylphenidate and dextroamphetamine, corticosteroids, sympathomimetics, isoniazid, levodopa, cimetidine, bromocriptine, procarbazine, and others. Withdrawal from CNS depressants such as barbiturates and benzodiazepines can produce manic symptoms. Recreational drugs include cocaine, amphetamines, and withdrawal from alcohol. In addition, antidepressant medications, bright light treatment, and ECT can precipitate a manic episode in vulnerable individuals.

○ **How is a manic episode distinguished from a hypomanic episode?**

In addition to the duration criteria, the episodes differ in severity. A hypomanic episode is described as symptoms that comprise a change in behavior and functioning that is noticeable to others; however, if symptoms are severe enough to produce marked impairment in social or occupational functioning or to warrant hospitalization, then a diagnosis of manic episode is more appropriate. Additionally, the episode is considered manic if psychotic symptoms are present.

○ **What is the difference between bipolar I and bipolar II disorders?**

Bipolar disorder, in general, refers to an episodic mood disorder characterized by episodes of major depression and by episodes of mood elevation (hypomania or mania). Bipolar I disorder describes a mood disorder characterized by one or more manic episodes, as opposed to bipolar II disorder in which one or more hypomanic episodes have occurred, but no full-blown manic episodes have ever occurred.

○   **What is a bipolar mixed episode?**

According to *DSM-IV*, a mixed episode is a period of mood disturbance lasting 1 week that meets criteria for both MDE (except for the 2-week duration) and manic episode. Many clinicians employ a more flexible definition of a mixed state, which includes meeting some but not all criteria for both MDE and manic episode. A mixed episode is sometimes difficult to distinguish from an MDE with agitation.

○   **What is meant by the bipolar disorder specifier "with rapid cycling"?**

Four or more episodes of mood disturbance within the past year. These episodes can be major depression, mania, hypomania, or mixed states. Rapid cycling is associated with a complicated course, incomplete response to lithium, and poor prognosis. It may be precipitated by overzealous treatment with antidepressant medication, and may be more common in individuals with hypothyroidism and possibly other medical/neurological illnesses (e.g., multiple sclerosis).

○   **According to *DSM-IV*, what would be the correct diagnosis for a patient with a history of multiple MDEs who becomes manic during treatment with a tricyclic antidepressant (TCA), a selective serotonin reuptake inhibitor (SSRI), or a serotonin norepinephrine reuptake inhibitor (SNRI)?**

Substance-induced mood disorder with manic features. Major depressive disorders or recurrent episodes of mood disturbance (including mania) that are precipitated by medications or other somatic treatments cannot be considered primary. Therefore, they are not counted as contributing to a diagnosis of bipolar disorder. However, the historical presence of a substance-induced mood disorder, particularly one precipitated by an antidepressant, does constitute a risk factor for bipolar disorder, and further use of similar medications is essentially contraindicated.

○   **What would be the most appropriate diagnosis for a person who experiences multiple episodes of hypomania and of subsyndromal depression?**

Cyclothymia. These disorders do not frequently come to the attention of clinicians, but since the mood changes are so chronic and unpredictable, they may be associated with significant distress and impairment.

○   **What are some risk factors for suicide completion?**

Caucasian, ethnicity, male gender, age between 18- and 25-year-old or age older than 65 years, comorbid medical problems, living alone, or with poor social support. The strongest risk factor for suicide is psychiatric illness. Mood disorders have the highest incidence of completed suicide, while Schizophrenia and substance dependence have a high incidence of suicide as well. In patients with major depression, comorbid panic attacks, anxiety, insomnia, alcohol use, and feelings of worthlessness are predictors of imminent risk. Finally, suicidal ideation, a past history of suicide attempts, and a family history of successful suicide are also predictors of risk.

○   **As of 2004, which antidepressants are required by the FDA to carry a "black box" warning for suicide risk?**

All antidepressants. The phenomenon of increased suicidal ideation (and risk for completion of suicide) after initiation of treatment with an antidepressant has been observed for many years, and is revisited occasionally when new agents or uses come into practice. Prozac® was nailed for this phenomenon about a year after it was introduced, while the use of antidepressants in children and adolescents became quite controversial because of the increased attention in the press (2004), with a resultant decrease in prescribing of antidepressants for children and adolescents and a coincidental increase in suicide rates for this population after 2004. As the numbers are quite small, the actual risk for suicide after initiation of a trial of antidepressants is difficult to determine. The bottom line is to closely follow up with your patients after initiation of treatment, develop a safety plan, and strengthen community support. Furthermore, the presence of any indication that safety cannot be maintained in the community should prompt a recommendation for inpatient hospitalization. This includes, but is not limited to high risk for substance use, anxiety and panic attacks, inability to contract for safety, and a high degree of social isolation.

○ **Do antidepressants cause congenital malformations?**

Studies have failed to show an increased rate of malformations with prenatal tricyclic exposure, suggesting that prenatal use is safe. However, study sizes have been small (most have been chart reviews), and the lack of difference between exposed and unexposed groups does not allow firm conclusions that tricyclic use is safe in early pregnancy. Similar results and limitations have stemmed from studies on prenatal exposure to other antidepressants, although some studies have found a slight increase in minor perinatal complications after third trimester use of various SSRI's such as fluoxetine and citalopram, and increased risk of cardiac malformations with the use of paroxetine during pregnancy has been noted.

○ **How long should a patient remain on antidepressants after resolution of a major depression episode?**

If the MDE is a patient's first episode, there is no underlying dysthymic disorder, and recovery is complete (i.e., no residual symptoms), the rule of thumb is to treat for 6 to 9 months, after the resolution of symptoms. However, a history of previous episodes, dysthymia, or an incomplete response, all call for longer treatment periods.

○ **When is maintenance treatment indicated?**

Full dose maintenance treatment should be considered in anyone who has a history of highly recurrent depressions. Data show that individuals with three or more episodes within 5 years should be treated for at least 5 years, maybe longer. In addition, maintenance treatments should be considered when there have been two relatively severe episodes associated with high suicide risk, or associated with comorbid psychiatric or medical conditions. Patients with underlying dysthymic disorder and/or incomplete remission are also candidates for maintenance treatment. Data show that the risk for relapse is substantially higher if the maintenance dose is less than the dose required for initial improvement of symptoms.

○ **If the patient does not respond to a therapeutic dose of an antidepressant after 2 to 3 weeks of treatment, what should you do?**

Wait. It may take 4 to 8 weeks before the patient begins to respond. The more chronic the depression, the longer it may take for the patient to respond.

○ **If the patient does not respond to a therapeutic dose after 8 weeks, what should you do?**

If no response at all, switch to another agent, probably to a medication from a different class (especially if there are side effects). If a patient partially responds, and there are significant side effects, switch to another medication within the same class. If a patient partially responds by week 8 of treatment and there are minimal or no side effects, either optimize the dose (e.g., 400 mg of bupropion, 150 mg of venlafaxine, and 100 mg of sertraline) and wait another 2 weeks or augment with another agent and continue to observe.

○ **If you choose to augment with another agent, what are some of the choices?**

Many augmentation agents are used currently. The most common include lithium, thyroid hormone (T_3 believed to be more efficacious than T_4), other antidepressants from different classes, buspirone, and stimulants.

○ **Is one class of antidepressant medication more effective than another?**

No. All classes are about equally effective. In general, one initially chooses one antidepressant over another on the basis of differential side effect profiles.

○ **How is cognitive therapy used to treat depression?**

Cognitive theory postulates that depression arises from maladaptive negative cognitions about oneself, others, and the future. Cognitive therapy seeks to identify these negative cognitions (sometimes called "hot thoughts") and replace them with healthier adaptive cognitions. This process frequently involves looking at the evidence that the patient has found to support his/her negative cognition, developing more adaptive cognitions and looking at evidence to support the more adaptive cognitions, and systematically helping the patient solidify the more adaptive ways of thinking. Evidence indicates good efficacy of cognitive therapy in the treatment of mild depressions and its positive role augmenting response to medication for acute treatment, as well as possibly preventing further episodes in the future.

○ **What type of therapy treats depression based on the theory that depression largely or in part stems from deficits in relationships and social bonds?**

Interpersonal therapy (IPT), developed by Harry Stack Sullivan, seeks to treat depression by improving relationships, communication, and socialization by addressing both present and past significant relationships. Intrapsychic processes are less emphasized than in traditional psychoanalysis or psychodynamic therapy.

○ **What are the two classes of tricyclic antidepressants according to molecular structure?**

Tertiary amines (two methyl groups on the N atom of the side chain) include imipramine, amitriptyline, clomipramine, and doxepin. *Secondary amines (one methyl group)* include desipramine, nortriptyline, protriptyline, and amoxapine. The first step of metabolism of the tertiary amines is monodemethylation in the liver, yielding secondary amines. For example, imipramine is converted to desipramine, and amitriptyline is converted to nortriptyline. The secondary amines tend to have fewer anticholinergic side effects, are less sedating, and are less likely to be associated with orthostatic hypotension.

○ **What are the most common side effects of tricyclic antidepressants?**

Sedation, weight gain, anticholinergic effects (dry mouth, constipation, urinary retention, confusion), tremor, orthostatic hypotension, excessive sweating, and impotence. Generally, these side effects are dose related. Additionally, tricyclics have the tendency to slow intracardiac conduction by quinidine-like effects, and may be associated with decreased heart rate variability. A screening ECG is warranted on patients with suspected cardiac disease and all patients older than 40 years before initiating treatment with tricyclics. Bifascicular block, left bundle branch block, and a prolonged QT interval are considered as strong relative contraindications to tricyclic use. Sexual dysfunction can also be seen with tricyclic use.

○ **What are the symptoms of serious tricyclic toxicity?**

Antimuscarinic symptoms (dry mucous membranes, decreased bowel motility, mydriasis, blurry vision, urinary retention, confusion), CNS depression from drowsiness to coma, cardiac arrhythmias and conduction block, hypotension, and seizures. Death often occurs from arrhythmia, hypotension, or seizures. The minimum fatal dose of tricyclics is considered to be between 1 and 2 g. Thus, it is not advisable to prescribe more than 1-week supply of TCA to a depressed patient at risk for suicide.

○ **What is the treatment of a significant tricyclic overdose?**

Induce emesis if the patient is awake, intubate and administer gastric lavage if the patient is stuporous or comatose. To block the absorption of tricyclic, activated charcoal (30 mg) is given as well. Ventilatory support and vasopressors may be required. Arrhythmias may require emergent treatment, and continuous telemetry is indicated for patients who experience arrhythmias, a QRS duration above 0.1 second, or those patients who have a serum tricyclic level above 1,000 ng/mL. Seizures may require intravenous anticonvulsants.

○ **What can occur when desipramine and citalopram are coadministered?**

Tricyclic toxicity, as citalopram, can increase the concentration of desipramine by almost 50%. As an aside, citalopram and its derivative, escitalopram, have a higher risk for cardiotoxicity in overdose than other SSRIs. The cardiotoxicity is actually somewhat delayed and is characterized by a prolonged QTc interval and possible arrhythmias, such as torsades de pointes. Doses of over 2 g (a 90-day prescription of 20 mg tablets) can cause serious symptoms, while doses of over 4 g can be lethal.

○ **Which tricyclic antidepressant serum levels have been most studied?**

Nortriptyline. A therapeutic window of blood level between 50 and 150 ng/mL has been correlated with clinical improvement.

○ **In summary, what are the major pros and cons of tricyclic antidepressants?**

Pros: the TCAs are at least as effective for MDE as any other class of medications, are inexpensive, and have a long, thorough record of use behind them.

Cons: the TCAs are anticholinergic (causing dry mouth, blurring vision, constipation, urinary retention, confusion), antiadrenergic (causing orthostasis and reflex tachycardia), and antihistaminic (causing sedation and weight gain). In addition, they have sexual side effects and several drug–drug interactions. Most importantly, they can be cardiotoxic and can be lethal in overdose. Finally, most TCAs can lower the seizure threshold.

○ **What is the chief pharmacodynamic difference between the available selective serotonin reuptake inhibitors (SSRIs)?**

Half-life. Fluoxetine has a relatively long half-life of 48 to 96 hours and an active metabolite, norfluoxetine, has a half-life of 7 to 14 days. Sertraline has a half-life of 24 hours and an active metabolite with a half-life of 62 to 100 hours. Paroxetine has a half-life of 24 hours at a dose of 20 mg a day and no active metabolites. Fluvoxamine has a half-life of 12 to 24 hours. Escitalopram has a half-life of 30 hours and no active metabolites. Agents with relatively longer half-lives take longer to "wash out," but are less likely to produce withdrawal symptoms upon discontinuation.

○ **What are the symptoms of SSRI withdrawal (or discontinuation syndrome)?**

Anxiety, irritability, dizziness, and flu-like symptoms (rhinorrhea, malaise, myalgia, nausea and vomiting, chills, diarrhea), vivid dreams, mood lability, and paresthesias (tingling in the extremities, "electric shocks" shooting down arms and legs). These symptoms resolve if the original or a substitute SSRI is resumed and slowly tapered.

○ **Which SSRI inhibits the cytochrome P-450 system?**

All of them. Fluvoxamine inhibits the 1A2 isoenzyme system, thus potentially interfering with the breakdown of theophylline and caffeine, among other drugs. Both fluoxetine and sertraline inhibit 2C isoenzymes, thus potentially increasing blood levels of phenytoin, diazepam, warfarin, barbiturates, and propanolol. To varying degrees, fluoxetine, sertraline, and paroxetine inhibit 2D6, and therefore may inhibit blood levels of TCAs, antipsychotics, type 1C antiarrhythmics and β-blockers. Finally, norfluoxetine (a metabolite of fluoxetine) is a modest inhibitor of 3A4, thus potentially interfering with the metabolites of carbamazepine, alprazolam, triazolam, terfenadine, astemizole, and cisapride.

○ **What commonly used analgesic can lose efficacy when combined with 2D6 inhibitors?**

Codeine. This inactive opiate is demethylated to an active form of morphine by 2D6.

○ **What is the treatment of SSRI-induced ejaculatory delay?**

Sexual side effects of SSRIs are common, including ejaculatory delay and anorgasmia. These side effects tend to be dose related, and lowering the dose of the SSRI can sometimes reverse the side effect. Some investigators advocate drug holidays, but SSRI withdrawal symptoms and worsening of depression limit this strategy's usefulness. Addition of certain medications has been shown to improve the sexual side effects of SSRIs. These medications include bupropion, buspirone, amantadine, bethanechol, yohimbine, stimulants, and some herbal products. However, many of these medications have significant side effect profiles of which one needs to be aware. Discontinuation of the SSRI, possibly in favor of a different antidepressant not associated with sexual side effects (e.g., bupropion, nefazodone, mirtazapine), should be considered as well.

○ **In summary, what are the pros and cons of selective serotonin reuptake inhibitors?**

Pros: the SSRIs are effective, safe, tolerable, and easy to use. The starting dose is often a therapeutic dose, they can be given once daily, and they are effective for anxiety disorders as well as depression.

Cons: The SSRIs have gastrointestinal side effects (nausea, diarrhea), are activating (anxiety, insomnia), and cause sexual side effects (delayed ejaculation, anorgasmia). The shorter-acting SSRIs have withdrawal symptoms. The SSRIs, to varying degrees, inhibit the cytochrome P-450 system. When combined with other classes of medications that are serotonin agonists (e.g., the MAOIs), they can cause a serotonin syndrome.

○ **What antidepressants are considered the "gold standard" for the treatment of major depression with atypical features?**

Monoamine-oxidase inhibitors.

○ **What is the potentially fatal side effect of monoamine oxidase inhibitors (MAOIs) when they are combined with tyramine-containing foods?**

Hyperadrenergic crisis. When MAOIs are ingested, they inhibit intestinal and hepatic monoamine oxidase, leading to absorption of noncatabolized dietary vasoactive amines (particularly tyramine, but also dopamine and phenylethylamine). These amines induce release of catecholamines from sympathetic neurons, leading to hypertension, tachycardia, hyperpyrexia, diaphoresis, and other sympathetic sequelae, including cardiac arrhythmia. Tyramine-free diets should be continued for 10 to 14 days after discontinuation of MAOIs.

○ **What is the potentially fatal consequence of combining MAOIs with SSRIs, tryptophan, venlafaxine, meperidine, and certain other serotonin agonists?**

Serotonin syndrome, which ranges from mild tremor, hypertension, tachycardia, and fever to a dangerous cluster of severe hyperthermia, seizures, coma, and even death. Because of this risk, SSRIs should not be used concomitantly with MAOIs. In fact, fluoxetine should be "washed out" for 5 weeks prior to initiating treatment with an MAOI, and shorter-acting SSRIs and venlafaxine should be "washed out" for the equivalent of approximately four to five half-lives (1–2 weeks) to play it safe. When switching from an MAOI to an SSRI, the MAOI should be "washed out" for 2 weeks prior to initiating SSRI treatment. Because the tricyclic, clomipramine, is predominantly serotonergic, similar restrictions apply with this medication as with the shorter-acting SSRIs. Other tricyclics can be used with caution with MAOIs if indicated.

○ **What other medications should be rigorously avoided in patients being treated with MAOIs?**

Hyperadrenergic crisis can occur when MAOIs are coadministered with sympathomimetics including amphetamines, methylphenidate, pseudoephedrine, phenylpropanolamine, levodopa, and others. Opiates must be used with caution; meperidine and dextromethorphan should be avoided due to reports of delirium, autonomic instability, and death associated with the use of these agents with MAOIs.

○ **In summary, what are the major pros and cons of MAOIs?**

Pros: the MAOIs are effective for a broad spectrum of mood and anxiety disorders and are especially effective for depression with atypical features and anergic bipolar depression. Additionally, MAOIs are less cardiotoxic and less epileptogenic than TCAs.

Cons: the MAOIs can be activating or sedating, have gastrointestinal and sexual side effects, and may cause weight gain. Most significantly, they can interact with certain foods (containing high amounts of tyramine) and medications (e.g., stimulants) to cause hypertensive crisis or other medications (e.g., SSRIs or narcotics) to cause serotonin syndrome.

○ **What is believed to be the mechanism of action of venlafaxine (Effexor®)?**

Serotonin and norepinephrine reuptake inhibition. In this way, venlafaxine is similar to tricyclic antidepressants, but tends to have fewer side effects. A common side effect that should be screened for and followed is diastolic hypertension.

○ **What are the pros and cons of venlafaxine?**

Pros: because it inhibits reuptake of both norepinephrine and serotonin (thus imparting "dual activity," hence the mnemonic, SNRI, or **S**erotonin **N**orepinephrine **R**euptake **I**nhibitor), it can be beneficial in some patients who have not done well with SSRIs and patients with melancholic features.

Cons: it tends to have activating side effects, and conversely, in some patients, may be sedating. As a potent serotonin reuptake inhibitor, it may cause gastrointestinal, discontinuation symptoms, and sexual side effects. A unique side effect is elevation of diastolic blood pressure.

○ **Duloxetine (Cymbalta®) is another SNRI that has FDA approval for what other condition besides major depression?**

Diabetic neuropathic pain. In fact, the evidence for long-term relief of chronic pain may be more robust than for relief of depressive symptoms. The mechanism of action for pain relief is believed to be related to improved serotonin and norepinephrine activity in the descending neurons of the caudal dorsal raphe nucleus that terminate in the spinal cord.

○ **What populations may represent relative contraindications to bupropion (Wellbutrin®) treatment?**

Patients with eating disorders are possibly a high-risk population for bupropion-induced seizures. This stems from a study testing bupropion in bulimic patients, which yielded an increased seizure incidence as an adverse event. Also, patients vulnerable to seizures (e.g., history of head injury, alcoholics with history of withdrawal, and primary seizure disorders) should not be treated with bupropion as a first-line agent. Finally, as bupropion has dopaminergic activity and has been associated with induction of hallucinations and delusions, it should be used cautiously, or not at all, in individuals with a history of psychosis.

○ **In summary, what are the pros and cons of bupropion?**

Pros: bupropion is effective, safe, tolerable, and may be particularly effective in ADHD and smoking cessation as well as for depression. In addition, it doesn't cause sexual side effects or disrupt sleep architecture, and drug–drug interactions are minimal.

Cons: bupropion has activating and gastrointestinal side effects and may not be as effective for anxiety disorders as some of the other antidepressants. Also, in some populations, the risk for seizures or psychotic episodes may be increased (as previously described). Rashes are a relatively common side effect for this drug.

○ **Which antidepressant exerts its primary effect at central alpha-2 adrenergic receptors?**

Mirtazapine (Remeron®). This antidepressant also has weak 5HT-2 reuptake inhibiting activity.

○ **What are the pros and cons of mirtazapine?**

Pros: effective for depression and anxiety symptoms, single daily dosing, lack of significant sexual side effects, and minimal serotonergic side effects.

Cons: potent anticholinergic effects (e.g., somnolence, weight gain), and 0.3% of patients in premarketing studies have developed blood dyscrasias.

○ **What are the pros and cons of nefazodone (Serzone®)?**

Pros: it is effective and has rapid-acting anxiolytic properties. It does not cause sexual side effects and does not disrupt sleep architecture.

Cons: it causes dizziness, gastrointestinal side effects, sedation, and visual trails. An inhibitor of cytochrome P-450 3A4, it should not be used with terfenadine, astemizole, or cisapride, and should be used cautiously with alprazolam or triazolam. Finally, the risk for hepatotoxicity (∼1 in 250,000) led to discontinued sales of the brand name drug in 2003.

○ **What laboratory studies should be obtained before implementing therapy with lithium?**

Baseline laboratory studies to obtain before initiating treatment with lithium include urinalysis, blood urea nitrogen, and creatinine to assess kidney function, a TSH (and possibly full thyroid panel), urine pregnancy test if indicated (due to the risk of teratogenesis), and an ECG if the patient is older than 50 years, or if cardiac disease is suspected.

○ **What are some medications that can alter lithium levels if taken concomitantly with lithium?**

Lithium levels are increased by most NSAIDS, tetracyclines, metronidazole, ACE inhibitors, and some diuretics (thiazides, spironolactone, triamterene, ethacrynic acid). Levels are decreased by theophylline, osmotic diuretics (mannitol), and acetazolamide.

○ **How does lithium toxicity typically present?**

The first signs of lithium toxicity tend to be coarse tremor, ataxia, and slurred speech. As toxicity progresses, neurological symptoms of dizziness, weakness, nystagmus, and excitement appear, along with gastrointestinal symptoms of nausea, vomiting, and abdominal pain. With moderate to severe toxicity, neurological symptoms advance to stupor/coma or delirium, seizures, fasciculations and hyperactive reflexes, and blurred vision, culminating in symptoms of circulatory collapse, including hypotension, arrhythmia, and conduction abnormalities.

○ **How is lithium toxicity managed clinically?**

Mild-to-moderate toxicity with serum levels less than 3 mmol/L, mild symptoms, and adequate urine output can be managed with correction of electrolyte disturbances and intravenous hydration. If serum level is above 3 mmol/L and severe symptoms are present, prompt dialysis should ensue. If the level is above 4 mmol/L, dialysis should ensue regardless of clinical symptoms.

○ **What teratogenic cardiac abnormality has been associated with lithium treatment during pregnancy?**

Ebstein's anomaly. The risk increases from 1 in 20,000 (0.005%) in the general population to 1 in 1,000 (0.1%) when exposure to lithium occurs during the first trimester.

○ **Which congenital malformations have been linked to in utero exposure to anticonvulsant mood stabilizers, particularly valproic acid and carbamazepine?**

Studies report a 15-fold increase in spina bifida in first-trimester exposed fetuses, increasing the incidence to 0.5% to 1.0%. Minor physical anomalies have also been reported to occur at higher rates.

○ **What are the known side effects of valproic acid treatment?**

Common side effects that are relatively benign include weight gain, alopecia, gastrointestinal effects including nausea/vomiting/diarrhea, sedation, tremor, thrombocytopenia, and benign elevation of hepatic transaminases (except in children younger than 2 years). Infrequent, but concerning side effects include hepatitis, bleeding disorders, neutropenia, pancreatitis, and drug-induced rashes. There is no standard set of prerequisite laboratory studies before beginning treatment with valproic acid, but baseline hepatic transaminases and a complete blood count are routinely obtained. Some clinicians also obtain a baseline serum amylase.

○ **What congenital metabolic disorders are associated with fulminate hepatitis following a trial of valproic acid?**

Urea cycle disorders, in particular ornithine transcarbamylase deficiency. Urea cycle disorders may account for the occurrence of hepatotoxicity of valproic acid in children younger than 2 years and that is why the use of valproic acid is essentially contraindicated in this age group.

○ **What is the typical effect of carbamazepine treatment on blood levels of concomitantly administered medications?**

Carbamazepine induces hepatic microsomal enzymes, leading to increased metabolism of itself and other hepatically metabolized drugs. This interaction leads to reduced blood levels of itself and other medications, necessitating administration of larger doses to maintain therapeutic serum levels.

○ **What is the pharmacokinetic interaction between lamotrigine and valproic acid when administered concomitantly?**

Valproic acid inhibits the metabolism of lamotrigine and thus increases the blood level of lamotrigine, whereas lamotrigine induces the metabolism of valproic acid, thereby decreasing valproic acid levels. When coadministered, the dose of lamotrigine should be utilized at one-half of the standard dose, and valproic acid levels should be closely monitored.

○ **What mood stabilizers have a high incidence of weight gain as a side effect?**

Lithium and valproic acid. Carbamazepine and lamotrigine are considered to have a relatively low incidence of weight gain.

○ **When are antipsychotic medications appropriate in the treatment of mood disorders?**

DSM-IV contains a specifier "severe with psychotic features" for both MDE and manic episode. Patients with these mood states sometimes present with psychotic symptoms in addition to the depressive or manic symptoms. It is appropriate to treat these patients with antipsychotic medications to expedite recovery to baseline.

○ **What is meant by "mood congruent" psychotic symptoms?**

Hallucinations and delusions can be mood congruent, meaning the content of the symptom is consistent with either depressive or manic ideation. For example, derogatory command auditory hallucinations of "You're no good, you should kill yourself" are consistent with depression, whereas auditory hallucinations of an angel's voice singing and telling the patient that they are close to God are consistent with mania. Similarly, nihilistic delusions of being punished for some terrible act of transgression are consistent with depression, whereas delusions of grandeur are consistent with mania. Of note, somatic delusions (e.g., body parts not working, stomach is rotting) are not uncommon in depression, particularly in the elderly.

○ **Electroconvulsive therapy can be traced back to which original work?**

Ladislaus von Meduna's original experiments in 1934 used pharmacologic agents to induce seizures, while in 1938, Cerletti and Bini were the first investigators to use electric shock to treat patients with psychiatric illnesses.

○ **What is the mechanism of action of ECT?**

The mechanism of action is still not fully understood. Possible neurochemical mechanisms include changes in the concentration or ratio of neurotransmitters (noradrenergic, serotonergic, and cholinergic), downregualtion of β-adrenergic receptors and/or muscarinic acetylcholine receptors, decreased GABA activity, and increased opioid activity, while neurophysiologic mechanisms may include increased slow-wave activity over the prefrontal lobes (i.e., ECT increases seizure threshold).

○ **What are the most compelling indications for the use of electroconvulsive therapy (ECT)?**

MDE with psychotic symptoms has been shown to respond well to ECT, and often this disorder requires a rapid resolution because of the risk that the psychotic symptoms present to the patient. This makes ECT a suitable choice. Other situations in which a rapid response is necessary and warrant ECT as a treatment option include debilitating MDE with failure to maintain adequate caloric intake (particularly in the geriatric population), acute suicide risk, refractory mania, and neuroleptic malignant syndrome. ECT is often the treatment of choice in situations where contraindications to antidepressants exist, with some clinicians considering pregnancy to be in this category. Depressive disorders that are refractory to pharmacotherapy and psychotherapy should lead clinicians to consider ECT as well.

○ **Should ECT ever be used as a primary treatment?**

Primary use of ECT, prior to a trial of medications, may be considered (after careful evaluation and discussion of risks and benefits) in the following situations:

- When the need for a rapid, definitive response exists on either medical or psychiatric grounds (refractory mania or psychosis, neuroleptic malignant syndrome, or catatonia).
- When the risks of other treatments outweigh the risks of ECT (pregnancy).
- When a history of a poor drug response and/or good ECT response exists from previous episodes of the illness.
- Patient preference.

○ **What is the primary indication for electroconvulsive therapy (ECT)?**

Affective illnesses.

○ **What are the contraindications to ECT?**

There are no absolute contraindications to ECT. Increased intracranial pressure (because of an intracranial mass or an impending stroke) is a relative contraindication as intracranial pressure in increased during ECT. Recent myocardial infarction is also a relative contraindication as postictal bradycardia can occur, as can arrhythmias, because of the tachycardia that is induced during the seizure. Blood pressure before, during, and after ECT should be carefully monitored, and if hypertension occurs, it should be appropriately treated. Overall, the most important side effects of ECT are those of cognitive deficits and cardiovascular decompensation.

○ **True/False: Osteoporosis is a relative contraindication for ECT.**

False. When first used for the treatment of depression and other psychiatric disorders in the 30s and 40s, ECT was associated with long bone fractures or dislocations caused by the induction of seizure activity without concurrent anesthesia and muscle relaxation. However, use of anesthesia and muscle relaxants during the procedure has essentially eliminated fractures as a side effect, even when osteoporosis is present.

○ **Which psychiatric medications should be discontinued prior to the initiation of a course of ECT?**

Benzodiazepines and **anticonvulsants** should be discontinued due to their interference with seizure induction. **Lithium** should be stopped due to the risk of increased postictal delirium.

○ **True/False: Seizure duration is considered a reliable guideline for determining the effectiveness of ECT treatment.**

False. Seizure duration has not been shown to be a reliable guideline for the effectiveness of ECT. It is recommended that an induced seizure have a duration of at least 15 to 25 seconds, as measured by either EEG tracing or tonic–clonic extremity movements. Prolonged seizures of above 180 seconds warrant termination with IV barbiturate or benzodiazepine. Shorter duration of a seizure may occur in older patients and later in a course of ECT. A relationship between postictal suppression and clinical improvement has been shown in studies. Note: seizure duration is not a measure of seizure threshold.

○ **Is it important to consider seizure threshold when administering ECT?**

Yes, as stimulus intensities will need to be adjusted depending on whether bilateral or unilateral treatments are administered. Unilateral ECT requires stimulus intensities that are 2.5 to 6 times the seizure threshold, while bilateral ECT requires stimulus intensities that are 1.5 times the seizure threshold. While unilateral ECT, which is most often applied to the nondominant hemisphere, has less cognitive impairment associated with it, it is considered to be less effective than bilateral ECT, and as noted above, requires a higher stimulus intensity to induce a seizure.

○ **What type of electrical current do most ECT machines used in the United States deliver?**

Brief pulse current, which is associated with less cognitive impairment, and induces a seizure with less energy than a sine-wave current of electricity. The electrical stimulus is generally in the neighborhood of 800 milliamps, with duration of flow for 1 to 6 seconds.

○ **How can EEG changes as a result of electroconvulsive treatment be summarized?**

As the number of electroconvulsive treatments increase, EEG slowing begins to persist.

○ **What is considered the biggest problem after successful acute ECT treatment?**

The biggest problem after ECT is high relapse rates. High relapse rates are not surprising given that most patients are treatment resistant, and ECT is often stopped the moment it is effective. Continuation or maintenance ECT is an option in preventing relapse.

○ **How does maintenance ECT compare to pharmacotherapy for maintenance treatment of depression after successful induction of remission by ECT?**

As many patients are treatment resistant to begin with, relapse rates after successful induction of remission by ECT are high in both groups. Combined maintenance ECT and pharmacotherapy may offer the best protection against relapse.

○ **What is the relationship of seizure threshold and electroconvulsive treatment?**

Maintenance ECT can be associated with an increased seizure threshold.

○ **What is the mortality rate for electroconvulsive treatment?**

Approximately 1 per 1,000 to 1 per 10,000 (similar to the risk of mortality associated with general anesthesia).

○ **What are patients' attitudes regarding electroconvulsive treatment (based on recent research)?**

Patients who have received a course of ECT generally report favorable results and are willing to undergo the treatment if needed again.

○ **In expressing antielectroconvulsive views, what organized group is most often quoted?**

The Scientology organizations, not the American Medical Association.

○ **What are the current trends in malpractice litigation in regard to electroconvulsive treatment?**

Surveys indicate that ECT accounts for only a minimal amount of malpractice claims and generally results in decisions favorable to the psychiatrist.

○ **Which medical–legal issues about ECT should always be followed?**

Never do involuntary ECT unless court ordered. This generally occurs only when ECT is considered lifesaving. Informed consent for ECT is, of course, *absolutely* mandatory, and should include information regarding the risk for the potential of permanent memory loss, as well as for the more probable retrograde and anterograde amnesia for events occurring shortly before, during, and after ECT, as well as risk for adverse cardiac events, and anesthesia-related side effects. Finally, the risks and benefits of other treatments or no treatment must be reviewed and understood.

○ **What is the most common indication for phototherapy in psychiatry?**

Major depressive disorder with seasonal pattern (seasonal affective disorder). Phototherapy involves exposing the retina to visible light. This treatment is also effective in shifting the sleep–wake cycle in patients with delayed sleep phase disorder.

CHAPTER 9 Anxiety Disorders

○ **What is anxiety? What are its clinical symptoms?**

Anxiety is a diffuse, unpleasant feeling of apprehension, the source of which cannot be clearly identified. Its clinical symptoms include tremors, pounding heart, tightness in the chest, perspiration, an uncomfortable feeling in the abdomen, inability to relax or sleep, and sometimes the urge to void.

○ **What is the difference between fear and anxiety?**

Fear is the emotional and physiological response to a recognized external threat. Anxiety is an unpleasant emotional state, the source of which is less readily identified. Patients use the terms fear and anxiety interchangeably.

○ **What is the prevalence of anxiety disorders?**

Anxiety disorders are the most common psychiatric disorders. In NIMH-ECA study, the prevalence in the preceding 6 months was found to be 8.3%. The lifetime prevalence is unknown, but estimated to be in the range of 15% to 25%.

○ **What is the psychoanalytic view of anxiety?**

Freud proposed that anxiety is a signal to the ego that an unacceptable drive is pressing for conscious representation and discharge.

○ **What is a panic attack? How long does it last?**

Panic attacks are episodes of sudden, intense periods of anxiety. The severity of symptoms leads to the fear of having a heart attack, fainting, "going crazy," or dying. These episodes usually abate within 10 minutes and rarely last more than an hour, but for the person experiencing the attack, it may seem like a very long time.

○ **What foods, drugs, and maneuvers can precipitate panic attacks?**

Caffeine, alcohol, marijuana, thyroid supplements, sympathomimetics, stimulants, and yohimbine can precipitate panic attacks. Sodium lactate infusion provokes panic attacks in approximately 70% of patients with panic disorders. Exercise, carbon dioxide inhalation, and cholecystokinin administration can also precipitate panic attacks.

○ **What cardiac disorders are associated with panic disorder?**

Mitral valve prolapse is seen in approximately 50% of patients with panic disorder. There is also a high association between cardiac arrhythmia, hypertension, and panic disorder.

○ **What are some medical conditions that mimic the symptoms of panic attacks?**

Myocardial infarction, arrhythmia, congestive heart failure, angina, pulmonary embolism, asthma, and irritable bowel syndrome.

○ **Which endocrine disorders may be associated with panic attacks?**

Diabetes, hypothyroidism, hyperthyroidism, parathyroid disease, Cushing's disease, and pheochromocytoma.

○ **How would you treat a patient with panic disorder?**

In the short term, cognitive–behavioral treatment (CBT) compares well to pharmacological treatment. CBT consists of an information component, somatic management skills, cognitive restructuring, and exposure. A combination of pharmacotherapy and CBT may have some short-term synergistic effects. The drugs most commonly used for the treatment of panic disorder are SSRIs, tricyclic antidepressants (imipramine, clomipramine), MAOIs, and benzodiazepines. Other less commonly used agents are venlafaxine, buspirone, and propranolol. The benefits of treatment with CBT tend to last longer compared to pharmacotherapy or combined treatment.

○ **What is a phobia?**

A phobia is an irrational fear resulting in a conscious avoidance of the specific feared object, activity, or situation. The patient consciously realizes that the fear is unfounded and experiences the fear as ego-dystonic. There are three groups of phobias. They are agoraphobia, social phobia, and simple phobias.

○ **In simple phobias, what are the common feared objects and situations?**

Fear of animals, storms, heights, illness, and injury are commonly seen in patients with simple phobias.

○ **What is the prevalence of agoraphobia?**

The NIMH-ECA study reported a 6-month prevalence of agoraphobia of 3.8% for women and 1.8% for men.

○ **What is the relationship between panic disorder and agoraphobia?**

Panic disorder may exist with or without agoraphobia. Most cases of agoraphobia are thought to be due to panic disorder. If panic disorder is treated, the agoraphobia often improves.

○ **What comorbid conditions are commonly associated with social phobia?**

Major depression, alcoholism, and avoidant personality disorder are common among persons with social phobia.

○ **How is social phobia treated?**

Exposure therapy in fantasy and with videotape feedback is helpful to many individuals. The exposure can be graded in hierarchy from the least to the most frightening. Muscle relaxation, hypnosis, and tranquilizing drugs may be used to reduce the level of anxiety. In some cases, supportive therapy, family therapy, and insight-oriented therapy may be beneficial. Monoamine oxidase inhibitors and β-blockers are most commonly used. Other useful drugs are benzodiazepines, tricyclics, and SSRIs.

○ **What are the differential diagnoses for social phobias?**

Schizophrenia, major depression, obsessive–compulsive disorder (OCD), and paranoid and avoidant personality disorders.

○ **What are obsessions and compulsions?**

An obsession is a recurrent intrusive thought, feeling, idea, or impulse. A compulsion is a conscious recurrent behavior such as counting, checking, hand washing, or avoiding. A patient with OCD realizes the irrationality of the obsession and experiences both the obsession and the compulsion as ego-dystonic, at least at some point in the course of the illness. When minimal distress is present, the specifier, "with poor insight" is applied to the diagnosis.

○ **What themes are common in the obsessive thoughts of individuals affected by OCD?**

Contamination themes, fears of harming self or others, fear of making an error, fears of violating religious or societal norms, and fears of various sexual thoughts or desires are common obsessive thoughts.

○ **What do you know about the epidemiology of OCD?**

The 6-month prevalence of OCD is approximately 1.5% and the lifetime prevalence is 2.5%. Men and women are affected equally. In one-third of individuals, the disorder starts by the age of 15 years; a second peak occurs in the third decade of life.

○ **What do you know about the pathophysiology of OCD?**

There is evidence to suggest dysfunctional serotonin neurotransmission in the orbital cortex and caudate nuclei.

○ **What defense mechanisms play important roles in OCD?**

Three defense mechanisms are considered important. They are isolation, undoing, and reaction formation.

○ **What are obsessive–compulsive spectrum disorders?**

A wide range of psychiatric and medical disorders have been hypothesized to be related to OCD. Included in this group are body dysmorphic disorder, hypochondriasis, eating disorders, impulse control disorders, paraphilias, nonparaphilic sexual addictions, and Tourette's disorder.

○ **How common are OCD symptoms in schizophrenia?**

Up to 20% of patients with schizophrenia exhibit symptoms suggestive of OCD.

○ **What personality disorders are frequently associated with OCD?**

Avoidant, dependent, histrionic, or passive–aggressive personality disorders are the most frequent Axis II diagnoses in OCD patients. Relatively few patients with OCD meet criteria for obsessive–compulsive personality disorder.

○ **How is OCD differentiated from OCPD?**

In general, persons experiencing symptoms of OCD tend to be distressed by their thoughts and behaviors, while individuals diagnosed with OCPD experience little to no distress in how they interact with others (i.e. their way or no way). In addition, the person diagnosed with OCPD tends to apply their rules to all interpersonal interactions, while the individual with OCD tends to have thoughts and behaviors that are restricted to a limited number of themes or fears.

○ **How is OCD differentiated from hypochondriasis?**

Hypochondriasis symptoms are focused exclusively on misinterpreted bodily functions and symptoms, while OCD symptoms are driven by fears of contamination.

○   **Differentiate OCD from body dysmorphic disorder.**

In body dysmorphic disorder, the recurrent thoughts are limited exclusively to beliefs of having a physical defect.

○   **What features of paraphilias and nonparaphilic disorders differentiate them from OCD?**

The behaviors observed in paraphilias and nonparaphilias are ego-syntonic, while the individual with OCD will experience considerable distress when they have recurrent thoughts of various sexual behaviors, and will go to great lengths to avoid engaging in those behaviors.

○   **How do tics differ from compulsions?**

Tics are not preceded by an uncontrollable impulse to vocalize, or to contract a muscle (or muscle group). At times complex, tics do not have any preceding anxiety or thoughts that are characteristic of obsessions, such as contamination themes.

○   **How common is depression in OCD?**

Approximately 50% of patients with OCD show symptoms of depression or dysthymia. EEG and neuroendocrine studies have suggested some commonality between depression and OCD.

○   **What anatomical and cerebral functional abnormalities have been noted in patients with OCD?**

Enlarged ventricles and decreased volumes of caudates have been noted in some patients with severe OCD. Several PET studies have suggested abnormalities in the caudate nuclei and prefrontal cortex.

○   **What symptom inventories and rating scales are often used during assessment and treatment of OCD?**

The Yale–Brown Obsessive Compulsive Symptom Checklist (Y-BOCS) or the Obsessive–Compulsive Inventory are useful tools to evaluate the number of different obsessive and compulsive thoughts, while the Yale–Brown Obsessive Compulsive Symptom rating scale can be used to monitor severity of symptoms at baseline and at various points during treatment. Assessing a patient's degree of insight may be of additional benefit, and can be measured using the Brown Assessment of Beliefs Scale and/or the Overvalued Ideas Scale.

○   **How effective is behavior therapy in OCD?**

Behavior therapy is considered the treatment of choice in OCD. Exposure and response prevention yields 60% to 80% reduction in symptoms in three-fourths of patients. Other helpful behavioral techniques include desensitization, thought stopping, flooding, implosion, and aversive conditioning.

○   **What pharmacological agents are useful in the treatment of OCD?**

In general, SSRIs are considered the first line of pharmacologic treatment for OCD. Generally, the SSRIs are considered equally efficacious. Clomipramine (Anafranil), and MAOIs can also be effective in treating OCD, but their side effect profiles may limit tolerability. Benzodiazepines such as alprazolam (Xanax), and clonazepam (Klonopin) may be useful in some patients. Psychotropic medications are used as either first line or as adjuvant to behavior therapy.

○   **What is the role of neurosurgery in the treatment of OCD?**

Stereotaxic limbic leukotomy and anterior capsulotomy have been shown to help a majority of severely ill OCD patients who have failed to benefit from other treatments.

○ **What is the prevalence of posttraumatic stress disorder (PTSD)?**

The NIMH-ECA study found a lifetime prevalence of 1% in both sexes; 15% of the general population had at least one symptom of PTSD.

○ **What kind of traumatic events can lead to symptoms of PTSD?**

DSM-IV has described two components related to the traumatic event. (1) The person experienced, witnessed, or was confronted with an event or events that involved actual or threatened death or serious injury or a threat to the physical integrity of self or others. (2) The person's response involved intense fear, helplessness, or horror. The threat does not always need to be external. Being diagnosed with a life-threatening illness, or learning about the sudden, unexpected death of a family member can also produce PTSD symptoms.

○ **What are the three major symptom clusters of PTSD?**

Persistent reexperiencing of the traumatic event, persistent avoidance of stimuli associated with the trauma (and numbing of general responsiveness), and persistent symptoms of increased arousal.

○ **How long must symptoms of PTSD be present before a diagnosis thereof can be made?**

One month. If symptoms are present for less than 3 months, the specifier of "acute" is applied; if symptoms are present for more than 3 months, the specifier of "chronic" is applied.

○ **What diagnosis is made when symptoms of PTSD are present in the first month following exposure to a traumatic event?**

Acute stress disorder. Symptoms must also be present at least 2 days following exposure to a traumatic event and must cause significant impairment of functioning before a diagnosis of acute stress disorder is made.

○ **Other than the chronological difference, how does a diagnosis of acute stress disorder differ from that of PTSD?**

The presence of dissociative symptoms during or after the traumatic event is required for a diagnosis of acute stress disorder. These include, but are not limited to, depersonalization, numbing, detachment, derealization, dissociative amnesia, reduced awareness, or dissociative amnesia. In addition, at least one symptom of each of the core symptoms of PTSD (reexperiencing, avoidance, and increased arousal) must also be present.

○ **Describe factors that increase the risk for developing PTSD.**

In general the severity, duration, and proximity to the traumatic event are factors that increase the risk for PTSD symptoms.

○ **Which urinary catecholamine levels are increased in patients with PTSD?**

The 24-hour urinary excretion of epinephrine, norepinephrine, and dopamine are increased when compared to healthy controls.

○ **What neuroanatomic abnormality has been most consistently observed in patients with PTSD?**

Reduction in the volume of the hippocampus by 8%, as measured by MRI, has been noted in patients with PTSD. This is associated with deficits in short-term memory.

○ **What comorbid conditions are commonly associated with PTSD?**

Major depression, minor depression, generalized anxiety disorder, panic disorder, substance abuse, somatoform disorder, and personality disorders are common comorbid conditions associated with PTSD.

○ **What groups of drugs are considered useful in the treatment of PTSD?**

SSRIs, antiadrenergic agents (propranolol, clonidine), MAOIs, and tricyclic antidepressants are most commonly used in PTSD. Anticonvulsants (carbamazepine, valproate) are less commonly used and benzodiazepines are useful in some patients.

○ **Describe the course and prognosis of chronic PTSD.**

The full syndrome of PTSD usually develops some time after the trauma. Symptoms can fluctuate over time and may be most intense during periods of stress. Approximately 30% recover, 40% have mild symptoms, 20% have moderate symptoms, and 10% remain unchanged or get worse. A good prognosis is predicted by a rapid onset of symptoms, short duration of symptoms, good premorbid functioning, strong social support, and the absence of other psychiatric or medical problems.

○ **How common is generalized anxiety disorder (GAD) in the general population?**

Generalized anxiety disorder is thought to be quite common, affecting 5% of the population with a female to male ratio of 2:1.

○ **What comorbid conditions are commonly associated with GAD?**

It is estimated that at least 50% of patients with GAD have coexisting conditions. GAD frequently coexists with major depression or dysthymia, although the more common comorbidity is with another anxiety disorder such as social phobia or panic disorder.

○ **What is the most common anxiety disorder in childhood?**

Separation anxiety disorder is very common in childhood. It is characterized by developmentally inappropriate and excessive anxiety concerning separation from home or from loved ones.

○ **How common are symptoms of anxiety in depressive disorder?**

Approximately 60% of patients with depression have some anxiety symptoms, with 20% to 30% having frank anxiety attacks.

○ **What common medications or substances can produce symptoms of anxiety in the elderly?**

Alcohol (intoxication or withdrawal), stimulants (caffeine, sympathomimetics), steroids, thyroid preparations, anticholinergic medications, and antidepressants commonly produce anxiety symptoms in the elderly.

○ **Name some nonpharmacologic treatments available for treating generalized anxiety disorder.**

Reassurance, environmental manipulation, relaxation, biofeedback, meditation, cognitive behavior therapy, and supportive and dynamic psychotherapy are some of the nonpharmacologic treatments available for treating GAD.

○ **Apart from benzodiazepines, what other drugs are used in the treatment of GAD?**

Buspirone, tricyclic antidepressants, β-adrenergic antagonists, and antihistamines are used in the treatment of GAD.

○ **Describe the course and prognosis of GAD.**

GAD commonly persists for many years. Untreated, it usually waxes and wanes in response to common stressors. With treatment, symptoms are reduced, but usually recur when treatment is stopped.

○ **How are benzodiazepines classified?**

On the basis of the duration of half-life, benzodiazepines are classified into short acting and long acting. Examples of short acting are triazolam, alprazolam, and lorazepam. Examples of long acting are diazepam, chlordiazepoxide, and flurazepam.

○ **Describe some of the common side effects of benzodiazepines.**

Common side effects of benzodiazepines include over sedation, impairment of memory, paradoxical stimulant effects, depression, tolerance, dependence, and respiratory depression when combined with other sedatives.

○ **How do benzodiazepines work?**

Benzodiazepines bind with γ-aminobutyric acid (GABA) receptors, which increases their affinity for GABA, thereby increasing the flow of chloride ions into the neurons. This hyperpolarizes and inhibits the neuron. BZ-1 receptors are believed to be involved in the mediation of sleep and BZ-2 receptors are believed to be involved in cognition, memory, and motor control.

○ **Which benzodiazepine has antidepressant effects?**

Alprazolam has antidepressant effects comparable to those of the tricyclic antidepressants.

○ **What are the advantages of using buspirone over benzodiazepines in the treatment of GAD?**

Buspirone does not have sedative effects, does not interact with alcohol, and does not lead to dependence.

○ **How long does it take for buspirone to show its full therapeutic effects?**

Two to three weeks.

○ **Can buspirone be used in the treatment of alcohol or benzodiazepine withdrawal?**

No. Buspirone is ineffective in the treatment of alcohol or benzodiazepine withdrawal.

○ **What are the side effects of propranolol?**

Bronchospasm, worsening of congestive heart failure, hypotension, peripheral vasospasm, depression, confusion, and hallucinations.

○ **What are the indications for using benzodiazepines?**

Generalized anxiety disorder, insomnia, panic disorder, agitation, akathisia, and alcohol withdrawal.

○ **Which antihistamine is sometimes used as an anxiolytic?**

Hydroxyzine

○ **In which anxiety disorders are MAOIs used?**

Social phobia, OCD, and posttraumatic stress disorder.

CHAPTER 10 Somatoform Disorders

○ **What is somatoform disorder?**

Somatoform disorder is a psychological condition in which patients have physical symptoms that cannot be fully explained by medical findings or known physiological mechanisms. There must be strong evidence that psychological factors play an important role in the onset, severity, exacerbation, or maintenance of the physical symptoms.

○ **What are the six major somatoform disorders according to the *DSM-IV*?**

Somatization disorder, conversion disorder, hypochondriasis, body dysmorphic disorder, pain disorder, and undifferentiated somatoform disorder.

○ **What is the common name for somatization disorder?**

Briquet's syndrome, which is named after the French physician who first described it in 1859.

○ **What are the typical symptoms associated with somatization disorder?**

Somatoform disorder is characterized by a history of multisystem physical complaints beginning before the age of 3 years, occurring over several years, which results in either the seeking of treatment or in clear psychosocial dysfunction. There must be four separate pain symptoms, two different gastrointestinal symptoms, one sexual symptom, and one pseudoneurological symptom experienced by the patient over several years. After appropriate medical workup, there are few or no objective findings to support the symptoms.

○ **What is the typical clinical presentation of a patient with somatization disorder?**

Patients rarely are seen initially by a mental health clinician. They are usually encountered in primary care fields. Patients will generally have a long list of complicated medical problems and medications. They tend to overdramatize their present and past symptoms. Chronological and descriptive histories of their problems are often vague and nondescript, with criticism of past health care providers.

○ **What is a typical treatment plan for patients with somatization disorder?**

Patients are generally best managed in primary care settings rather than mental health settings. Clinicians should avoid direct confrontation, but provide empathic support for the patient's genuine distress and pain. Focused, physical exams should be performed at each visit, similar to other medical patients. The patient should be seen regularly, every 2 to 4 weeks, regardless of the number and severity of complaints. Limits should be set on excessive use of telephone triage and length of visits. The goal of treatment is to improve functioning and coping with symptoms, not necessarily curing them. At times, intensive case management by payors can prevent unnecessary procedures and duplication of previous medical work-ups.

○ **What are the epidemiological characteristics of somatization disorder?**

Somatization disorder is usually diagnosed in women. It occurs in 0.1% of the general population, and is more often diagnosed in minorities, lower socioeconomic groups, and less formally educated groups. First-degree female relatives of patients with somatization disorder have a 20% increased rate of somatization disorder, while first-degree male relatives have an increased incidence of antisocial personality disorder, alcohol dependence, and somatization disorder.

○ **What is the psychodynamic explanation of somatization disorder?**

Somatization is considered a defense against painful, intense affect. The experience of physical pain allows for the avoidance of intense affect. Alexithymia is also associated with somatization disorder.

○ **In comparison to the general public, do patients with somatoform disorders undergo more surgeries?**

Yes, somatoform disorder patients have three times the body weight of internal organs removed by surgery.

○ **What is the typical psychological dilemma that patients with somatoform disorder usually encounter with health professionals?**

A "no-win situation" where patients distrust clinicians they must rely on for continued care. Most medical clinicians consider these patients to have psychogenic or psychological illnesses that do not respond to typical medical modalities. Both parties are frustrated when the patient continues to have medical symptoms despite full-scale efforts by the clinician. The patient senses the clinician's frustration and skepticism and then trust and compliance decrease.

○ **What are frequent complications of somatization disorder?**

Substance abuse, excessive laboratory tests, medications, surgeries, work and social impairment, chronic demoralization with the medical system, depression, anxiety, marital problems, and divorce are associated with this disorder.

○ **What is hypochondriasis?**

Hypochondriasis is a chronic and persistent disorder where patients are preoccupied with excessive misinterpretations of common somatic symptoms that they feel will have a severe and negative outcome. This over-worry about physical sensations continues despite adequate medical interventions.

○ **What is the difference between hypochondriasis and somatization disorder?**

Patients with somatization disorder complain about multiple physical symptoms, whereas patients with hypochondriasis are preoccupied with worry and fear about getting or having a serious disease.

○ **What is the current psychopharmacological management suggestion for hypochondriasis?**

Hypochondriasis may be a variant of obsessive–compulsive disorder (OCD), where patients obsess about the fear of having a medical illness and are driven by compulsion to overuse medical treatments. High doses of serotonergic agents, such as selective serotonin reuptake inhibitors, can be effective. Response requires high doses and is slower when compared to treating depression, again consistent with an OCD pattern.

○ **What is the current suggested psychotherapeutic approach to hypochondriasis?**

Clinicians should give patients facts about their difficulties, clarify the difference between pain and the experience of pain, describe how emotions affect the perception of physical sensations, demonstrate how selective attention and suggestion contribute to amplifying a symptom's seriousness, work on psychological coping with physical symptoms, and convey empathy.

○ **What is conversion disorder?**

Patients with conversion disorder have symptoms suggesting a neurological or medical functional loss. Psychological factors are associated with the onset of the functional deficit. While patients do not intentionally feign the deficit, medical or neurological findings that could explain the functional loss are absent.

○ **What are some typical conversion disorder symptoms or signs?**

Blindness, paralysis, tunnel vision, seizures, dyscoordination, anosmia, anesthesia, and paresthesia have been associated with conversion disorder. Often, there is symbolic meaning to the functional losses noted above. Conversion disorders usually are characterized by one physical symptom, whereas somatization disorder and hypochondriasis are characterized by many symptoms.

○ **Which somatoform disorder is associated with "la belle indifference"?**

Conversion disorder. "La belle indifference" refers to an attitude of relative unconcern about the pseudoneurological symptoms associated with conversion disorder. Note: this condition is also found in stoic individuals with genuine medical findings, and therefore is not pathognomonic of conversion disorder.

○ **What is the difference between pain disorder and conversion disorder?**

Patients must have neurological symptoms other than pain to qualify for the diagnosis of conversion disorder. Conversion disorder is typically seen in late childhood or early adulthood and is associated with childhood trauma and dissociation. Pain disorder occurs when patients have pain in one or more anatomical sites, and this causes marked psychosocial impairment. Like conversion disorder, psychological factors are thought to predate, exacerbate, or maintain the pain symptoms.

○ **What are some characteristics of patients with pain disorder?**

Sixty percent of these patients have a first-degree relative with chronic pain. Thirty-eight percent of patients with pain disorder misuse alcohol, 30% have mood disorders, and approximately 50% will respond to antidepressants, suggesting that for some individuals, pain disorder is a depression spectrum illness.

○ **What is a typical treatment plan for patients with pain disorder?**

Treatment options for patients with pain disorder include appropriate pain management, use of longer-acting analgesics on a scheduled basis, and avoidance of *prn* dosing. Antidepressants, cognitive–behavioral therapies, and biofeedback have been shown to be effective for some individuals. Supportive psychotherapy is also helpful.

○ **What is body dysmorphic disorder?**

This disorder occurs when there is preoccupation with an imagined anatomic defect in appearance, or if there is a slight physical anomaly, the patient's concern is excessive. This preoccupation causes psychosocial distress and inhibits functioning.

○ **Does cosmetic surgery improve body dysmorphic disorder symptoms?**

No. Plastic surgery usually leads to new problems. Patients may not feel that the surgery was a complete success or will focus on another anomaly. Behavior therapy with exposure and desensitization has been shown to be a successful psychotherapeutic intervention.

○ **When is the *DSM-IV* definition of "psychological factors affecting medical conditions" applicable?**

This term is used when the presence of one or more specific psychological or behavioral factors (including comorbid mental disorders) adversely affects a general medical condition.

○ **What are some medical conditions commonly exacerbated by stress?**

More than 40 "psychosomatic illnesses" have been identified. Common ones include acne, eczema, psoriasis, asthma, coronary artery disease, essential hypertension, peptic ulcer disease, arrhythmias, migraine headaches, urticaria, and irritable bowel syndrome.

○ **What are the five life events considered most stressful on the Social Readjustment Rating Scale (1994)?**

In descending order of severity: death of a spouse, divorce, death of a close family member, marital separation, serious injury or illness.

○ **Who coined the term "biopsychosocial"?**

George Engel, Professor of Medicine and Psychiatry at the University of Rochester, New York, 1977.

○ **What are the five major theories explaining the association between psychological factors and medical conditions?**

Concomitant effects, somatopsychic causation, psychosomatic specificity, stress, and holistic models.

○ **Which of the above theories reflects the traditional biomedical view that disease is always biophysical in origin?**

The somatopsychic causation model understands psychological changes as reactive to biological events.

○ **Which of the above theories views somatic and psychological distress as being linked by mutual constitutional or environmental causal factors?**

The concomitant effect theory, also referred to as "collateral transduction."

○ **Which theory from above holds that physical illness is exacerbated by nonspecific reactions to noxious psychosocial experiences?**

The stress theory rejects the notion that specific psychological factors are involved. Illness exacerbation is explained by the physiological effects of the stress response.

○   **What is telogen effluvium?**

Telogen effluvium occurs when there is sudden and diffuse loss of hair in response to psychological or physical stress. The differential diagnosis includes thyroid disease, iron deficiency anemia, alopecia areata, and iatrogenic causes, such as the use of valproic acid.

○   **Which primary skin disorders are commonly exacerbated by emotional stress?**

Stress can exacerbate psoriasis, acne vulgaris, alopecia areata, urticaria, psychogenic purpura, rosacea, lichen planus, atopic dermatitis, and other eczemas.

○

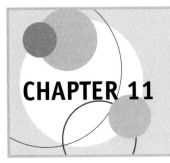

CHAPTER 11

Factitious and Dissociative Disorders

○ **Define factitious disorders.**

Factitious disorders are characterized by variable constellations of physical and psychological symptoms intentionally produced by an individual to assume the sick role. Literally, they are artificial, feigned, or sham symptoms. Common examples include contamination of urine sample with blood or feces, insertion of foreign bodies into joint cavities, or introduction of pathogens into the blood stream by patients to feign illness. Factitious disorders have been known since the second century when Galen wrote the earliest description of these disorders.

○ **How common are the factitious disorders?**

Some studies estimate that 0.5% to 8% of patients admitted to psychiatric units have a diagnosis of factitious disorders. A study in 1990 reported that these disorders may often be missed and consequently underreported. Conversely, these may be overreported as some of the same affected individuals may seek care from different institutions and providers under different names.

○ **What is the differential diagnosis of factitious disorders?**

The differential diagnosis of factitious disorder includes true physical/medical or general medical conditions, somatoform disorders, antisocial personality disorder, borderline personality disorder, schizophrenia, and malingering.

○ **What is the usual age of onset of factitious disorders?**

Various studies report the median age of onset to be early adulthood or early twenties, with a range varying between 16 and 64 years old.

○ **Are there any sex differences in prevalence of factitious disorders?**

Yes. Contrary to popular belief that the factitious disorders are more common in males (probably because of the well-known example of Munchausen's syndrome), a number of old and new reviews of literature including a 10-year retrospective study of patients revealed that factitious disorders are more common in females.

○ **Is there any known genetic basis for factitious disorders?**

No known genetic basis exists for these disorders. Although not infrequently, these patients have comorbid conditions, e.g., mood disorders, substance-related disorders, and personality disorders, which are known to have some genetic basis.

O **What kinds of jobs or employment situations are associated with the diagnosis of factitious disorders?**

The diagnosis is strongly associated with persons who are employed as laboratory personnel, nurses, physicians, or others who are intimately familiar with health and medically related fields such as medical secretaries, hospital volunteers ambulance drivers, and emergency medical technicians.

O **What are the characteristics of factitious disorder with predominantly psychological symptoms?**

These highly suggestible patients commonly present symptoms according to their own concept of mental illness. They may endorse symptoms mentioned in a review of systems, and their symptoms appear to worsen when under perceived observation. They may present with symptoms of bereavement, dissociation, or psychosis. Finally, these individuals may be pleasant and overly cooperative, or they may be extremely uncooperative and negativistic.

O **What are the characteristics of factitious disorder with predominantly physical symptoms?**

As the name implies, physical symptoms dominate the clinical picture suggesting the presence of a general medical condition(s). Patients may seem to spare no effort at attempts to secure admission or stay in hospital. They may present with a multitude of physical symptoms limited only by the patient's sophistication and imagination. They may show multiple scars and commonly present with acute abdominal pain, hematuria, fever, seizures, rashes, abscesses, and any other combination of symptoms.

O **What are the features of factitious disorder with combined psychological and physical signs and symptoms?**

In presentation of this category, neither the physical nor psychological symptoms predominate, and motivation to attain the sick role remains as in other categories. The patients may present their illness with dramatic flare, but still remain vague and inconsistent. They lie in one form or the other and may make their stories intriguing to the listener, whose interest may unwittingly reinforce the patient's behavior. As an extensive workup usually remains negative, they may modify their symptoms depending on their knowledge of medical or mental illness. They rarely have visitors and may frequently demand analgesics. They may be very defensive and may suddenly leave the hospital when they feel challenged by the lack of clinical data supporting their reported illness. To perpetuate their sick role, they may attempt to gain admission to different hospitals across various cities, states, and even countries.

O **What psychodynamic factors are considered in the etiology of factitious disorders?**

Several postulates exist in an attempt to explain apparently senseless, often intriguing, puzzling, and sometimes highly risky behavior of patients suffering from these disorders. Some patients may be expressing their masochistic behavior and fantasies through the medium of medical setting(s), while others may be reliving their earlier experience of being a patient, when they might have felt valued or loved. Some suggest that the patient may find hospitals to be a psychological substitute for a "confusing parental figure." These patients may also be reacting to the need for mastery of previous experiences where hospital personnel may have played a traumatic role in early personality development. Alternatively, through hostility and deception, a patient may be seeking love and approval from an idealized but devalued physician figure. Additionally, in the patient role, he or she may be symbolically fulfilling the need for an illusory sense of being "in control." The choice of medical field by many of these patients may be an expression of identification with the aggressor and merger with an ambivalently held ego ideal. Finally, others believe that patients may be attempting to minimize the impact of some unconscious guilt feelings derived from reaction to conflicts caused by traumatic childhood experiences.

O **What is "pseudologia phantastica"?**

This is an interesting phenomenon that occasionally occurs in some patients presenting with complaints suggestive of factitious disorders with predominantly physical symptoms. They present their personal and clinical histories in outrageously grandiose manners and may engage in pathologic lying. They usually excite curiosity and intrigue in the listener who may unwittingly gratify the patient's need for attention, ironically reinforcing the symptoms.

○ **What is a "Gridiron abdomen"?**

Patients with chronic factitious disorder with predominantly physical symptoms may acquire multiple abdominal scars from repeated surgical procedures. These scars may resemble a gridiron pattern.

○ **What other psychiatric conditions are commonly associated with factitious disorders?**

Depressive disorders, substance-related disorders, somatization disorders, and dissociative disorders are commonly associated with factitious disorders.

○ **What features should help the psychiatrist to differentiate factitious disorders from other disorders?**

Several factors may alert the physician to a possible diagnosis of factitious disorder. These include a history and description of symptoms that represents a patient's perception of his/her psychiatric/medical disorder and not a clinical picture consistent with a recognized disorder; the worsening or presence of symptoms only during observation; the ongoing appearance of new symptoms that are inconsistent with existing diagnoses, especially when an extensive workup is reported as negative to the patient; the occurrence of new symptoms similar to those of other patients in the vicinity; consistent and repeated poor response to conventional treatment for a given diagnosis; and an overly dramatic, flamboyant, graphic, unverifiable presentation of history.

○ **How are factitious disorders differentiated from acts of malingering?**

The underlying motives for patient behavior distinguish these disorders from each other. However, the symptoms are intentionally produced in both cases. In factitious disorders, it is the psychological need for assumption of the sick role, while in malingering there is usually an obvious external incentive, e.g., avoidance of conscription, or a prisoner feigning illness to avoid physical labor. Factitious disorders are always considered to be psychopathologic in nature, while malingering may be an adaptive response in certain circumstances, e.g., a person held hostage simulates illness to avoid physical labor.

○ **What psychological tests may be of help in differentiating factitious disorders from true psychiatric disorders?**

Projective tests, and in particular, the Bender Gestalt test may be helpful.

○ **Briefly describe the course and prognosis of factitious disorders.**

The onset of these disorders usually occurs in early adulthood, and it commonly follows real illness, real or imagined loss, or estrangement. Outcomes vary from resolution after one episode to recurrent hospitalizations and lifelong incapacitation. Patients hopping from one hospital to another seem to have the worse prognosis.

○ **What treatment approaches are available for the treatment of these patients?**

Once a diagnosis of factitious disorder is certain, combined medical psychotherapeutic measures are indicated. An early psychiatric consultation may prevent any unnecessary medical/surgical procedures. Opinions differ on whether, when, and how a patient should be informed of the diagnosis. Most investigators suggest disclosure in a supportive and nonaccusatory manner, indicating assurance of further treatment and care. Psychiatric hospitalization is usually recommended after confirmation of the diagnosis to the patient and treatment of any associated medical or psychiatric conditions continues. Others suggest that symptoms should be treated as they are, and the patient should be given plausible technical or scientific explanations of symptoms. The same physician should follow the patient's treatment.

○ **Per the *DSM-IV*, give an example of factitious disorder NOS.**

Munchausen by proxy is a well-known example of factitious disorder NOS.

○ **What features characterize Munchausen by proxy?**

In this disorder, a care provider intentionally feigns or produces signs and symptoms of an illness in the person under her or his care. Typically, a parent (usually mother) causes illness in her child to indirectly assume the sick role.

○ **In Munchausen by proxy, who is most frequently the perpetrator?**

The mother is reported to be the perpetrator in 95% of the cases, and in the remaining 5% of the cases, it may be the father or baby sitter.

○ **What is the usual profile of a parent perpetrator in Munchausen by proxy?**

The usual profile of a parent perpetrator is that of an apparently very caring, overly concerned, articulate, and intelligent person (usually mother) with knowledge and sophistication commensurate with that person's experience in health and child care fields.

○ **What psychiatric disorders are often seen in perpetrators of Munchausen by proxy?**

Depression, personality disorders, and factitious disorders are commonly found in perpetrators of Munchausen by proxy.

○ **How high is the mortality rate in child victims of Munchausen by proxy?**

Mortality rates as high as 9% have been reported in these cases.

○ **Is Munchausen by proxy considered a form of child abuse?**

Yes. And it is reportable within the limits of state and local laws. A treating physician who fails to report a child victim of this disorder is liable for medical malpractice.

○ **What is the key factor in diagnosing Munchausen by proxy in children?**

If the symptoms disappear promptly once the child victim is removed from the custody of a suspected perpetrator, this should prompt any physician to consider the diagnosis of Munchausen by proxy.

○ **In order of frequency, what are the most common presenting symptoms in cases of Munchausen by proxy?**

According to the literature review by D. A. Rosenberg (1987), the most common presenting symptoms are bleeding (44%), seizures (42%), CNS depression (19%), apnea (15%), diarrhea (11%), vomiting (10%), fever (10%), and rash (9%).

○ **What special challenges are encountered in the treatment of patients with Munchausen by proxy?**

Once the diagnosis is suspected, treatment will be similar to any other child abuse case. Treatment priorities include prevention of further abuse, treatment of the victim, and counseling of the perpetrator, usually the mother. Parents must be informed, and the case must be reported to authorities. As the perpetrator usually becomes depressed and even suicidal after acknowledging child abuse, particular care should be taken in providing proper counseling and follow-up. Treatment of the victim will depend upon the type and severity of symptoms. Hospitalization for an intensive workup is usually indicated, while the placement issues are carefully considered. The child is usually removed from the family. Long-term follow-up studies of these cases indicate a poor prognosis, and many children reportedly themselves develop factitious disorders in adult life.

○ **Describe dissociative disorders.**

A usually sudden, often dramatic, disruption of memory, consciousness, identity, or perception of the environment, with variable duration, characterizes dissociative disorders. The disturbance is in the organization or structure, but not in the contents of these mental processes.

○ **How common are dissociative disorders?**

There is a general lack of good epidemiologic studies on these disorders. Estimates of prevalence of dissociative disorders vary widely between 1/10,000 and 5% to 10% of the general population and from 0.5% to 2% in psychiatric populations, with a female-to-male ratio of 9:1. Recently, these cases have been reported with increased frequency, attributed possibly to the availability of diagnostic criteria and to increased awareness among mental health care providers.

○ **What are some etiologic concepts underlying dissociative disorders?**

Dissociative phenomena are considered to be an adaptive response to overwhelming trauma. Dissociation caused by fragmentation of memory, consciousness, perception, or identity allows the affected individual to escape from the traumatic events in their present and future life contexts. Dissociation in humans as a defense mechanism has been likened by some to phenomenon of "sham death" in lower animal species.

○ **How are repression and dissociation similar?**

They both are ego defense mechanisms and "lock" traumatic information out of awareness.

○ **What features distinguish dissociation from repression?**

In dissociation, relevant information is stored untransformed, while in repression, it is "buried" and transformed. Information is usually directly and easily accessible in dissociation, e.g., through hypnosis. In repression, retrieval necessitates translation. "Out-of-awareness" information in dissociation is for specific time periods, while in repression the information "black out" may be regarding an episode or event over an indefinite span of time. Dissociation is almost invariably associated with trauma, while repression is associated with inner conflicts, wishes, and fears.

○ **What are the common characteristics of memory loss in dissociative amnesia?**

Memory loss in dissociative amnesia is typically retrograde and for episodic or explicit memory affecting some specific autobiographical, painful, or traumatic experience. It may involve minutes to years of time. Semantic or implicit memory pertaining to languages, skills, or social behavior remains unaffected. The memory losses associated with dissociated amnesia are described in *DSM-IV* as localized, selective, generalized, continuous, or systematized.

○ **In what age group does dissociative amnesia occur?**

It occurs in any age group.

○ **What comorbid conditions are associated with dissociative amnesia?**

Common comorbid conditions include conversion disorders, bulimia nervosa, alcohol abuse, depression, and Ganser's syndrome.

○ **What is the differential diagnosis of dissociative amnesia?**

The differential diagnosis is fairly wide ranging and includes epilepsy, head trauma, transient global amnesia, dementia, delirium, substance-induced persisting amnesia, substance intoxication, PTSD, acute stress disorder, somatization disorder, age-related cognitive deficits, and malingering.

○ **What are the diagnostic criteria for the diagnosis of dissociative fugue?**

Travel away from one's usual environment with inability to recall details from one's past and confusion regarding identity. The behavior is generally associated with a traumatic event and generally occurs in adulthood.

○ **What differentiates dissociative fugue from dissociative amnesia?**

Travel. In dissociative fugue, the individual is not only amnestic for traumatic events but also travels out of their usual environment, and in rare cases, the patient may assume a new identity.

○ **How common is dissociative fugue?**

The prevalence of dissociative fugue is estimated to be 0.2% in the general population, with notable increases in its incidence during natural catastrophes and in wartime.

○ **What commonly happens after recovery from a dissociative fugue?**

Recovery from dissociative fugue may be followed by lack of recall of what transpired during the fugue state, as well as amnesia of the precipitating trauma. Disruption in marriage, social, and occupational life can occur, while the presence of anger, shame, guilt, and even that of suicidal ideation is not uncommon.

○ **What comorbid conditions are associated with dissociative fugue?**

Mood disorders, PTSD, and substance abuse frequently co-occur with dissociative fugue.

○ **Does schizophrenia predispose to fugue states?**

No. Schizophrenia is not known to be a predisposing factor for dissociative fugue, but heavy alcohol abuse is considered to be a predisposing factor in the development of dissociative fugue.

○ **Are there any culture-specific variations in the presentation of dissociative fugue?**

Yes. Various presentations that may meet the criteria of fugue states are seen in several different ethnic groups. Examples include "frenzy," "amok," and "piblokto" in Navajo, Indonesian, and Eskimo tribes, respectively.

○ **What are the most common dissociative disorders?**

Dissociative trance and possession trance are the most common disorders with worldwide distribution. Their prevalence is higher in industrially less-developed countries. Dissociative identity disorders (formerly multiple personality disorders) are more common in industrialized nations.

○ **What is the course and prognosis of dissociative fugue?**

This disorder affects adults. Onset is usually sudden, and the fugue sudden onset, may last for hours to days or months. Recovery is usually rapid and complete with rare recurrences. In some cases, dissociative amnesia may persist indefinitely as a residual symptom.

○ **How common is dissociative identity disorder?**

There is a great deal of controversy over "true" prevalence of this disorder. But it is generally accepted that there is an upsurge in the number of diagnosed cases of this disorder in the last two decades. Some studies estimate the prevalence to be approximately 1% of psychiatric inpatients, and others have reported rates of 3.3% of all inpatient psychiatric units. The increase in the number of reported cases is attributed to an increased awareness among providers, and a decreased possibility of misdiagnosing dissociative identity disorder as schizophrenia or bipolar disorder. Usually, 6 to 7 years elapse between the first manifestation of symptoms and confirmation of the diagnosis of dissociative identity disorder.

○ **What is the association between child abuse and dissociative identity disorder?**

A consistently high positive correlation is known to exist between dissociative identity disorder and physical or sexual abuse in childhood. Some studies reveal a history of abuse in 90% of these cases.

○ **What is the usual age range of presentation of dissociative identity disorder?**

The usual age range for presentation of this disorder is between adolescence and the third decade of life. Although in recent years, increasing numbers of diagnoses have been made in childhood. This disorder is rare after the fourth decade of life.

○ **What precautions should be observed when diagnosing dissociative identity disorder?**

Awareness of the following factors may help increase diagnostic accuracy:
- Questionable accuracy of childhood traumatic memories.
- Apparent difficulties in verifying the details of historical data.
- Potentially highly suggestible or hypnotizable patients with a propensity for dissociation.

○ **What comorbid conditions are associated with dissociative identity disorder?**

In decreasing order of frequency, dissociative identity disorder may coexist with the following: depressive disorders, substance abuse disorders, borderline personality disorder, sexual disorders, sleep disorders, and posttraumatic stress disorder.

○ **What features of psychological testing help distinguish dissociative identity disorders from schizophrenia?**

Patients with dissociative identity disorder score very high on the hypnotizability scale in contrast to schizophrenic patients who reveal very low scores or indicate the absence of hypnotizability.

○ **What treatment options are available to patients with dissociative identity disorder?**

Extended psychotherapy is the mainstay of treatment. Eventual integration of multiple alters into one is the ultimate goal of the treatment. Psychoactive drugs seem to be of little help in the treatment of comorbid depression, although impulse control disorder or aggressive behavior often shows response to antidepressants or anticonvulsants, respectively.

○ **What is the most common subordinate personality in dissociative identity disorder?**

A childlike personality is the most common subordinate personality in this disorder.

○ **What is the prevalence of depersonalization disorder?**

There is no data available on lifetime prevalence, but it is a common phenomenon as an isolated occasional experience. It is estimated that approximately 50% of the adult population may have experienced brief episodes, usually under stressful situations, and in itself, it is not considered pathologic.

○ **What age range is usually affected by depersonalization disorder?**

It usually presents in adolescence or adulthood.

○ **What causes depersonalization disorder?**

The cause of this disorder remains unknown, despite many proposed psychological, physiological, and psychodynamic theories, with little agreement among the experts.

○ **Is derealization a symptom of depersonalization disorder?**

No. Derealization is a symptom of anxiety, panic attacks, acute stress disorder, and PTSD. Derealization and depersonalization may often coexist.

○ **What comorbid conditions are associated with depersonalization disorder?**

Major depressive disorder, hypochondriasis, and substance-related disorders often co-occur with depersonalization disorder.

○ **What is the usual course and prognosis of depersonalization disorder?**

It usually occurs between the ages of 15 and 30 years and is rarely a presenting complaint. It usually accompanies complaints associated with anxiety, panic attacks, or depressive disorder. An episode may last from seconds to years, rarely remitting spontaneously. Long-term studies show that in more than 50% of cases, it is a chronic problem with a poor prognosis.

○ **Does the classification of dissociative disorders include amnestic disorders?**

No. Amnestic disorders are included in the classification of cognitive disorders.

○ **Are culturally sanctioned dissociative trance and possession trance pathologic?**

No. They are not considered pathologic as long as they are within culturally sanctioned limits and do not cause dysfunction in the individual's social and occupational life.

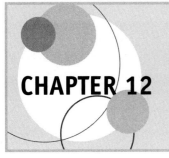

CHAPTER 12 **Sexuality Disorders**

○ **How are disorders involving sexual behaviors classified in the *DSM-IV*?**

The *DSM-IV* groups sexual disorders as Sexual Dysfunctions, Paraphilias, and Gender Identity Disorders.

○ **On which Axis in the multiaxial system are sexuality disorders listed?**

Usually Axis I. If the disorder is biogenic, it is coded on Axis III, unless there is substantial evidence that the dysfunctional episodes are not related to the onset of physiological or pharmacologic influences.

○ **According to the *DSM-IV* there are four phases in the sexual response cycle. In which phase(s) may sexual dysfunction occur?**

Sexual dysfunction can occur in any phase.

Phases	Examples of Dysfunction
Desire	Hypoactive sexual desire disorder; sexual aversion disorder
Excitement	Female sexual arousal disorder; male erectile disorder
Orgasm	Male and female orgasmic disorders; premature ejaculation
Resolution	Postcoital dysphoria; postcoital headache

○ **Define hypoactive sexual desire disorder.**

Hypoactive sexual desire disorder is the lack of sexual fantasies and the lack of desire for sexual interactions. It occurs in approximately 33% of women and 15% of men.

○ **How does sexual aversion disorder differ from hypoactive sexual desire disorder?**

Individuals with a sexual aversion disorder will experience considerable anxiety (aversion) in situations when genital sexual contact is possible and will go to great lengths to avoid such contact. There is a high incidence of sexual aversion disorder in individuals diagnosed with anorexia nervosa.

○ **How common is female sexual arousal disorder?**

It is estimated that approximately 20% of women experience difficulty in attaining and/or maintaining sexual excitement.

○ **What types of medications may cause female arousal disorder?**

Any medicine that influences hormonal patterns may cause arousal difficulty. Of note is that antihistaminic and anticholinergic properties can cause a decrease in vaginal lubrication.

○ **What factors contribute to continued potency in men older than 80 years of age?**

Factors related to continuing potency include availability of a partner, consistency in sexual activity, and absence of vascular disease.

○ **Define male erectile disorder.**

Male erectile disorder is the inability to attain or maintain an erection. Etiology is multifactorial.

○ **What is the mechanism of sildenafil (Viagra®), tadalafil (Cialis®), and vardenafil (Levitra®) in improving erectile function?**

These drugs inhibit phosphodiesterase type 5 (PDE5), an enzyme found in the tissue of the corpus cavernosum. This reduces the degradation of cGMP and keeps smooth muscle relaxed, thereby allowing inflow of blood to the corpus cavernosum. There may be some difference in duration of action among these medications, with tadalafil reportedly having the longest effect.

○ **Why is concurrent usage of organic nitrates contraindicated in the use of PDE5 inhibitors?**

Although PDE5 inhibitors are specific for phosphodiesterase type 5 (PDE5), they may have a minor inductive effect on other PDEs, and this may potentiate the systemic hypotensive effects of nitrates.

○ **In the United States, what drugs are used in penile injections as a therapy for erectile dysfunction?**

Papaverine, phentolamine, alprostadil, and prostaglandin E.

○ **What are the possible hazardous sequelae of penile injections with vasoactive substances?**

Priapism and sclerosis of the small veins of the penis.

○ **What is the role of nitric oxide and cGMP in the male sexual response?**

Nitric oxide relaxes the peripheral vascular smooth muscle through induction of cGMP synthesis and allows blood inflow to the corpus cavernosum, thereby facilitating erection. A decreased cGMP level facilitates the flaccid state.

○ **How is cGMP level regulated locally in the erection process?**

The synthesis of cGMP is catalyzed by guanylate cyclase, while the degradation of cGMP is catalyzed by phosphodiesterase (PDE). Both guanylate cyclase inducers (e.g., nitric oxide) and PDE inhibitors (e.g., sildenafil) may raise cGMP levels, thus promoting erection.

○ **What is the mechanism of gonadotropic-releasing hormone (GnRH) treatment for sexual dysfunction?**

GnRH stimulates the release of luteinizing hormone (LH). LH can increase testosterone in both sexes. However, an excess of GnRH will suppress both estrogen and testosterone. Therefore, GnRH treatment has a narrow therapeutic window.

○ **What percent of men experience recurrent premature ejaculation?**

Thirty-three percent.

○ **What condition is often misdiagnosed as male orgasmic disorder?**

Retrograde ejaculation.

○ **What percent of women experience female orgasmic disorder?**

Twenty-four percent.

○ **Does dyspareunia have an organic basis?**

In women, organic causes of dyspareunia, such as vaginitis, endometriosis, Bartholin gland infection, and episiotomy scars, should be ruled out before being deemed as secondary to dynamic causes. Much less common in men, dyspareunia is usually organic.

○ **What is Peyronie's disease?**

A disease of unknown etiology, Peyronie's disease is a condition in which sclerotic plaques are formed surrounding the corpus cavernosum, causing dyspareunia.

○ **What is vaginismus?**

Vaginismus is the involuntary tightening or spasm of vaginal muscles to the extent that sexual intercourse is not possible or extremely painful.

○ **How do the following antidepressants influence erectile function: imipramine, desipramine, clomipramine, amitriptyline, and trazodone?**

All but trazodone may have inhibitory effects on erectile function, specifically during the excitement and orgasm phases. Trazodone is associated with priapism.

○ **With which phase of sleep is nocturnal penile tumescence associated?**

Rapid eye movement phase.

○ **What general medical conditions may cause female sexual dysfunction?**

Hypothyroidism, diabetes mellitus, and primary hyperprolactinemia are some medical conditions that may cause female sexual dysfunction.

○ **MAOIs may interfere with female orgasmic capacity. If sexual dysfunction occurs, should the MAOI dosage be reduced?**

Not necessarily. In one study, the side effect disappeared after 16 to 18 weeks, without decreasing the dosage of the MAOI.

○ **What are the two stages of substance-induced sexual dysfunction?**

   1. Prolonged erection without ejaculation

   2. Gradual loss of erectile capability.

○ **What antipsychotics can cause retrograde ejaculation?**

   Theoretically, potent anticholinergics, which include most antipsychotics, can cause retrograde ejaculation. Medications commonly reported to have this effect include chlorpromazine, thioridazine, and trifluoperazine.

○ **Most TCAs may interfere with erection and delay ejaculation. Which TCA has the fewest sexual side effects?**

   Desipramine, as it has the fewest anticholinergic effects of any TCAs.

○ **SSRIs and SNRIs are reported to cause difficulty in reaching orgasm. Is there any medicine that can reverse this negative effect?**

   Cyproheptadine (Periactin) and methylphenidate (Ritalin) have been used to reverse orgasmic inhibition.

○ **Are there any antidepressant drugs that may improve libido?**

   Yes. Clomipramine and bupropion have been reported to increase sex drive. The phosphodiesterase type 5 inhibitors, testosterone, and estrogen replacement may also be of benefit when treating hypoactive sexual desire disorder.

○ **Can psychostimulants improve sexual function?**

   Amphetamines and methylphenidate may raise norepinephrine and dopamine level, and increase libido (phase 1). However, prolonged use may cause loss of desire and erectile function.

○ **Diphenhydramine (Benadryl) and cyproheptadine (Periactin) are both antihistamines. Why is only cyproheptadine used to treat sexual side effects produced by SSRIs?**

   While both agents are antihistamines, they do have different effects on other neurotransmitter systems. Diphenhydramine is hypnotic and also anticholinergic—effects that inhibit sexual function—while cyproheptadine has potent antiserotonergic effects, and therefore is used to reverse the serotonergic sexual side effects caused by SSRIs.

○ **SSRIs may inhibit arousal and can cause difficulty in reaching orgasm. Can these side effects be used therapeutically?**

   Yes. SSRIs administered 6 to 12 hours before intercourse can reduce the frequency of premature ejaculation. TCAs, PDE5 inhibitors, and topical anesthetics can also be of benefit. Nonpharmacologic interventions include use of condoms and masturbation 1 to 2 hours before sexual intercourse.

○ **Benzodiazepines are hypnotic. Can this effect decrease sexual function?**

   Theoretically, yes. But clinically, more people have found that benzodiazepines improve sexual function that may otherwise be inhibited by anxiety.

○ **Does administration of androgens enhance sexual function in men?**

   This treatment has been successful only in men with decreased testosterone levels.

○   **Does oxytocin play a role in male sexual response?**

Yes, it is believed so. The plasma level of oxytocin has been found to rise before ejaculation.

○   **What is the National DES Education Program?**

Diethylstilbestrol (DES), an androgenic steroid, was used in the 1950s and 1960s to prevent abortion. However, it may cause reproductive tract disorders in children born to DES-treated mothers. Grown "DES daughters and sons" organized the program, which is also sponsored by NCI, to provide information on potential medical problems caused by DES use.

○   **Anatomically, which part of the brain is believed to be directly involved in sexual function?**

The limbic system, which includes the hippocampus, mamillary bodies, anterior thalamic nuclei, and amygdala.

○   **What are the effects of dopamine and serotonin on sexual function?**

It is believed that dopamine increases libido, while serotonin inhibits sexual function.

○   **What is orgasmic anhedonia?**

Normal physiological response to sexual stimulation without erotic sensation.

○   **How do the α-adrenergic receptors influence sexual function? How do α-blockers modify these effects?**

Activated α-receptors inhibit erection but promote ejaculation. Some α-blockers may cause priapism (e.g., trazodone), while others lead to impaired ejaculation (e.g., TCAs, MAOIs, and thioridazine).

○   **How do the β-adrenergic receptors influence sexual function? How do β-blockers modify these effects?**

As activation of β-receptors promotes erection, use of β-blockers may lead to impotence.

○   **What are the normal ranges of penis size?**

According to Masters and Johnson, 7 to 11 cm in the flaccid state and 14 to 18 cm in the erect state.

○   **How many sperm cells are contained in one ejaculation?**

Approximately 120 million.

○   **What is the G-spot?**

First described by Ernst Graefenberg, it is an area in the anterior wall of the vagina. It was reported that stimulation of the area can induce orgasm, though experimentation failed to verify this claim.

○   **Is masturbation considered psychopathologic?**

Masturbation is a psychopathologic symptom only when it becomes a compulsion.

○   **What is the effect of alcohol on sexual function?**

Small amounts of alcohol may slightly increase the testosterone level in women, thereby increasing libido. In men, alcohol decreases libido in two ways: it reduces testosterone levels, and it reduces the hepatic metabolism of estrogenic compounds. The latter effect causes feminization in long-term users.

○ **What are the effects of opioids, hallucinogens, cannabis, and barbiturates on sexual function?**

In general, all these addictive substances may occasionally enhance the sexual experience mainly due to alteration of consciousness or reduction of anxiety. But in the long term, they all negatively affect sexual function.

○ **What are some specific therapeutic techniques for the disorders of vaginismus, premature ejaculation, sexual desire disorder, and male orgasmic disorder, respectively?**

Dysfunction	Therapeutic Techniques
Vaginismus	Vaginal dilation
Premature ejaculation	Squeeze technique
Sexual desire disorder	Masturbation
Male orgasmic disorder	Extravaginal ejaculation followed by gradual vaginal entry

○ **What is the difference between sexual identity and gender identity?**

Sexual identity describes the biologic characteristics (genotype, secondary sexual characteristics) that define one's sex. Gender identity is a psychological state that reflects the self-awareness of being male or female.

○ **What is the difference between gender identity and gender role?**

Gender identity is a psychological state that reflects the self-awareness of being male or female. Gender role is a social behavior pattern by which one identifies oneself to others as being male or female.

○ **Define sexual orientation.**

Sexual orientation refers to one's gender preference for a sexual partner, or in other words, the sex that one experiences heightened sexual desire for. Generally, sexual orientation is classified as homosexual, bisexual, or heterosexual. The age of the desired partner is also a consideration, as in the pedophilias.

○ **When and how is gender identity established?**

Gender identity is established by the age of 3 years. It generally depends on the sex that an individual is reared to be, regardless of biologic factors. In gender identity disorder, the child or adolescent identifies his/her self as one sex, but have an intense desire to be the other sex, and are uncomfortable in their assigned gender role.

○ **What is the difference between a homosexual and a transsexual?**

Homosexuals are comfortable with their own biologically assigned sex and have a sexual orientation toward the same sex. Transsexuals are uncomfortable with their biologically assigned sex and may have sexual attraction to males, females, or both sexes.

○ **What is the sexual orientation of transsexuals?**

Female transsexuals usually have a sexual orientation toward women. Male transsexuals are predominately orientated toward men, but 25% are sexually attracted to women, and may become "lesbian" after reassignment.

○ **What are intersex conditions?**

Intersex conditions include a variety of syndromes in which people have anatomic or physiological aspects of both sexes.

○ **Why does the presence of testes not guarantee the development of male genital structures?**

The development of genital structures depends on presence or absence of androgen, from whatever source. If fetal androgen is missing (enzyme deficiency) or androgen receptors are defective (testicular feminization), female genitalia will develop.

○ **Can fetal hormones influence the development of gender identity?**

Fetal hormones have been demonstrated to play a part in gender role and sexual orientation, but no influence on gender identity has been discovered.

○ **How are paraphilias classified in the *DSM-IV*?**

Essentially according to the object, behavior, or person that induces sexual excitement.

○ **List the paraphilias.**

There are eight:

1. Exhihibitionism
2. Fetishism
3. Pedophilia
4. Sexual masochism
5. Sexual sadism
6. Transvestic fetishism
7. Voyeurism
8. Paraphilias not otherwise specified.

○ **Among legally identified cases, what is the most common form of paraphilia?**

Pedophilia.

○ **Paraphilias occur mostly in what age and sex group?**

Paraphilias are most commonly diagnosed in men, between the ages of 15 and 25 years. The *DSM-IV* reports that approximately 50% of individuals diagnosed with paraphilias are married.

○ **What characteristics are positive prognostic factors for paraphilias?**

The victim must be 13 years or younger. The perpetrator must be 16 years or older. The difference in ages between the victim and the perpetrator must be at least 5 years. The diagnosis for individuals in late adolescence requires clinical judgment that takes into account the age difference, cultural setting, and the sexual maturity of the alleged perpetrator and victim. Nonconsensual/coerced participation of a child victim warrants a diagnosis of pedophilia, regardless of age.

○   **What are the two types of pedophilia?**

Exclusive (sexual attraction to only children) or nonexclusive (sexually attracted to both children and adults).

○   **What are the gender and age characteristics of children victimized by pedophiles?**

Female victims are the most frequently reported cases, and are usually around the age of 8 to 10 years. Male victims tend to be slightly older. Pedophiles who are attracted to males tend to have a recurrence rate that is twice as high as those who prefer females.

○   **What is the difference between sexual masochism and sexual sadism?**

Sexual masochism is characterized by feelings of sexual arousal during thoughts or acts that are psychologically or physically abusive to self, while sexual sadism is characterized by sexual arousal during thoughts or behaviors psychologically or physically abusive to a sexual partner, who may or may not be consenting.

○   **What particular type of sexual masochism has a high potential for lethality?**

Autoerotic hypoxia or hypoxyphilia (gaspers).

○   **A man demands that his partner wear high-heeled shoes during sexual intercourse. Can this be diagnosed as fetishism?**

Not necessarily. To be diagnosed as any paraphilia, the sexual urges and fantasies involving unusual objects or activities must be recurrent, intensive, and cause clinically significant distress or impairment in social, occupational, or other important areas of functioning.

○   **Cross-dressing is typical for both transvestic fetishism and male gender identity disorder. What is the difference between these two disorders?**

In transvestic fetishism, cross-dressing causes sexual excitement, while in gender identity disorder it does not.

○   **Describe the difference between exhibitionism, frotteurism, and voyeurism.**

Exhibitionists experience sexual arousal when exposing their "privates" to strangers, while the frotteurist experiences sexual arousal when touching a nonconsenting victim, generally in a public place whereby they can readily escape and not be identified. In voyeurism, the unsuspecting victim is not touched, but is observed while undressing or having sex, which causes increased sexual arousal in the observer.

○   **What are necrophilia, coprophilia, and klismaphilia?**

Necrophilia is a sexual desire toward cadavers and an obsession with obtaining sexual gratification from cadavers. Coprophilia is the derivation of sexual pleasure by defecating on a partner, or being defecated on, or eating feces. Klismaphilia is the use of enemas as part of sexual stimulation. They are classified as Paraphilias Not Otherwise Classified, as are telephone scatologia (obscene phone calls), zoophilia, and urophilias to name a few.

○   **What characteristics are positive prognostic factors for paraphilias?**

Having a history of normal coitus and high motivation for change.

○ **What are the mainstream treatments for paraphilias?**

Insight-oriented psychotherapy, behavior therapy with self-administered noxious stimuli, antipsychotic or antidepressant medication if comorbid with schizophrenia or depressive disorders, and antiandrogens for hypersexual paraphilias.

○ **What are SA, SLAA, and SAA?**

The above mnemonics stand for **S**ex**a**holics **A**nonymous, **S**ex and **L**ove **A**ddicts **A**nonymous, and **S**ex **A**ddicts **A**nonymous, respectively. These are self-help groups that adopted the philosophies and methods of AA to help people with sex addictions.

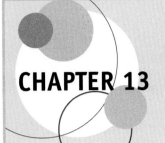

CHAPTER 13 Eating Disorders

○ **What are the essential criteria for a diagnosis of anorexia nervosa?**

Weight less than 85% of ideal body weight (or failure to grow at expected rates); intense fear of being fat; disturbance in body image; and amenorrhea for at least three cycles.

○ **What are the two subtypes of anorexia nervosa?**

Restricting type and binge eating/purging type.

○ **What are the essential criteria for a diagnosis of bulimia nervosa?**

Recurrent episodes of binge eating, recurrent inappropriate compensatory behavior, self-evaluation unduly influenced by body shape and weight, and frequency of binge/purge episodes of at least twice a week for 3 months.

○ **What are the two subtypes of bulimia nervosa?**

Purging type and nonpurging type.

○ **List examples of compensatory behaviors individuals utilize to prevent weight gain.**

- Self-induce emesis
- Excessive use of laxatives or other purgatives
- Use of diuretics or other medications
- Fasting
- Excessive exercise

○ **What is the mortality rate for anorexia nervosa?**

Ten to twenty percent over 10 to 30 years.

○ **What are the most common causes of death secondary to anorexia nervosa?**

Severe and chronic starvation, sudden death due to cardiac failure, and suicide.

○ **What professions and/or activities are associated with a higher risk of eating disorders?**

Dancers (especially ballet), fashion models, gymnastics, long-distance runners, cheerleaders, male jockeys, and wrestlers.

○ **What treatment modalities have been shown to be effective for anorexia nervosa?**

Nutritional rehabilitation. For patients with comorbid conditions, medications specific for that disorder can be considered. Supportive therapy is generally superior to cognitive behavioral therapy or interpersonal therapy. Fluoxetine and/or cognitive behavioral therapy after weight restoration may prevent relapse.

○ **What is the role of group therapy in the treatment of eating disorders?**

Group therapies are generally useful, especially for bulimia nervosa. The group may take various forms including psychodynamic, behavioral, feminist, or self-help orientations.

○ **What is the role of expressive therapies in the treatment of eating disorders?**

During psychotherapy for eating disorders, a patient learns to identify different feeling states and to respond appropriately.

○ **What is the efficacy of cognitive-behavioral therapy (CBT) in the treatment of bulimia nervosa?**

Numerous controlled studies have demonstrated the efficacy of CBT in bulimia nervosa for symptom reduction and relapse prevention. CBT has been found to be more effective when compared with treatment with antidepressants alone, self-monitoring plus supportive psychotherapy, and behavioral treatment without the cognitive treatment component.

○ **What are the primary foci for cognitive-behavioral therapy when used in the treatment of bulimia nervosa?**

CBT, when used to treat bulimia nervosa concentrates on distorted ideas about weight and shape, rigid rules regarding food consumption and pressure to diet, and recognition of the events that trigger episodes of binge eating.

○ **What types of medications have been shown to be effective for bulimia nervosa?**

Selective serotonin reuptake inhibitors (particularly fluoxetine), tricyclic antidepressants, and monoamine oxidase inhibitors.

○ **What other psychiatric disorders have a high rate of comorbidity with anorexia nervosa?**

Major depression and obsessive-compulsive disorder.

○ **What psychiatric disorders are present at increased frequencies in the family members of patients with anorexia nervosa?**

Family studies of anorexia nervosa have shown an increased frequency of mood disorders in the first-degree relatives of the anorexic probands compared with the first-degree relatives of normal control subjects. Mothers of anorexic patients also have been found to have a significantly greater prevalence of obsessive-compulsive disorder than mothers of controls.

○ **What psychiatric disorders have a high rate of comorbidity with bulimia nervosa?**

Major depression, substance abuse, and anxiety disorders.

○ **What are the criteria for hospitalization in a patient with an eating disorder?**

Medical hospitalization is indicated when vitals signs and metabolic status are unstable. Admission to an inpatient psychiatric unit is warranted when the patient is suicidal, excessively depressed, manic, or psychotic. Admission to an inpatient eating disorder unit is considered when body weight <85%, or when acute loss of weight with food refusal occurs at a lower level of care. Other factors that indicate the need for referral to an eating disorder inpatient unit include inability to gain weight during outpatient treatment, inability to control purging behaviors, need for supervision at all meals, and poor motivation.

○ **How rapidly should weight gain occur for anorexic patients during a refeeding treatment?**

A clinician should aim for an average weight gain of 1 to 2 pounds per week.

○ **How is body mass index (BMI) calculated?**

$$BMI = \frac{weight \ (kg)}{Height^2 \ (m)}.$$

○ **Is the BMI useful in estimating nutritional status?**

Generally not, except at either end of the spectrum. A BMI of <18.5 kg/m^2 is considered underweight while a BMI of >27 kg/m^2 is considered obese.

○ **How is ideal body weight calculated?**

In many different ways. The Devine formula, published in 1974 and based on estimates, was originally designed to calculate dosages for various medications, but has become widely used as a measure of IBW.

The Devine formulas:

$$IBW \ (for \ men) = 50 \ kg + 2.3 \ kg \times [height \ (in) - 60]$$

$$IBW \ (for \ women) = 45.5 \ kg + 2.3 \ kg \times [height \ (in) - 60]$$

Please note that the Devine formula is applicable to people taller than 5 ft (60 in).

○ **What medical complications may occur if an anorexic patient is refed too rapidly?**

Acute gastric dilation, fluid retention, congestive heart failure, cardiac arrhythmias, rhabdomyolysis, and death.

○ **What metabolic abnormalities are associated with the refeeding syndrome?**

Hypophosphatemia, hypocalcemia, hypomagnesemia, and thiamine deficiency.

○ **What is the age of onset for bulimia nervosa?**

Bulimia nervosa usually begins between the ages of 12 and 35 years, with the average age of onset being 18 years.

○ **What is the mean age of onset for anorexia nervosa?**

Age 17 years, with some data suggesting bimodal peaks at ages 14 and 18 years. The onset of this disorder rarely occurs after the age of 40 years.

○ **What cardiac changes occur with anorexia nervosa?**

Cardiac changes include loss of cardiac muscle, and cardiac arrhythmias, including atrial and ventricular premature contractions, prolonged QT interval, and ventricular tachycardia.

○ **What skeletal changes occur as complications of anorexia nervosa?**

Osteoporosis, which may be irreversible, is a serious complication of anorexia nervosa.

○ **What is "Russell's sign"?**

Russell's sign is the presence of callouses on the knuckles secondary to repeated self-induction of emesis.

○ **What percentage of patients with eating disorders are female?**

Ninety to ninety-five percent.

○ **What changes occur in the teeth with bulimia nervosa?**

Dental erosion, especially of the front teeth, with corresponding decay.

○ **What changes occur in amylase levels with bulimia nervosa?**

Mild elevation in salivary subtype of amylase.

○ **What are the most common electrolyte disturbances with bulimia nervosa?**

Hypokalemia, hyponatremia, and hypochloremic alkalosis occur in bulimia nervosa secondary to excessive emesis and consequent loss of hydrogen and chloride ions.

○ **How often should binge eating and inappropriate compensatory behaviors occur to meet criteria for a diagnosis of bulimia nervosa in the *DSM-IV*?**

At least twice a week for 3 months.

○ **What is the most common skin change that is associated with anorexia nervosa?**

Presence of lanugo hair.

○ **What is the functional status of each of the following neurotransmitters and peptides in anorexia nervosa: norepinephrine, serotonin, corticotropin-releasing factor (CRF), neuropeptide Y, and cholecystokinin (CCK)?**

Norepinephrine is decreased, serotonin is increased, CRF is increased, neuropeptide Y is increased, and CCK is also increased.

○ **What is the recommended effective dose for fluoxetine in the treatment of bulimia nervosa?**

Fluoxetine at a dose of 60 mg/d is favored by many investigators.

○ **What is a good way to follow reduction of vomiting in eating disorder patients who deny purging episodes?**

Getting a serum amylase level; this level is commonly elevated in patients who binge and vomit.

○ **How do you differentiate bulimia nervosa from the binge/purge subtype of anorexia nervosa?**

These conditions are differentiated by the characteristic low body weight and amenorrhea in anorexia nervosa.

○ **Which personality disorder may be associated with bulimia nervosa?**

Borderline personality disorder.

○ **What is the concordance rate for anorexia nervosa in monozygotic twins versus dizygotic twins?**

Fifty percent for monozygotic versus 10% for dizygotic twins.

○ **What is the approximate lifetime prevalence of obsessive-compulsive disorder in anorexia nervosa?**

Twenty-five percent.

○ **What is the response-prevention technique for bulimia nervosa?**

Binging and purging patients are required to stay in an observed dayroom area for 2 to 3 hours after every meal to prevent purging. Bathroom doors may also be locked to prevent access for purging.

○ **What abnormalities in hematopoiesis are seen in acutely emaciated anorexic patients?**

Leukopenia, relative lymphocytosis; normochromic, normocytic anemia of mild-to-moderate severity.

○ **What changes in blood chemistry are seen in anorexia nervosa?**

Elevated serum liver enzymes; elevated serum cholesterol; carotenemia; elevated blood urea nitrogen (BUN), creatinine, hemoglobin, and hematocrit secondary to dehydration.

○ **What changes in the thyroid system occur in anorexia nervosa?**

Diminished plasma thyroxine without elevation of thyroid-stimulating hormone (TSH).

○ **What changes in the gastrointestinal system are seen in anorexia nervosa?**

Diminished motility, delayed gastric emptying, bloating, constipation, acute gastric dilation or gastric rupture, and abdominal pain.

○ **What role may fluoxetine play in the treatment of anorexia nervosa?**

Fluoxetine may reduce the risk of relapse among patients with anorexia nervosa who have gained weight. It may also be used to treat comorbid depression.

○ **What changes have occurred in the epidemiology of anorexia nervosa in the last 50 years?**

The incidence has increased 10-fold, and it appears to be becoming more widespread in terms of sociocultural groups who are affected.

○ **What compensatory behaviors are used by bulimic patients after binging?**

Self-induced vomiting, abuse of laxatives, diuretics, diet pills, enemas, excessive exercise, and fasting.

○ **What compensatory mechanism is most frequently used by bulimic patients after a binge?**

Self-induced vomiting is employed by 80% to 90% of patients with bulimia nervosa.

○ **What abnormalities in thinking are observed in patients with eating disorders?**

Dichotomous (all-or-none) thinking, decreased concentration, disturbed body image, disturbed perception (e.g., lack of recognition or denial of fatigue, weakness, or hunger), and a sense of ineffectiveness.

○ **What percentage of patients with anorexia nervosa develop bulimic symptoms?**

Up to 50%.

○ **What is the lifetime prevalence of anorexia nervosa?**

Approximately 0.5% to 3.7%.

○ **What is the lifetime prevalence of bulimia nervosa?**

Lifetime prevalence of bulimia nervosa is 1.1% to 4.2% of young women in United States.

○ **In family studies, how are mothers of individuals with anorexia nervosa often described?**

Overprotective, intrusive, perfectionistic, and fearful of separation.

○ **How are fathers of anorexic patients often described?**

Withdrawn, passive, emotionally constricted, obsessional, moody, and ineffectual.

○ **What is the most common finding during CT of the head in individuals with anorexia nervosa?**

Enlarged ventricles that improve with weight gain.

○ **What has been found to be elevated in the CSF of patients with anorexia nervosa?**

The serotonin metabolite, 5-hydroxyindole acetic acid (5-HIAA).

○ **How have antidepressants been found to be helpful for bulimia nervosa?**

All trials have demonstrated a significantly greater reduction in binge eating under antidepressant medication compared with placebo.

○ **What is the probable mechanism behind stress-induced eating?**

Stress-induced eating is probably driven by activation of the opioid system.

○ **In studies done on anorexia nervosa cases, what factors point to poor outcome and prognosis?**

Generally speaking, poor outcome has been associated with longer duration of illness, older age of onset, previous admission to a psychiatric hospital, poor childhood social adjustment, premorbid personality difficulties, and disturbed relationships between patients and family members.

○ **Who was the first to describe the syndrome of anorexia nervosa as a medical condition?**

Sir William Gull in England and Charles Laségne in France described this condition almost simultaneously in the late 19th century.

○ **What are the cognitive and perceptual developmental defects postulated by Hilde Bruch (1973) as the core features of anorexia nervosa?**

Disturbance of body image, disturbance of perception, and a sense of ineffectiveness.

○ **Who first described bulimia nervosa and when?**

Gerald Russell in 1979.

○ **How does cyproheptadine work in anorexia nervosa?**

The weight gain induced by cyproheptadine is thought to be related to its potency as a serotonin antagonist, because animal studies suggest that decreases in hypothalamic serotonin are usually associated with increases in food consumption.

○ **What is the first step in the treatment of an anorexic patient?**

The first step in treatment is to obtain the anorexic patient's cooperation in the treatment program.

○ **What are some risk factors for the development of reduced bone density in anorexia nervosa?**

A decreased level of estrogen, high levels of cortisol, and poor nutrition (e.g., decreased calcium intake).

○ **What event usually precedes the onset of both anorexia nervosa and bulimia nervosa?**

Both illnesses typically follow a period of dieting.

○ **What test can be done to assess the risk for pathologic fractures secondary to osteoporosis in anorexia nervosa?**

Bone mineral densitometry.

○ **What is the role of enteral tube feedings and parenteral alimentation in the treatment of anorexia nervosa?**

These interventions are used only rarely, when indicated by the patient's medical condition, for as brief a period of time as is necessary, while normal eating is developed.

○ **What medical complications may develop if ipecac is ingested?**

Cardiomyopathy and toxic myopathy. Cardiac failure caused by cardiomyopathy from ipecac intoxication may occur and usually results in death.

○ **What are the signs and symptoms of ipecac intoxication?**

Symptoms of precordial pain, dyspnea, generalized muscle weakness associated with hypotension, tachycardia, abnormalities in the electrocardiogram, elevated liver enzymes, and elevated erythrocyte sedimentation rate.

○ **What endogenous stimulant of eating behavior has been found to be significantly elevated in the cerebrospinal fluid of emaciated anorexic patients?**

Neuropeptide Y.

○ **How do anorexic patients who binge and purge differ from anorexic patients who merely restrict food intake?**

Anorexic patients with bulimic behaviors show a relatively frequent association with impulsive behavior such as suicide attempts, self-mutilation, stealing, and substance abuse. They are less likely to be regressed in their sexual activity and may be promiscuous, and are more likely to have discrete personality disorder diagnoses.

○ **What emotional symptoms may occur due to starvation?**

Irritability, depression, preoccupation with food, and sleep disturbance.

○ **What effect does immigration play in the development of eating disorders?**

Immigrants from cultures in which eating disorders are rare and who emigrate to cultures in which the disorders are more prevalent may develop eating disorders as thin-body (Western) ideals are assimilated.

○ **What is the relationship between amenorrhea and weight loss in individuals with anorexia nervosa?**

Amenorrhea is usually a consequence of weight loss in anorexia nervosa, but in a minority of individuals, the amenorrhea may precede the weight loss. Menarche may be delayed in prepubertal females with anorexia nervosa.

○ **What is the typical weight of individuals with bulimia nervosa?**

Individuals with bulimia nervosa are usually within the normal weight range, although some may be slightly overweight or underweight. The disorder may occur, but is uncommon, among moderately and morbidly obese individuals.

○ **What are the diagnostic criteria for binge-eating disorder and how is it classified?**

Binge-eating disorder is currently listed as an example of Eating Disorder Not Otherwise Specified in the *DSM-IV.* Criteria for this diagnosis include recurrent episodes of binge eating in the absence of regular use of inappropriate compensatory behaviors characteristic of bulimia nervosa, with binge eating occurring, on the average, at least 2 days a week for 6 months.

○ **What are the characteristics of a binge?**

A binge is characterized by eating more within a discrete period of time than most people would eat in a similar time period; feeling a sense of lack of control over eating during the episode; eating much more rapidly than normal; eating until feeling uncomfortably full; eating large amounts of food when not feeling physically hungry; eating alone because of being embarrassed by how much one is eating; and feeling disgusted with oneself, depressed, or very guilty after overeating.

○ **What is the difference between bulimia nervosa and binge-eating disorder in the requirements for diagnosis in terms of binge-eating behavior?**

Binge eating for bulimia nervosa should occur at least twice a week for 3 months versus 2 days a week for 6 months in binge-eating disorder. Also, in binge-eating disorder, there are no associated inappropriate compensatory behaviors after a binging episode.

○ **What is the usual age of onset of binge eating?**

The onset of binge eating is typically in late adolescence or in the early 20s, often coming soon after significant weight loss from dieting, but binge eating can occur before a period of dieting in some individuals. Hence, there appear to be at least two distinct patterns of onset in binge-eating disorder.

○ **True/False: Binge-eating disorder is a risk factor for bulimia nervosa.**

False. Only a minority of individuals with the diagnosis of binge-eating disorder develop bulimia nervosa at a later time (<10% according to Striegel-Moore et al., 2001). An early age of onset, however, increases the risk of developing bulimia nervosa.

○ **What risk factors exist for binge-eating disorder?**

Negative self-concept, a family history of depression and/or obesity, childhood obesity, and challenging environmental factors increase the risk for binge-eating disorder. The earlier age of onset subgroup frequently has a greater number of risk factors.

○ **What is the prevalence of binge-eating disorder?**

In community samples, a prevalence rate of 0.7% to 4% has been reported.

○ **What percentage of individuals in weight-control programs have binge-eating disorder?**

Approximately 15% to 50%, with a mean of 30%.

○ **What is the gender ratio of binge-eating disorder?**

Females are approximately 1.5 times more likely to have this eating pattern than males.

○ **How do you define obesity?**

Obesity can be defined as a body mass index (BMI) more than 30, or body weight greater than 20% more than the upper limit for height.

○ **Is obesity an eating disorder?**

Generally not, as obesity is more likely a result of genetic and activity factors. Dietary intake does however play a role, and changes thereof can be of benefit.

○ **Obesity has a definite familial component. What percentage of offspring of two obese parents will have a tendency to be obese?**

Eighty percent.

○ **What percentage of offspring of one obese parent will have a tendency to be obese?**

Forty percent.

○ **What types of cancer are found at a higher rate in obese males?**

Prostate and colorectal cancer.

○   **What types of cancer are found at higher rates in obese females?**

Gallbladder, breast, cervical, endometrial, uterine, and ovarian cancer.

○   **To date, what is the most efficient treatment of mild obesity?**

Behavior modification in groups, a balanced diet, and exercise.

○   **What is the most effective treatment for severe obesity?**

Severe obesity is most effectively treated by surgical procedures that reduce the size of the stomach.

CHAPTER 14   Sleep Disorders

○ **How are normal sleep and wakefulness regulated?**

Normal sleep and wakefulness are regulated by three mechanisms, the ultradian rhythm of rapid eye movement (REM) and non-REM sleep, the circadian rhythm of sleep and wakefulness, and the homeostatic regulation of sleep–wake cycles.

○ **What is the ultradian rhythm of REM and non-REM sleep?**

The ultradian rhythm of REM and non-REM sleep is the alternation of these two major phases of sleep in cycles more frequent than every 24 hours. Sleep begins normally with a non-REM period that is between 70 and 90 minutes in duration and is followed by the first REM period, which lasts for approximately 10 minutes. Thereafter, the sleep architecture alternates between these two phases with a total of 80 to 110 minutes in one complete cycle. REM periods, which occur four to five times a night, become progressively longer in duration, with the final REM period occurring just prior to awakening.

○ **What are the stages of non-REM sleep?**

Non-REM sleep is divided into four stages. Stage 1 is a brief transition stage between wakefulness and sleep, characterized on EEG by the disappearance of α waves, and the predominance of theta waves. Stage 2 is marked by theta waves, K-complexes, and sleep spindles on EEG, while muscle tone and eye movements diminish. Stages 3 and 4 are marked by high amplitude, slow delta waves on EEG (stage 3 has less than 50% of delta waves and Stage 4 has more than 50% delta waves), with atonic muscle tone and no eye movements. Stages 3 and 4 are the most refreshing stage of sleep.

○ **What is REM sleep?**

REM sleep is rapid eye movement sleep. The amount of ocular activity per minute is called REM density. Most skeletal muscles are atonic and the autonomic nervous system is hyperactive during REM sleep. Dreams are common, and are more abstract than the dreams formed during non-REM sleep.

○ **What is REM latency?**

The amount of time from the onset of sleep to onset of the first REM period is called REM latency. This period is normally 60 to 90 minutes. REM latency is decreased in depression, narcolepsy, and with the use of certain medications.

○ **What is the circadian rhythm of sleep and wakefulness?**

The activity–rest or sleep–wake cycle is an example of a circadian rhythm, a biologic cycle occurring within a 24-hour period of time. Examples of other circadian rhythms include the daily variations of growth hormone and thyroid hormone secretion, and the daily variations in core body temperatures.

○ **What is the role of the suprachiasmatic nucleus (SCN) in the regulation of sleep?**

The SCN plays an important role in the regulation of most circadian rhythms in humans and animals. The endogenous activity rhythm of the SCN is synchronized with the environment primarily by ambient light. The light energy reaches the SCN by traveling through the retina, retinohypothalamic tract, and geniculate body.

○ **What is the role of light in regulating sleep?**

Exposure to light and darkness can change the phase position of the underlying biological oscillator. Bright light at the beginning of the day advances the phase position of the underlying biological oscillator, while bright light in the evening delays it.

○ **What are the normal age-related changes in sleep and wakefulness?**

The newborn spends nearly 50% of total sleep time (up to 20 h/d) in REM sleep, with short bouts of sleep and wakefulness throughout a 24-hour period. At around 3 months of age, the infant begins to sleep through the night, and from thereon, total sleep time and total REM sleep progressively diminish. In middle and older age, sleep becomes shallow, fragmented, and phase advanced. REM latency and stages 3 and 4 decline, and daytime napping becomes common.

○ **What is the neurophysiology of sleep?**

The non-REM/REM sleep cycle is regulated within the brain stem. Isolated brain stem preparations have been shown to generate REM sleep, while isolated forebrains (thalamus, hypothalamus, dorsal raphe nucleus, and solitary nucleus) generate non-REM sleep and wakefulness.

○ **What is the neurochemistry of sleep?**

Although no specific "sleep neurotransmitters" have been identified yet, acetylcholine induces REM sleep and cortical activation, while serotonin and norepinephrine inhibit REM sleep. This may explain the short REM latency observed in depression and related disorders.

○ **How are sleep disorders broadly classified according to the *DSM-IV*?**

Sleep disorders are broadly divided into primary sleep disorders (dyssomnias and parasomnias), sleep disorders related to another mental disorder, and other sleep disorders.

○ **How are dyssomnias (disorders of initiating and maintaining sleep) subtyped according to the *DSM-IV*?**

The dyssomnias are subtyped as primary insomnia, primary hypersomnia, narcolepsy, breathing-related sleep disorder, circadian rhythm sleep disorder, and dyssomnia not otherwise specified.

○ **How are the parasomnias (disorders of sleep-related abnormal behaviors) subtyped according to the *DSM-IV*?**

Parasomnias are subtyped as nightmare disorder, sleep terror disorder, sleep walking disorder, and parasomnia not otherwise specified.

○ **List examples of sleep disorders associated with medical or psychiatric disorders.**

Sleep disorders associated with psychiatric disorders include:

- psychotic disorders
- mood disorders
- anxiety disorders
- panic disorder
- alcohol/substance abuse disorders

Sleep disorders associated with neurologic conditions include:

- dementia
- Parkinsonism
- sleep-related epilepsy
- headaches

Sleep disorders associated with other medical disorders include:

- sleeping sickness
- COPD
- asthma
- gastrointestinal reflex
- peptic ulcer disease
- fibrositis

○ **What is primary insomnia?**

In primary insomnia, the predominant complaint is difficulty initiating or maintaining sleep, or nonrestorative sleep, for at least 1 month. The impairment causes significant distress or impairment in functioning. The impairment is not due to other sleep, medical, psychiatric, or substance-related problems. The etiology is unclear. It appears to be a conditioned response. Approximately 1 in 3 people report insomnia, while 1 in 6 describe it as serious, and approximately 1 in 12 call it chronic. The rates are higher in women, elderly, and in lower socioeconomic classes. Diagnosis is difficult, usually arrived at by exclusion. Simple solutions are rare. Clinical management is multidimensional involving psychosocial, behavioral, and pharmacologic interventions.

○ **What is primary hypersomnia?**

In primary hypersomnia, the predominant complaint is that of excessive sleepiness for at least one month. The impairment causes significant distress or decline in functioning and is not due to other sleep, medical, psychiatric, or substance-related problems. The patient usually complains of long, nonrefreshing sleep, daytime sleepiness, and difficulty awakening. No other symptoms of narcolepsy are experienced. Approximately 5% to 10 % of patients with sleep disorders complain of primary hyperinsomnia. The diagnosis should be made by polysomnographic confirmation of hypersomnia and not by subjective reports. Primary hyperinsomnia must be differentiated from Kleine-Levin syndrome. Treatment includes use of stimulants, e.g., methylphenidate, or stimulating antidepressants, e.g., SSRIs or MAOIs.

○ **What is Kleine-Levin syndrome?**

Kleine-Levin syndrome is a rare condition usually seen in adolescent boys. Periods of hypersomnia (18–20 h/d) occur, as well as episodes of aggressive or inappropriate sexual behavior and compulsive overeating. Treatment is with stimulants, e.g., methylphenidate, or stimulating antidepressants, e.g., SSRIs or MAOIs.

○ **What is narcolepsy?**

Narcolepsy is a sleep disorder manifested by sudden, repeated intrusion of REM sleep into periods of wakefulness. The classic narcoleptic tetrad consists of sleep attacks, cataplexy (brief episodes of generalized muscle weakness, often precipitated by intense emotions), sleep paralysis, and sleep hallucinations (hypnagogic or hypnopompic). The disorder is usually lifelong, first developing in twenties, with the full syndrome unfolding over several years. Patients usually have "sleep-onset REM periods," rather than the usual non-REM sleep phases. REM onset at sleep, documented by multiple sleep latency tests, is consequently, the most valid diagnostic test, although not essential to make a diagnosis of narcolepsy, especially when cataplexy is present.

○ **How is narcolepsy treated?**

Treatment includes use of stimulants or modafinil for sleep attacks. Tricyclic antidepressants (TCAs) and norepinephrine-containing SSRIs can prevent or lessen cataplexy. Sodium oxybate or γ-hydroxybutyrate (GHB) is remarkably effective in controlling both the excessive daytime sleepiness and cataplexy of narcolepsy. The potential for abuse of either stimulants or sodium oxybate (GHB) warrants careful monitoring of use.

○ **What are breathing-related sleep disorders (BRSDs)?**

BRSDs are sleep disorders caused by either sleep apnea or alveolar hypoventilation, which results in disruption of sleep and daytime sleepiness.

○ **What is central sleep apnea?**

Central sleep apnea results from the failure of the CNS respiratory neurons to activate the phrenic and intercostal motor neurons that mediate respiratory movement. There is no attempt to breathe. A diagnosis of central sleep apnea is made by documenting cessation of breathing for 10 to 120 seconds, with five or more episodes of apnea per hour.

○ **What is obstructive sleep apnea (OSA)?**

OSA results from the collapse of pharyngeal airways during inspiration resulting in interrupted sleep, hypoxemia, hypercapnia, and hypertension. It is associated with snoring, cognitive decline, and daytime sedation. Patients are usually overweight. Lifetime prevalence is between 4% and 9%, and it is more prevalent in males.

○ **How are oral appliances, sleep position restriction, and continuous positive airway pressure (CPAP) used in the treatment of breathing-related sleep disorders?**

A variety of oral appliances that manipulate the position of the mandible or tongue can reduce snoring or sleep apneas, while tennis balls placed into pockets or on back of night gowns can keep people from sleeping supine, thereby also reducing snoring or sleep apnea. Nasal CPAP is the most effective treatment for obstructive sleep apnea. The results can be dramatic and its use has made surgery a second line of treatment for breathing-related sleep disorders.

○ **What surgical procedures are used in the treatment of breathing-related sleep disorders?**

Tracheostomy was used in the 1970s to treat obstructive sleep apnea, but simpler procedures such as uvulopalatopharyngoplasty and maxillomandibular corrections have been developed since to increase posterior airway space.

○ **What is circadian rhythm sleep disorder?**

Circadian rhythm sleep disorder results from a mismatch between the biologic rhythms of the sleep–wake cycle and the external demands upon the sleep–wake system. Examples include delayed sleep phase disorders, shift work, and jet lag. The diagnosis is based on careful review of history, including review of sleep patterns, napping, alertness and behavior. Symptoms can include insomnia, hypersomnia, and fatigue.

○ **What is delayed sleep phase disorder?**

Delayed sleep phase refers to a delay of the circadian rhythm in the sleep–wake cycle. The rhythm is shifted to a later clock time relative to conventional rest–activity patterns. These individuals sleep late and wake-up late pattern are considered "night owls," and often choose careers to suit their sleep pattern.

○ **What is the treatment of delayed sleep phase disorder?**

The treatment includes chronobiologic strategies to shift the phase position of the endogenous circadian oscillator in the right direction. For example, exposure to bright light in the early morning advances the delayed sleep phase, while exposure to bright light in the evening will delay the sleep phase. Approximately 2500 to 10,000 lux of light for 2 h/d or spending time outdoors is required to achieve these goals. Use of "Zeitgebers" (indicators of time) can facilitate synchronization to a 24-hour cycle, with a regular wake-up time being perhaps the most powerful Zeitgeber.

○ **What is shift work sleep disorder?**

Nearly a quarter of all Americans work nonconventional shifts (i.e., other than 8 AM to 5 PM). This requires the internal circadian oscillator to constantly readjust to these external demands. These individuals are often sleep deprived and prone to accidents. Indeed, many industrial and traffic accidents are thought to have been caused by these shift demands. Chronobiologic techniques, sleep hygiene, napping, and moving the shifts in a clockwise fashion, e.g., day to evening to night, are helpful.

○ **What is jet lag associated sleep disorder?**

Jet lag occurs when an individual travels across several time zones. Traveling east advances the cycles and traveling west delays the cycle. This can lead to sleepiness, insomnia, mood changes, and gastrointestinal disturbances. Management includes advance preparation for the time zone changes, sleep hygiene, and quick synchronization with the clock at the destination by either taking a nap or remaining awake for extra time. A short course of hypnotic medication may be helpful.

○ **What is periodic limb movement sleep disorder?**

Periodic limb movement sleep disorder (PLMS), previously denoted as nocturnal myoclonus, is a disorder in which repetitive, brief, and stereotypic limb movements occur during sleep, in 20- to 40-second intervals. The bed partner often reports that the patient is restlessness, kicks, has cold feet, and has daytime sleepiness. Polysomnographic recordings that document five or more tibialis muscle jerks per hour in stages 1 and 2 of sleep, and is associated with arousal, make the diagnosis. The cause of PLMS is unclear. Treatments include trials of L-dopa/carbidopa, baclofen, and benzodiazepines.

○ **What is restless leg syndrome?**

Restless leg syndrome is a condition wherein paresthesias of the lower legs, feet, or thighs in the recumbent position cause an irresistible urge to move the legs, resulting in sleep-onset insomnia. Almost all patients with restless leg syndrome have PLMS but not all patients with PLMS have restless leg syndrome. Treatment strategies are the same as for PMLS.

○ **What is nightmare disorder?**

This disorder is characterized by extremely frightening dreams leading to awakening. The individual can recall the dream in detail. It occurs during REM sleep and, therefore, it is more common in the second half of the sleep period. The person is generally oriented and alert after awakening. The disorder leads to considerable distress, and is not part of another psychiatric disorder, e.g., PTSD. More common in children, it is usually self-limiting but psychotherapy, desensitization, and support is helpful.

○ **What is sleep terror disorder?**

This disorder is characterized by abrupt awakening from sleep, usually occurring in the first 1 to 2 hours after the onset of sleep. The individual experiences intense fear, panic, tachycardia, rapid breathing, and sweating. The individual has difficulty recalling the details of the dream, is amnestic for the incident, and is unresponsive to comfort or support. Sleep terrors usually occur during sleep stages 3 and 4, and is seen in 1% to 6% of children (much less in adults). Onset usually begins at around 4 to 6 years of age and resolves by adolescence. Benzodiazepines suppress delta sleep and therefore are helpful.

○ **What is sleep walking disorder?**

Sleep walking disorder is characterized by repeated episodes of rising from bed during sleep and walking about, usually during the first third of the sleep period. The person has a bland, staring face, is relatively unresponsive to others, and can be difficult to awaken. Once awake, the person is alert and oriented, but has amnesia for the episode. Treatment includes maintaining safety of the environment and the use of benzodiazepines or sedating antidepressants.

○ **What is REM sleep behavior disorder?**

The disorder is characterized by the presence of complex behaviors, e.g., walking, running, singing, and talking during REM sleep usually in the second half of the sleep episode. Apparently, there is a lack of muscle atonia during REM sleep so that the individual engages in complex activities. Recall of dreams is also good. It occurs mostly in elderly men and is associated with a variety of degenerative neurologic conditions and use of tricyclic antidepressants, alcohol, sedative hypnotic withdrawal, and biperiden. Clonazepam 0.5 to 1.0 mg at bedtime is effective in controlling the symptoms.

○ **What psychiatric disorders are associated with sleep disorders?**

Psychiatric disorders associated with sleep disorders include depression, alcohol abuse, panic disorders, generalized anxiety disorder, PTSD, schizophrenia, and substance abuse.

○ **What changes in sleep are characteristic of depression?**

Sleep changes characteristic of depression include shortened REM latency, redistribution of REM toward the early part of the night, and increased REM density. The amount of sleep in stages 3 and 4 is reduced, and patients experience difficulty initiating and maintaining sleep, with a low arousal threshold. Blunted levels of melatonin, testosterone, and growth hormone have been noted, as well as increased levels of cortisol. Total sleep deprivation and selective REM deprivation, paradoxically, have a transient antidepressant effect.

○ **What is substance-induced sleep disorder (SISD)?**

This disorder is characterized by a prominent disturbance in sleep, sufficiently severe to warrant independent clinical attention. It occurs during or within 1 month of substance intoxication or withdrawal, and the substance abuse is etiologically related to sleep disturbance. This disorder may include insomnia, hypersomnia, parasomnias, or a mixed clinical picture.

○ **What substances are associated with SISD?**

Common substances associated with SISD include alcohol, nicotine, amphetamines, cocaine, caffeine, opioids, sedatives, and hypnotics. Some adrenergic, dopaminergic, and cholinergic agonists and antagonists, antihistamines, SSRIs, and steroids can also cause sleep disorder.

○ **List some sleep-promoting pharmacologic agents.**

Sleep-promoting pharmacologic agents include:

- benzodiazepine receptor agonists
- imidiazopyridines (e.g., Ambien)
- chloral hydrate

Nonprescription sleeping aids include:

- sedating antihistamines
- protein precursors (e.g., L-tryptophan)

○ **What are the principal guidelines for the pharmacologic treatment of sleep disorders?**

The principal guidelines of pharmacologic treatments for sleep disorders include use of prescription medications instead of over-the-counter medications when possible (because they have been vigorously tested) and use of the lowest possible dose for the shortest possible time to achieve relief of symptoms. The patient should take the medication for two or three nights consecutively and repeat the sequence no more than two or three times. Chronic continuous use should be avoided, as all benzodiazepine receptor agonists have the potential for abuse, reduced driving ability, and respiratory suppression. Abrupt withdrawal will cause some degree of rebound anxiety and insomnia. The rationale for using hypnotics, and consent for use, should be carefully documented in the patient's medical records, especially for the elderly, as they are more susceptible to the sedative and cognitive side effects of benzodiazepine receptor agonists, thus increasing the risk for falls and hip fractures.

○ **What is the role of stimulant medications in the treatment of sleep disorders?**

Stimulant medication is used for the treatment of certain intrinsic dyssomnias, e.g., narcolepsy and idiopathic hypersomnia, and for sleep-related asthma. They should not be used for sleep apneas or extrinsic dyssomnias, e.g., jet lag. Methylphenidate is considered a first-line agent, but use has limited their increased potential for abuse. Self-administration of caffeinated beverages, nicotine, and chocolate is also common in these disorders.

○ **What is the role of antidepressant medications in sleep disorders?**

Sedating antidepressants taken at bedtime can be very helpful for a depressed patient. Tricyclic antidepressants are also useful in treating cataplexy, as the anticholinergic action of these medications suppresses REM intrusion during wakefulness.

○ **Can antidepressant medications worsen sleep disorders?**

Yes. Some tricyclic antidepressants and SSRIs can produce or exacerbate sleep-related movement disorders, e.g., periodic limb movement disorder, restless leg syndrome, and myoclonus.

○ **What is the role of melatonin, L-dopa, and anticonvulsants in the treatment of sleep disorders?**

Additional medications used in the treatment of sleep disorders include melatonin, L-dopa, and anticonvulsants. Trials using melatonin to treat circadian rhythm disorder in blind patients have been successful, as melatonin advances the sleep phase. Its use in sighted individuals is being explored. L-dopa can be used to treat periodic limb movement disorders, while anticonvulsants have been tried to treat nocturnal paroxysmal dystonia, PTSD-related nightmares, and restless leg syndrome.

○ **What is the role of bright light treatment in sleep disorders?**

Exposing a patient to bright light (greater than 10,000 lux) can alter the intrinsic circadian rhythm. Early morning bright light therapy can be used to phase advance individuals. Similarly, exposure to bright light in the evening can help individuals with advanced sleep phase syndrome. Light therapy in the morning is also being utilized to treat seasonal affective disorder, shift workers, astronauts, and jet lag.

○ **What is the role of behavior modification in the treatment of sleep disorders?**

Many behavior techniques including sleep hygiene, stimulus control therapy, sleep restriction therapy, relaxation therapy and biofeedback, cognitive restructuring, and chronotherapy are useful modalities available for the treatment of sleep disorders. Up to 70% to 80% of patients with insomnia will respond to behavioral interventions alone.

○ **What is sleep hygiene?**

Sleep hygiene refers to good sleep rules and rituals. Some examples include maintaining a regular sleep–wake schedule; avoidance of naps; keeping a steady program of daily exercise; insulating the room against excessive noise, light, cold, and heat; eating a light snack before retiring if hungry; avoiding stimulants such as caffeine and nicotine; setting time aside for emotionally laden issues before sleep; and avoiding conditioned arousal associated with the bed and bedroom.

○ **Describe stimulus control therapy.**

Stimulus control attempts to enhance stimulus cues for sleeping and decrease stimulus cues associated with sleeplessness. Examples of some principles include going to bed only when sleepy, use of the bed only for sleeping, not watching TV or reading in the bedroom, not lying in bed if unable to sleep within 15 minutes, and awakening at the same time every-day.

○ **What is sleep restriction therapy?**

For patients who find themselves lying awake in bed unable to sleep, restricting time in bed can consolidate sleep. To enhance sleep at night, sleep at other times during the day should be avoided except with the elderly, and a strict wake-up time should be adhered to. When sleep efficiency reaches 85% (time asleep as a percentage of time in bed), the time in bed is increased by 15 minutes. This produces a gradual decline in wakefulness and promotes sleep.

○ **How are relaxation therapy and biofeedback used in the treatment of sleep disorders?**

In relaxation therapy, self-hypnosis, progressive relaxation, visual imagery, and deep breathing exercises are utilized to produce relaxation. Biofeedback methods provide stimulus cues for physiological markers of relaxation, thereby increasing self-awareness and enhancing relaxation. These techniques are often combined with other modalities to enhance sleep.

○ **How does the use of cognitive restructuring improve sleep patterns?**

Cognitive restructuring addresses insomnia by identifying false assumptions about sleep (i.e., a fear that sleep will be hard to initiate or interrupted.

○ **What is chronotherapy?**

When individuals are deprived of environmental cues, the typical day lasts 25 to 26 hours. In chronotherapy, progressive phase delaying is utilized to synchronize the biologic clock with the internal circadian oscillator. Thus, phase delaying each night for 2 to 3 hours proceeds, until the sleep onset coincides with the desired time. During this process, the patient has to cope with an odd sleep–wake cycle for a week or two. Therefore, chronotherapy is not a popular strategy in treating sleep disorders.

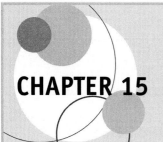

CHAPTER 15

Impulse Control Disorders

○ **What are the features common to all impulse control disorders?**

Failure to resist an impulse to perform a self-destructive act; escalating tension prior to committing the act; and during commission of the act, the person feels pleasure or release.

○ **What are the categories of impulse control disorders classified in *DSM-IV*?**

Intermittent explosive disorder, kleptomania, pyromania, pathological gambling, trichotillomania, and impulse control disorder NOS.

○ **What region of the brain is associated with impulsive and violent behavior?**

The limbic system.

○ **Which hormone has been most consistently associated with violent and aggressive behavior?**

Testosterone.

○ **An association has been reported between impulsive violent behavior and which type of epilepsy?**

Temporal lobe epilepsy.

○ **What childhood disorder is frequently associated with impulse control disorders?**

Attention deficit hyperactivity disorder.

○ **Brain stem and cerebrospinal fluid (CSF) levels of which neurotransmitter are often decreased in patients with impulse control disorders?**

5-hydroxyindoleacetic acid (5-HIAA), a metabolite of serotonin.

○ **Are impulse control disorders ego-dystonic or ego-syntonic?**

Ego-dystonic symptoms or behaviors are not viewed as a part of the self and are generally recognized by the patient as pathologic. Ego-syntonic behaviors, on the other hand, are perceived as a normal part of the personality and are less likely to be perceived as maladaptive. Most impulse control disorders are ego-syntonic; patients fail to recognize the pathologic nature of their behavior. This observation helps to explain why these individuals do not seek treatment. In some cases, however, patients may experience transient feelings of anxiety, depression, or remorse (consistent with an ego-dystonic quality), but this is an inconsistent finding.

○ **What is intermittent explosive disorder?**

Intermittent explosive disorder is characterized by discrete episodes of failure to resist aggressive impulses that result in serious assaultive acts or destruction of property.

○ **To what extent is the aggressive behavior seen in intermittent explosive disorder a reaction to external psychosocial stressors?**

According to the *DSM-IV*, the degree of aggression seen in intermittent explosive disorder is "grossly out of proportion to any . . . precipitating psychosocial stressors."

○ **Do patients with intermittent explosive disorder show signs of increased impulsivity or aggression in between episodes?**

No. There is no increase in aggressiveness or impulsivity in between episodes of intermittent explosive disorder.

○ **In what ways does intermittent explosive disorder resemble seizure disorders?**

Patients with intermittent explosive disorder may experience an aura. Other features suggesting an epileptoid state include postictal changes in sensorium, partial amnesia, and hypersensitivity to photic or auditory stimuli. These patients may also have soft neurologic signs and nonspecific EEG findings.

○ **How common is intermittent explosive disorder?**

The exact incidence of intermittent explosive disorder is not known. Although the disorder is thought to be rare, it may be underreported in the general population. It is more common in men than in women.

○ **Describe the familial linkage of intermittent explosive disorder.**

Intermittent explosive disorder is more common in first-degree biological relatives of persons with the disorder than in the general population.

○ **List four psychosocial factors that are thought to contribute to the development of intermittent explosive disorder.**

1. Alcohol dependence in the family.
2. A history of physical abuse during childhood.
3. Frequent exposure to violence.
4. Parental promiscuity.

○ **Following an episode of violence, what emotional reactions are commonly seen in patients with intermittent explosive disorder?**

Patients are generally unable to explain their behavior and react with feelings of guilt, depression, and anxiety.

○ **According to *DSM-IV*, what conditions must be ruled out before a diagnosis of intermittent explosive disorder can be made?**

Impulsivity or aggression related to another psychiatric disorder precludes a diagnosis of intermittent explosive disorder. Examples include the psychotic disorders, the manic phase of bipolar disorder, antisocial personality disorder, borderline personality disorder, conduct disorder, and attention deficit hyperactivity disorder. Aggression related to substance abuse or a general medical condition (e.g., head trauma) must also be ruled out, as well as aggression that may occur during delirium or dementia. Finally, some individuals will attempt to use a diagnosis of intermittent explosive disorder in order to avoid legal consequences of their aggressive behaviors, i.e., malinger.

○ **Describe the course and prognosis of intermittent explosive disorder.**

The disorder most often begins during the second or third decade of life. By midlife the frequency and intensity of episodes begins to decline.

○ **What pharmacologic agents are used in the treatment of intermittent explosive disorder?**

Traditionally, anticonvulsants have been used to treat this disorder (e.g., carbamazepine and phenytoin). More recently, valproic acid has been found to be effective. Other medications used include lithium carbonate, propranolol, trazodone, and the selective serotonin reuptake inhibitors (e.g., fluoxetine).

○ **What are the characteristics of impulse control disorder not otherwise specified (NOS)?**

This is a category for impulse control problems that do not meet the criteria for a specific impulse control disorder. As with the other disorders in this class, the behavior is not better explained by another psychiatric condition. Examples of the NOS category include compulsive shopping and repetitive self-mutilation.

○ **What is trichotillomania?**

The recurrent pulling out of one's hair resulting in noticeable hair loss. Trichotillomania may either be a primary disorder or a symptom of some other condition (e.g., a form of self-mutilation associated with borderline personality disorder).

○ **Describe the behavioral sequence associated with trichotillomania.**

The patient experiences an increasing sense of tension prior to the behavior. This feeling intensifies until the patient cannot resist pulling his or her hair. Immediately after the hair pulling, the person feels a sense of relief. Over time, this sequence repeats itself until hair loss is noticeable. Many patients experience feelings of embarrassment or humiliation as a result of the behavior.

○ **What other psychiatric disorders may be associated with trichotillomania?**

Obsessive-compulsive disorder, compulsive personality disorder, borderline personality disorder, and depression.

○ **What etiologic factors have been linked to trichotillomania?**

Stress has been cited as a factor in many patients with the disorder, as hair pulling may represent a maladaptive attempt to cope with stress. Other factors include fear of abandonment and recent object loss. Self-stimulation to offset underlying feelings of emptiness may also be a factor.

○ **What is the most common anatomic site for hair pulling?**

The scalp is the most common area of the body affected. Eyelashes and eyebrows may also be involved. Other parts of the body (e.g., armpits, trunk, or pubic hair) are involved less frequently.

○ **List four other behaviors that may be associated with trichotillomania.**

1. Swallowing of hair (i.e., trichophagy).
2. Head banging.
3. Nail biting.
4. Scratching of the skin may be present.

Other forms of self-mutilation (e.g., self-cutting) may also be seen.

○ **In addition to alopecia, what other complications may occur as the result of trichotillomania?**

Superficial skin irritation or minor infections may occur as the result of hair pulling. When trichophagy accompanies hair pulling, bezoars, malnutrition, and intestinal obstruction may develop.

○ **To what extent are patients with trichotillomania aware of their behavior?**

During the early stages of the disorder the behavior may be entirely unconscious. Over time, as alopecia becomes noticeable, patients have increasing awareness of the behavior but feel unable to resist. Trichotillomania is ego-dystonic; patients experience the behavior as unwanted and feel subjective distress as a result of the hair pulling.

○ **What is the primary differential diagnosis for trichotillomania?**

Obsessive-compulsive disorder. Trichotillomania is a repetitive behavior that is associated with increased tension and anxiety when the individual attempts to resist. Unlike obsessive-compulsive disorder, however, trichotillomania is not associated with intrusive obsessional thoughts.

○ **Describe the course and prognosis of trichotillomania.**

The onset of trichotillomania is usually in childhood or adolescence, although it may occur at any age. The disorder tends to be chronic; exacerbations are often associated with external psychosocial stressors.

○ **What medications are used to treat trichotillomania?**

The selective serotonin reuptake inhibitors (e.g., fluoxetine, sertraline, and paroxetine) may be effective in the treatment of trichotillomania. Other drugs used to treat obsessive-compulsive disorder (e.g., clomipramine, and fluvoxamine) may also be effective. When depression is an associated finding, other antidepressants (e.g., the tricyclics) may decrease hair pulling. In general, drugs with serotonergic activity appear to be the most effective.

○ **What psychotherapeutic approaches have been used in the treatment of trichotillomania?**

Insight-oriented psychotherapy is of benefit for these patients, particularly when underlying issues related to depression or abandonment are present. Behavioral therapy (e.g., biofeedback) may also be useful. In most cases, a combination of psychotherapy and pharmacotherapy is most effective.

○ **What is the *DSM-IV* definition of pathological gambling?**

This disorder is defined as persistent and recurrent maladaptive gambling behavior.

○ **List the major characteristics of pathological gambling.**

These patients display an intense preoccupation with gambling that is characterized by a need to gamble progressively increasing amounts of money in order to achieve the desired level of excitement. Patients experience repeated unsuccessful attempts to stop gambling. The gambling behavior is often used as a means of escape from day-to-day problems. Following losses, patients will gamble larger amounts of money in an attempt to break even. Over time, patients will lie to conceal their losses and engage in various illegal activities to obtain money for gambling.

○ **How common is pathological gambling in the United States?**

The disorder is estimated to be present in 1% to 3% of the population.

○ **What is the sex distribution of pathological gambling?**

In general, the disorder is more common in men than women.

○ **Is there a familial link in pathological gambling?**

Yes. The parents of persons with pathological gambling are more likely to have the disorder than would be expected in the general population.

○ **What is the connection between alcohol abuse and pathological gambling?**

Men with pathological gambling have higher rates of alcoholism than the general population. Women with the diagnosis are more likely to be married to men with alcohol abuse problems.

○ **List five other psychiatric disorders that are associated with pathological gambling.**

1. Major depression.

2. Panic disorder.

3. Agoraphobia.

4. Obsessive-compulsive disorder.

5. Attention deficit hyperactivity disorder.

○ **What neurotransmitter is thought to be involved in pathological gambling?**

Catecholamine metabolism may be impaired in pathological gambling. Patients with the disorder may seek the activating effects of norepinephrine that accompany the tension associated with gambling.

○ **What psychosocial factors are associated with pathological gambling?**

Loss of a parent during childhood may contribute to the development of the disorder. Other factors include inappropriate parental discipline, exposure to excessive gambling early in life, family emphasis on money and material objects, and financial instability in the family.

○ **Describe the personality characteristics of patients with pathological gambling.**

Narcissistic and antisocial traits are often prominent in these patients.

○ **What psychiatric conditions should be considered in the differential diagnosis of pathological gambling?**

The two disorders most commonly considered in the differential diagnosis are antisocial personality disorder and the manic phase of bipolar disorder.

○ **How is pathological gambling distinguished from antisocial personality disorder?**

Criminal behavior associated with pathological gambling is almost always related to attempts to obtain money to support the gambling behavior, and is usually nonviolent. Examples include theft, fraud, and embezzlement. These persons also frequently lie to conceal their gambling. In all cases, however, antisocial behavior is directly related to the underlying gambling. In antisocial personality disorder, there is pervasive criminal behavior and a disregard for the rights of others in all areas of functioning.

○ **How is pathological gambling distinguished from the manic phase of bipolar disorder?**

Excessive gambling may be a symptom associated with manic episodes. A history of mood swings, impulsivity, and impaired judgment is usually present across a wide range of activities. Gambling and other impulsive behaviors are clearly *secondary* to the mood swings. Patients with pathological gambling, on the other hand, experience euphoria following periods of winning; episodes of depression may follow extended losing streaks. The mood swings in pathological gambling are reactions to events associated with gambling rather than the cause of the behavior.

○ **Describe the three phases commonly seen in pathological gambling.**

1. The first, or *winning*, phase consists of a series of successes, which generate large amounts of money; these early wins serve to "hook" the patient on gambling.

2. The first phase is followed by a series of *progressive losses* during which gambling becomes the central activity in the patient's life. During this phase the patient takes increasingly greater financial risks and becomes preoccupied with obtaining money for gambling.

3. The final phase consists of *desperation* in which gambling overshadows all other activities. The patient withdraws from other areas of life, engages in illegal activities to obtain money, and experiences the loss of important relationships. It may take up to 15 years to reach the final phase of this process.

○ **What type of treatment is most effective for pathological gambling?**

Group therapy is the most effective form of treatment for pathological gambling. The most widely recognized form of group therapy is Gamblers Anonymous, which is based on the model of treatment established by Alcoholics Anonymous. Various gambling institutions will allow individuals to have themselves "banned and barred" from their facility, but there always seems to be another casino in the area.

○ **What defense mechanisms are most prominent in patients with pathological gambling?**

Denial and rationalization. Patients with this disorder generally fail to recognize its severity. They will go to great lengths to explain or justify their behavior. At other times, patients will attempt to conceal their behavior from others. These defenses make patients reluctant to come forward for treatment; patients most often seek treatment secondary to family pressure or legal problems resulting from gambling.

○ **What is kleptomania?**

DSM-IV defines kleptomania as a recurrent failure to resist impulses to steal objects not needed for personal use or their monetary value.

○ **List the clinical features associated with kleptomania.**

The essential feature of kleptomania is the recurrent impulse to steal unneeded objects. In most cases, the theft is spontaneous with little or no advance planning. Patients usually have the money to purchase the objects taken. They report a feeling of tension and excitement prior to stealing, followed by a sense of relief after the act. Patients are frequently unable to explain why a particular object was stolen; the act of stealing is clearly more important than the object taken. Many patients fail to consider the possibility that they may be arrested for shoplifting. Feelings of guilt or shame may be experienced in between episodes of kleptomania but they fail to deter future thefts.

○ **What is the prevalence of kleptomania?**

The exact prevalence of the disorder is not known. According to *DSM-IV*, kleptomania is thought to occur in less than 5% of persons arrested for shoplifting.

○ **What is the sex distribution of kleptomania?**

Although the sex distribution of kleptomania is unknown, it appears to be more common in women than in men.

○ **What psychodynamic factors are commonly associated with kleptomania?**

A variety of psychodynamic factors have been implicated in kleptomania. Excessive aggressive and libidinal impulses have been cited in the etiology of the disorder. The disorder may appear, or worsen, following psychosocial stressors. For some patients, the act of stealing may represent a symbolic attempt to recover a lost relationship or deal with rejection. Finally, unconscious wishes for punishment may influence the behavior.

○ **Which psychiatric conditions are associated with kleptomania?**

Depression, obsessive-compulsive disorder, and eating disorders (e.g., bulimia nervosa) may be associated with kleptomania.

○ **Disturbances in which neurotransmitter system are implicated in kleptomania?**

Serotonin.

○ **To what extent are patients with kleptomania troubled or disturbed by their behavior?**

Some patients with kleptomania may not consider the risk of being caught. Others describe a feeling of excitement when they escape detection. In other cases, the patient may experience guilt and remorse after the act, and may attempt to return the stolen item.

○ **Which psychiatric conditions should be considered in the differential diagnosis of kleptomania?**

Kleptomania must be distinguished from stealing for financial gain or associated with other antisocial behaviors. Depression and anxiety may occur in patients with kleptomania, particularly if there are legal problems related to the behavior. Stealing in response to command hallucinations associated with schizophrenia or related to a manic phase of bipolar disorder must be differentiated from kleptomania. Persons with cognitive problems (e.g., Alzheimer's disease) may inadvertently steal because they forget to pay for objects.

○ **How is kleptomania differentiated from shoplifting?**

Kleptomania can be distinguished from shoplifting by the fact that the individual who shoplifts does so for monetary gain or other reasons (peer influence), while the kleptomaniac steals for the "thrill" rather than the gain.

○ **Describe the course and prognosis of kleptomania.**

Stealing may begin in childhood or adolescence. Once the behavior becomes apparent it tends to run a chronic course. Exacerbations and remissions may occur over time, and are often influenced by psychosocial stressors. The prognosis with treatment tends to be good.

○ **List the pharmacologic agents used in the treatment of kleptomania.**

The selective serotonin reuptake inhibitors have been used with some success in the treatment of kleptomania. This class of drugs includes fluoxetine (Prozac®), sertraline (Zoloft®), and paroxetine (Paxil®).

○   **What psychotherapeutic approaches have been used to treat kleptomania?**

Insight-oriented psychotherapy may be of benefit in the treatment of kleptomania, particularly when the disorder is associated with guilt and depression. Behavior therapy, such as aversive conditioning, may also be of benefit.

○   **What factors complicate the treatment of kleptomania?**

Many patients with the disorder are never arrested for shoplifting, and experience relatively little subjective distress as a result of the behavior. Thus, there is little motivation to seek treatment. For those persons who are arrested, the courts may mandate treatment. Lack of motivation and resentment over court-ordered treatment may retard the therapeutic process, but may be the only way individuals with a history of kleptomania ever address the stealing behavior. For some individuals, a few nights in jail serves as an effective aversive stimulus and the behavior stops.

○   **What is pyromania?**

Pyromania is the deliberate and purposeful setting of fires. According to *DSM-IV*, the behavior must occur on more than one occasion in order to the diagnosis to be made. This diagnosis excludes those persons who deliberately set fires to mask some other criminal activity or to express a social or political agenda (e.g., terrorists).

○   **List the clinical features associated with pyromania.**

Patients with pyromania display an intense fascination with fire and explosives. Many of these patients choose occupations in which they are exposed to fire (e.g., firefighter, demolitions, etc.). A sense of tension precedes the act, followed by relief after the fire is set. In many cases, the patient does not consider the potential for loss of life or property associated with the act. It is not uncommon for persons with this diagnosis to remain at the scene of the fire or to return to the scene to witness the consequences of their actions; many pyromaniacs experience a voyeuristic satisfaction from observing the results of their behavior.

○   **What is the prevalence of pyromania?**

No data are available on the prevalence of pyromania. The disorder is thought to be rare among adults.

○   **What is the sex distribution of pyromania?**

Pyromania is more common among men than women.

○   **What psychodynamic factors are commonly associated with pyromania?**

Pyromania may represent an aggressive act aimed at overcoming feelings of inadequacy. The act of fire-setting may symbolize a quest for power over others. Sigmund Freud viewed fire as a symbol of sexuality; thus, pyromania may represent an effort to assert one's sexuality or to overcome feelings of sexual inadequacy. Other theorists have postulated that pyromania emerges in response to childhood rejection.

○   **Which psychiatric conditions are associated with pyromania?**

Some studies have cited an increased incidence of alcohol abuse or mental retardation among fire-setters.

○   **What is the relationship between fire-setting and childhood behavior?**

Many children display a transient fascination with fire. In most cases, children outgrow this interest and do not display the behavior as adolescents or adults. A childhood history of conduct disorder is seen in many adult fire-setters. Childhood symptoms of truancy, running away from home, delinquency, and enuresis may predict adult pyromania.

○ **In which neurotransmitter system are disturbances implicated in pyromania?**

Low levels of 5-HIAA and 3-methoxy-4-hydroxyphenylglycol (MHPG), both metabolites of serotonin, have been found in the cerebrospinal fluid of patients with pyromania.

○ **Describe the behavioral sequence associated with pyromania.**

Persons with the disorder experience intrusive thoughts about fire-setting and an increasing sense of tension prior to the act. At some point the impulse becomes irresistible, culminating in the setting of fires. Immediately following the act, the patient experiences a sense of relief. Feelings of guilt or remorse may or may not occur following the act. This sequence tends to repeat itself over time.

○ **Which conditions should be considered in the differential diagnosis of pyromania?**

Among children or adolescents, conduct disorder is the most common differential diagnosis. Fire-setting may also occur in response to command hallucinations associated with schizophrenia or during the manic phase of bipolar disorder. The deliberate setting of fires to obtain monetary gain may be seen in antisocial personality disorder. Fire-setting to obtain revenge for some perceived social or interpersonal injustice must also be differentiated from pyromania.

○ **Describe the course and prognosis of pyromania.**

The disorder generally begins in childhood. It escalates over time and becomes increasingly destructive through the adolescent and adult years. The prognosis with early diagnosis and treatment is good; untreated adults have a poor prognosis.

○ **List the pharmacologic agents used in the treatment of pyromania.**

Little research exists on the effectiveness of pharmacologic agents for the treatment of pyromania. Medications used to decrease impulsivity, such as lithium or carbamazepine (Tegretol®), may be effective. The selective serotonin reuptake inhibitors, such as fluoxetine (Prozac®), may also be of benefit.

○ **What psychotherapeutic approaches have been used to treat pyromania?**

Most adults with the diagnosis are incarcerated. Group psychotherapy or behavioral therapy may be effective. Few studies exist on the effectiveness of treatment; therefore, caution should be exercised in assessing psychotherapeutic strategies.

CHAPTER 16 — Personality Disorders

○ **What is "personality"?**

Personality is the sum of an individual's emotional, cognitive, and behavioral traits as demonstrated under ordinary living conditions. Personality is relatively stable and leads to more or less predictable affective, cognitive, and behavioral responses to everyday events.

○ **What are personality traits?**

Personality traits are enduring patterns of perceiving, relating to, and thinking about the environment and oneself that are exhibited in a wide range of social and personal contexts. The way a particular person usually responds to a variety of situations or contexts reflects his or her personality traits.

○ **Are personality traits helpful or harmful?**

Personality traits are neither helpful nor harmful per se. They may be adaptive, maladaptive, or both, depending upon the situation or context in which they are expressed. For example, obsessive-compulsive traits may be adaptive for a physician in his work but maladaptive in his family life and interpersonal relationships.

○ **What are some of the important factors that help to determine an individual's personality?**

Personality is biopsychosocially determined. It is a combination of interrelated and interacting factors that include:

- innate temperament, as determined by constitution, heredity, and biology
- developmental experiences, especially within one's family
- role models, including family members, friends, teachers, etc.
- cultural and societal influences, such as socioeconomic status, living environment, educational opportunities, available role models, religious and cultural heritage, national character, and so forth.

○ **What did Sigmund Freud think about the etiology of personality?**

Freud believed that personality traits or disorders are related to fixation at various psychosexual stages of development. For Freud, what is now called dependent personality disorder is the result of fixation at the oral stage, whereas obsessive-compulsive personality disorder characteristics, such as stubbornness and conscientiousness, are the outcome of fixation at the anal stage of development.

○ **At what point in development is an individual's personality permanent and unalterable?**

At no point. Crucial components of personality appear to be genetically and biologically determined, and, in conjunction with one's environment, an individual's personality is typically well formed and stable by adolescence or early adulthood. Nevertheless, an individual's personality continues to evolve and change throughout life, in response to various biopsychosocial factors.

○ **How does stress affect an individual's personality?**

Stress may have multiple effects on personality. Personality traits are often exacerbated by stress, but one's personality usually reverts to its baseline after the crisis has passed. Stress may also cause long-lasting changes in personality although, as a general rule, recurrent stress over prolonged periods of time is more likely than single acute stressful episodes to produce significant long-term personality changes. Stress may elicit both positive and negative as well as adaptive and maladaptive personality changes.

○ **What is a personality disorder?**

A personality disorder is an enduring pattern of inner experience and behavior that has an onset in adolescence or early adulthood, is inflexible and pervasive across a broad range of personal and social situations, is stable and of long duration, and leads to clinically significant distress or impairment in social, occupational, or other important areas of functioning. The enduring pattern of a personality disorder is evident in an individual's cognition, affectivity, interpersonal functioning, and/or impulse control. Gabbard views personality disorders as being a composite of four components: temperament, an internalized set of object relations, an enduring sense of self, and a specific set of defense mechanisms.

○ **Are personality traits synonymous with personality disorders?**

No.

○ **Are strong personality traits synonymous with personality disorders?**

No.

○ **What is the relationship between personality traits and personality disorder?**

Personality traits, in themselves, do not constitute a personality disorder, even if such traits are very marked. It is only when personality traits become inflexible and maladaptive and cause significant functional impairment or subjective distress that they constitute a personality disorder.

○ **What is the prevalence of personality disorders?**

The prevalence is 10% to 15% in the general population. Borderline personality disorder is the most common, occurring in 2% of the general population and in 10% of all psychiatric outpatients.

○ **What are some of the key factors that distinguish Axis I psychiatric symptoms from Axis II personality disorder symptoms?**

Axis I psychiatric symptoms are usually ego-dystonic (the patient recognizes that he is symptomatic and does not wish to have the symptoms), often are more bothersome to the patient than to others, and are infrequently adaptive. In contrast, Axis II personality disorder symptoms are often ego-syntonic, typically more disturbing or problematic to others than to the patient, and may have adaptive components (e.g., compulsive traits in a physician).

○ **If Axis II personality disorder signs and symptoms are often ego-syntonic, do individuals with personality disorders suffer themselves rather than simply inflicting suffering on others?**

Yes, they often do. Personality disordered individuals are often unhappy with the adverse effects of their own behavior (e.g., rejection by others) and/or their inability to function effectively and achieve their goals. Furthermore, individuals with personality disorders also frequently suffer from comorbid Axis I mental illnesses.

○ **What is the relationship between *DSM-IV* Axis I and Axis II disorders?**

Axis I and Axis II disorders frequently coexist, so one should be alert for Axis I mental illnesses in those patients with personality disorders, and vice versa.

○ **What are some of the most common comorbid Axis I mental illnesses in personality disordered patients?**

Depressive disorders, anxiety disorders, and alcoholism/substance abuse are commonly comorbid with many personality disorders, but especially with the cluster B personality disorders. Posttraumatic stress disorder (PTSD) may also be a comorbid condition with borderline personality disorder. Anxiety disorders are frequently found in individuals with personality disorders from cluster C (e.g., social phobia with avoidant personality disorder).

○ **What is the "spectrum relationship" of personality disorders and Axis I mental illnesses?**

The "spectrum relationship" concept suggests that certain Axis I and Axis II disorders are related, based upon biologic marker correspondence, phenomenological similarities, or familial aggregation. Examples include the Axis I disorder schizophrenia and the Axis II schizotypal personality disorder as well as the Axis I disorder social phobia and the Axis II avoidant personality disorder.

○ **Is there any particular relationship between mood or anxiety disorders and personality disorders?**

Mood and anxiety disorders are often diagnosed in persons suffering from personality disorders, and their prevalence is also increased in the biologic relatives of those with personality disorders. These relationships again point to the likelihood of a spectrum, or continuum, of Axis I mental disorders, personality traits, and personality disorders, based upon the severity and pervasiveness of certain characteristics.

○ **What are some of the genetic links between, and familial associations among, Axis I and Axis II disorders?**

Patients with schizophrenia are more likely to have biological relatives with any of the cluster A personality disorders (especially schizotypal personality disorder) than are mentally healthy controls. Antisocial personality disorder is associated with an increased incidence of alcohol abuse in biological relatives, borderline personality disorder is correlated with an increased incidence of mood disorders in biological relatives, and there is a strong association between histrionic personality disorder and somatization disorder (Briquet's syndrome). Obsessive-compulsive traits are more common in monozygotic than dizygotic twins. Avoidant personality disorder patients often have high anxiety levels.

○ **How often do two or more personality disorders co-occur in the same person?**

Frequently. Most personality constellations are not as distinct as described in *DSM-IV*, and many personality disorders are on a continuum, or overlap, with one another.

○ **How are defense mechanisms related to personality and personality disorders?**

A person's characteristic defense mechanisms help define his or her personality. Indeed, certain defense mechanisms tend to be associated with each of the Axis II personality disorders. When these defense mechanisms are working effectively, a personality-disordered individual may be able to control various emotions and views the "symptoms" as ego-syntonic.

○ **When do personality disorders become evident?**

Personality disorders, by *DSM-IV* definition, require an onset no later than early adulthood; and many personality disorders can be diagnosed by this time. On the other hand, some personality-disordered individuals may not come to clinical attention until later in life. Such individuals may have negotiated a reasonably successful and happy life, effectively masking the presence of their personality disorder, until their maladaptive personality traits are exacerbated, often following a major stressor or loss (e.g., break-up of a marriage or loss of other significant supportive persons, disruption of previously stabilizing social structures such as job or career). Thus, a man with a narcissistic personality disorder might not come to clinical attention, and receive a personality disorder diagnosis until midlife (e.g., 45 years), but the symptoms of such a disorder must have been present since adolescence or young adulthood.

○ **What is the earliest age at which a personality disorder can be diagnosed?**

One must be very cautious in diagnosing personality disorders in childhood or adolescence because childhood traits of a personality disorder often change and may even disappear by adulthood. Nonetheless, personality disorders may be diagnosed in children or adolescents if an individual's particular maladaptive personality traits appear to be pervasive, persistent, and unlikely to be limited to a particular developmental stage. Personality disorders diagnosed in individuals younger than 18 years must have been present for at least 1 year. Antisocial personality disorder is the one exception to this rule; it cannot be diagnosed in individuals younger than 18 years.

○ **What about the apparent onset of a new personality disorder in middle age or later life?**

Although personality disorders may not come to clinical attention until later in life, the de novo development of a change in personality in middle adulthood or later life warrants a thorough evaluation to determine the possible presence of a personality change due to a general medical condition or an unrecognized substance-related disorder.

○ **What is the quickest and most reliable key to the diagnosis of personality disorders?**

Interpersonal relations. Indeed, it is in interpersonal relations that most aspects of personality disorders are evident, and as a result, it is difficult to make a personality disorder diagnosis without evidence of impaired interpersonal relations.

○ **What are some other clues to the diagnosis of personality disorders?**

Externalization of blame ("It's not my fault") and failure to learn from past mistakes.

○ **In addition to the above, what other clues might lead doctors, in particular, to suspect a personality disorder in a given individual?**

Physician countertransference is often an important, and not infrequently the earliest, clue. Another clue is splitting/polarization of the treatment team.

○ **How is countertransference manifested in work with personality-disordered patients?**

A physician finds himself or herself experiencing atypical thoughts or feelings toward a particular patient; or, the physician behaves in atypical ways with a particular patient. These atypical thoughts, feelings, and/or behaviors are unusual or exaggerated as compared to the physician's usual response to other patients.

○ **Give some examples of countertransferential thoughts or feelings with personality-disordered patients.**

Frustration, irritation, anger, a sense of defeat, and feeling manipulated are common. Unusual preoccupation with a particular patient is another frequent phenomenon. Countertransferential fantasies may include those of torturing or killing, having a sexual relationship with, or rescuing/saving a particular patient.

○ **How do physicians act out their countertransference with personality-disordered patients?**

There are innumerable behaviors including:
- avoidant (refusal to return telephone calls, inappropriate referral to other physicians)
- sadistic (being rude or condescending, ordering unnecessary and/or painful tests)
- sexual (being flirtatious or seductive, or engaging in frank sexual activity)
- rescue fantasy enactment's (giving excessive attention, time, or care; being uncharacteristically "drawn in" to a patient)

Countertransference to personality-disordered patients may lead a physician to ignore important symptoms of the patient or even unconsciously encourage a patient to act self-destructively. Physician boundary violations with a given patient should always suggest the possibility of physician countertransferential acting out.

○ **Describe the defining features of, and diagnostic entities within, each *DSM-IV* personality disorder cluster.**

- Cluster A (odd and eccentric): paranoid, schizoid, and schizotypal.
- Cluster B (dramatic and emotional): antisocial, borderline, histrionic, and narcissistic.
- Cluster C (anxious and fearful): avoidant, dependent, and obsessive-compulsive.

○ **What is the difference between paranoid personality disorder and schizophrenia?**

People with paranoid personality disorder do not have the abnormalities of thought process (e.g., loose associations), thought content (e.g., delusions), hallucinations, flattening of affect, deterioration in hygiene, or social withdrawal typical of schizophrenia.

○ **How would you distinguish between paranoid personality disorder and schizotypal personality disorder?**

Like persons with paranoid personality disorder, people with schizotypal personality disorder may be generally suspicious and have paranoid ideation; however, they also have odd or unusual beliefs, perceptual experiences, and odd thinking, speech, and behavior, unlike persons with paranoid personality disorder.

○ **How is paranoid personality disorder distinguished from delusional disorder?**

People with delusional disorder typically have single, circumscribed delusions, whereas those with paranoid personality disorder tend to be globally suspicious but not necessarily delusional (although individuals with paranoid personality disorder may have false paranoid beliefs that reach delusional intensity). A typical example of a delusional disorder: "My daughter is trying to poison me." A typical example of paranoid personality disorder: "You can't trust anyone; they're all out to get you."

○   **What are the most common defense mechanisms used by people with paranoid personality disorder?**

The classic defense mechanism involved in paranoia is projection. Other defense mechanisms are denial, reaction formation, and splitting.

○   **Which groups or organizations may have a high percentage of people with paranoid personality disorder?**

Paramilitary or survivalist groups and cults.

○   **Give some examples of the odd beliefs or magical thinking of schizotypal personality disorder.**

Superstitiousness, telepathy, clairvoyance, or an unexplained "sixth sense."

○   **How does schizoid personality disorder differ from schizotypal personality disorder?**

Both disorders have restricted interpersonal relationships, but the schizotypal has odd beliefs and behaviors as well.

○   **How would you distinguish between schizoid and schizotypal personality disorders at a party?**

You would not, because neither would go to a party. However, if they did attend, the schizotypal would be the one wearing odder clothes, having stranger ideas, and behaving more peculiarly. Whereas the schizoid would have no desire to interact with anyone at the party, the schizotypal would be anxious about having to do so.

○   **Is there a relationship between schizotypal personality disorder and schizophrenia?**

Schizotypal personality disorder was added to the *DSM* based on the concepts of latent or borderline schizophrenia. A certain percentage of people with schizotypal personality disorder go on to become frankly schizophrenic, and there is an increased likelihood of schizophrenia in family members of those with schizotypal personality disorder.

○   **What is adult antisocial behavior?**

It is a pattern of behavior that usually begins in childhood and persists throughout life characterized by activities that violate the society's legal and ethical systems. It is not due to a mental disorder.

○   **In what psychiatric disorders is violent behavior part of the diagnostic criteria in *DSM-IV*?**

Intermittent explosive disorder, antisocial personality disorder, borderline personality disorder, and conduct disorder.

○   **What mental disorders are included in the differential diagnosis of antisocial behavior?**

Intermittent explosive disorder, antisocial personality disorder, borderline personality disorder, conduct disorder, schizophrenia, other psychotic disorders, bipolar disorder, substance-related disorders, and cognitive disorders.

○   **What neurologic disorder must be distinguished from antisocial behavior in the differential diagnosis?**

Temporal lobe epilepsy.

○   **What laboratory tests and imaging studies can aid in the differential diagnosis of adult antisocial behavior?**

Routine lab tests including CBC, chemistry panel, TFTs, RPR, UA, B_{12}, folate, thiamine, drug screen and alcohol level, EKG, CXR, and EEG. An MRI is recommended for violent patients as better than CT at determining temporal lobe pathology.

○ **What distinguishes antisocial behavior from antisocial personality disorder?**

Antisocial personality disorder requires evidence of preexisting psychopathology such as a previous diagnosis of conduct disorder with onset before age 15 and a long-standing pattern of irresponsible and antisocial behavior since the age of 15.

○ **What associated psychiatric, neurologic, and intellectual vulnerabilities would suggest that a diagnosis other than antisocial behavior would be more appropriate?**

Neurologic impairment, below average general intellectual functioning, psychotic symptoms, and isolated discrete episodes of disinhibition.

○ **Who originally coined the term "psychopathic"?**

Koch, in 1891, first introduced the term. Although originally intended to describe a seriously impaired person, Kurt Schneider (1959) adopted the term to refer to antisocial people who were not considered to be psychiatrically ill.

○ **What social factors contribute to antisocial behavior?**

Availability of handguns, poverty, lack of education, and substance abuse.

○ **What family characteristics have been associated with the development of antisocial behavior?**

Lack of parenting skills, physical abuse and family discord, and a history of alcoholism in the parents.

○ **What psychotic symptom is most frequently associated with violent behavior?**

Paranoid ideation.

○ **What is the prevalence of adult antisocial behavior?**

The prevalence of antisocial behavior in the general population varies from 5% to 15%, depending on the criteria used. Within the prison population, prevalence figures of 20% to 80% are reported. Men account for more antisocial behavior than women.

○ **Is there a genetic basis for violent behavior?**

There appears to be no specific chromosomal abnormality that accounts for antisocial behavior (including sex chromosome abnormalities).

○ **How do you distinguish antisocial behavior from intermittent explosive disorder?**

Intermittent explosive disorder, an impulse control disorder, is manifested by discrete episodes of loss of control. There are few or no signs of general impulsiveness or aggressiveness between episodes. The person is remorseful and worried about the consequences of their actions.

○ **How is antisocial behavior manifested in schizophrenia and other psychotic disorders?**

Symptoms of psychotic disorganization and extreme agitation may result in antisocial behavior. Patients with psychotic disorders may have a low frustration level. Akathisia resulting as a side effect of antipsychotic medication may be a contributing factor. Antisocial behavior attributed to this would not receive a separate *DSM-IV* diagnosis.

○ **How is adult antisocial behavior differentiated from antisocial acts of substance-related disorders?**

In a substance-related disorder, the antisocial behavior only occurs in the context of disinhibition and impaired judgment from substance intoxication or emotional lability from substance withdrawal, and the behavior is not present during periods of sobriety.

○ **What diagnosis do you give to a 16-year-old patient with an antisocial personality?**

Conduct disorder. Although the diagnosis of antisocial personality disorder requires antisocial symptoms to have been present since the age of 15 years, the antisocial personality disorder diagnosis cannot be made until the age of 18 years.

○ **What is the difference between a psychopath, a sociopath, and a person with antisocial personality disorder?**

Basically none. Historically, these terms were distinguished from one another in various ways, but today they are mostly used interchangeably. Antisocial personality disorder, which is a behaviorally based diagnosis, is thought to be more reliable, and more inclusive, than the diagnoses of psychopath or sociopath.

○ **In order to be diagnosed with antisocial personality disorder, does an individual have to have a criminal record?**

No.

○ **What are the most common defense mechanisms used by people with borderline personality disorder?**

Splitting, denial, projection, projective identification, acting out, idealization, and devaluation.

○ **What CNS structure is consistently different in borderline personality-disordered patients with a history of trauma?**

The amygdala is consistently reduced in volume, which is associated with hyperactivity of the amygdala. The hypothalamic pituitary adrenal axis has also been shown to be hyperactive in these individuals.

○ **How can you distinguish the affective abnormalities in someone with borderline personality disorder from someone with bipolar disorder?**

The mood changes of bipolar patients typically take place over the course of days, weeks, or months, whereas borderline patients have affective instability with intense dysphoria, irritability, or anxiety that usually lasts a few hours and rarely more than a few days. While not always true, the affective changes in patients with borderline disorder are typically reactive to interpersonal events; the mood changes of bipolar disorder tend to be more independent of interpersonal relations.

○ **What does the "borderline" of borderline personality disorder mean?**

Historically, "borderline personality" was used to describe individuals with both neurotic and psychotic symptoms and who were considered to be on the borderline between neurosis and psychosis.

○ **Give some examples of the identity disturbance of borderline personality disorder.**

Examples of the unstable self-image of a person with borderline personality disorder may include such areas as sexuality (straight, gay, bisexual), occupation (lawyer, carpenter, astrophysicist, pizza chef), or politics (democrat, republican, socialist).

○ **What are the typical defense mechanisms operative in histrionic individuals?**

The three most prominent defense mechanisms are repression, sexualization, and regression.

○ **Give some examples of the grandiose fantasies of people with narcissistic personality disorder.**

"I'm the strongest, smartest, handsomest, richest, most gifted, most successful person on earth and you're not."

○ **Describe the feeling of being "special" that is typical of those with narcissistic personality disorder.**

"When I'm sick, which I almost never am, I never speak to a medical student or a resident, only the Chief of Staff" or "I'd never join that club; anybody can get in" or "You don't appreciate my thesis because only Stephen Hawking, Richard Feynman, or Albert Einstein could understand it."

○ **What is "entitlement"?**

Entitlement is an unreasonable expectation of especially favorable treatment or automatic compliance with one's expectations. "I want this book and you should give it to me without my having to pay for it" or "Only the little people have to pay taxes" or "Of course you'll play golf with me today as we planned, even though you broke both your arms yesterday in an auto accident."

○ **Describe Westen's three subtypes of narcissistic personality disorders (Russ et al. 2008).**

The high functioning/exhibitionist narcissist, the fragile narcissist, and the grandiose/malignant narcissist.

○ **How are the defense mechanisms of idealization and devaluation manifested in narcissistically disordered individuals?**

These defenses complement and mutually reinforce one another such that when the individual's self is idealized and other persons are devalued, and vice versa.

○ **What is the difference between persons with schizoid personality disorder and avoidant personality disorder?**

People with schizoid personality disorder live an isolated life style without any desire for close interpersonal relationships, and they appear to be indifferent to the praise or criticism of others. In contrast, people with avoidant personality disorder, while appearing shy and timid, very much want to have relationships with other people; they are, however, very sensitive to criticism or rejection and they view themselves as socially inept or personally unappealing.

○ **What is the difference between the abandonment fears of borderlines and those of persons with dependent personality disorder?**

Not much. They both fear being abandoned and both may engage in a whole range of maladaptive behaviors in order to prevent being left by another person. Persons with avoidant personality disorder, however, lack the other maladaptive features typically associated with borderline personality disorder.

○ **What is the relationship between obsessive-compulsive disorder (OCD) and obsessive-compulsive personality disorder (OCPD)?**

By definition, to be diagnosed with OCD, a person must have obsessions and/or compulsions; the preoccupation with orderliness, perfection, and mental and interpersonal control of OCPD is not required. Similarly, a diagnosis of OCPD does not require either obsessions or compulsions. In reality, however, OCD and OCPD symptoms can coexist in a given individual, and a person may be given both diagnoses if he or she meets the criteria for both.

○ **What are some of the defense mechanisms most frequently used by individuals with OCPD?**

Intellectualization, rationalization, isolation of affect, reaction formation, displacement, and undoing. Obsessive traits are particularly associated with isolation of affect, while compulsive traits are characterized by the defense mechanism of undoing. Individuals with OCPD often have difficulty recognizing or acknowledging their own anger, and they fear losing control of it; thus, reaction formation and displacement of anger are common OCPD defenses.

○ **If Sigmund Freud were alive today, what would he think of the *DSM-IV* diagnosis of OCPD?**

The *DSM-IV* OCPD diagnosis is the heir to Freud's anal character or anal personality, which consisted of the triad of orderliness, parsimony (reluctance to part with things), and obstinacy. Freud saw these traits as reaction formations to unconscious desires to be disorderly, dirty, messy, profligate, rebellious, and out of control.

○ **How does someone with OCPD feel about morals, ethics, and values?**

He is all for them and applies them rigidly.

○ **What is the principle issue for someone with OCPD in his or her interpersonal relationships?**

Control. People with OCPD are determined to remain in control themselves and to control those around them. They tend to be very sensitive to position and status, paying close attention to who is up and who is down and where they stand in relation to others.

○ **What is the course and prognosis of personality disorders?**

By definition, personality disorders are stable and enduring over time, but this does not mean that they are immutable. Even without therapeutic intervention, some personality disorders appear to become less evident or "burn out" over time (e.g., antisocial and borderline), whereas others remain more-or-less constant (e.g., obsessive-compulsive and schizotypal), and still others may become more marked with age (e.g., dependent and narcissistic). The decrease in severity of expression of certain personality disorders with aging is often the result of accumulating corrective experiences and/or biologic changes.

○ **Are there other things, besides age, that may favorably alter the symptoms and/or course of personality disorders?**

New experiences, fortunate interpersonal relationships, favorable life circumstances, good luck, and a desire to change for the better (either for oneself or for a loved one such as a child or significant other).

○ **How about psychotherapy?**

A variety of psychotherapeutic modalities have been used with varying success. Dialectical behavior therapy, supportive and cognitive-behavioral psychotherapy appear to be generally useful; and, with some personality-disordered individuals, psychodynamic psychotherapy, psychoanalysis, group therapy, and couples/family therapy may also be effective. As with all patients and all therapeutic interventions, psychotherapy techniques with personality-disordered patients may be unhelpful or even counterproductive if not appropriately chosen and applied.

○ **How about psychopharmacology?**

Psychotropic medications, like psychotherapeutic interventions, have been variably successful in the treatment of personality-disordered individuals. No medication has been shown, by itself, to specifically and significantly alter the symptoms or course of any given personality disorder. Nevertheless, various drugs may be beneficial in ameliorating particular symptoms. For example, neuroleptics may be of benefit in the treatment of thought abnormalities and dissociative symptoms; antidepressants and mood stabilizing drugs may control bothersome affective symptomatology; and anxiolytics may reduce anxiety symptoms. When psychotropic medications are considered for use with personality-disordered individuals, they should be targeted to specific, identifiable symptoms, and they should only be used in the dosages and duration necessary.

○ **Just how "treatable" are personality disorders?**

By definition, personality disorders are stable and enduring over time. Multimodal psychiatric interventions have been shown to bring considerable, and even long-lasting, relief to some personality-disordered individuals. However, there is no evidence at this time that personality disorders can be "cured." Treatment of personality disorders is often difficult and may require much time (e.g., years) for significant alterations to occur and become relatively permanent.

○ **What are some of the biopsychosocial management principles useful for treating personality-disordered individuals?**

- Clarification of short-term and long-term treatment goals.
- Provision of structure
- Appropriate limit setting
- Environmental manipulation
- Crisis intervention
- Psychiatric hospitalization
- Milieu therapy
- Psychotherapy (individual, group, and couples/family; dialectical behavior therapy, supportive, cognitive-behavioral, interpersonal, and dynamic).
- Diagnosis and treatment of comorbid conditions (e.g., Axis I disorders including alcoholism and substance abuse/dependence).
- Management of transference and countertransference
- Symptom-targeted pharmacotherapy

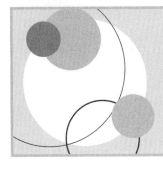

Section III

SPECIAL TOPICS

CHAPTER 17
Psychiatric Issues Related to Acquired Immunodeficiency Syndrome (AIDS)

○ **What are the characteristics of human immunodeficiency virus (HIV) encephalopathy?**

It is characterized by cognitive, affective, behavioral, and motor dysfunction, with impairments in attention, memory, motor speed, cognitive flexibility, time pressure, and problem solving.

○ **In what percentage of AIDS patients is HIV encephalopathy seen?**

Up to 75% by the time of death.

○ **What are the neuropathologic findings of HIV encephalopathy?**

Multinucleated giant cells, microglial nodules, diffuse astrocytosis, perivascular lymphocyte cuffing, cortical atrophy, white matter vacuolation, and demyelination.

○ **What do PET and SPECT scans show in HIV encephalopathy?**

Hypermetabolism of basal ganglia in early HIV; subcortical and cortical hypometabolism in the later stages.

○ **In autopsies performed on patients with AIDS, what percentages show involvement of the brain?**

It is 75% to 90%.

○ **Which agents may reverse or delay the progression of cognitive impairment seen in HIV encephalopathy?**

Zidovudine and possibly protease inhibitors.

○ **What are the major issues regarding counseling of persons about HIV serum testing?**

Issues regarding HIV serum testing include who should be tested, why a particular person should be (or not be) tested, what the test results signify, and what the implications are.

○ **What are the major psychodynamic themes for HIV patients?**

Guilt, punishment, and death.

○ **Should all HIV-positive psychotherapy groups be homogeneous?**

Not necessarily. In groups consisting of patients at various stages of HIV, sicker patients can act as role models by demonstrating coping skills for less ill members.

○ **What aspects of an HIV patient's premorbid history are important psychosocial factors to know prior to starting psychotherapy?**

Important psychosocial factors to inquire about include past suicide attempts, history of substance abuse, coping mechanisms, past and current sexual history, and available support systems.

○ **Name some medications used for HIV that can cause anxiety.**

Foscarnet, pentamidine (can induce hypoglycemia), atovaquone, amikacin, dronabinol, and interferon α-2a can all cause anxiety.

○ **Name some medications used for HIV that can induce mania.**

Medications used in the treatment of HIV-positive patients that can cause mania include zidovudine, dapsone, ciprofloxacin, isoniazid, didanosine, d4T, corticosteroids, ganciclovir, and procarbazine.

○ **Name some medications used for HIV that can induce psychosis.**

Medications that can induce psychosis include dapsone, pentamidine, trimethoprim/sulfamethoxazole, acyclovir, foscarnet, ganciclovir, ketoconazole/itraconazole, amikacin, ciprofloxacin, cycloserine, ethambutol, isoniazid, dronabinol, corticosteroids, thiabendazole, and vincristine.

○ **Name some medications used for HIV that may cause depression.**

Didanosine, zidovudine (AZT), dapsone, pentamidine, trimethoprim/sulfamethoxazole, acyclovir, foscarnet, ketoconazole/itraconazole, amikacin, ciprofloxacin, clofazimine, cycloserine, isoniazid, interferon α-2a, co-trimoxazole, corticosteroids, vincristine, and vinblastine may all contribute to a depressed state.

○ **Name some medications used for HIV that can induce a delirium.**

Pentamidine, trimethoprim/sulfamethoxazole, acyclovir, foscarnet, ganciclovir, amphotericin B, ciprofloxacin, ethambutol, procarbazine, isoniazid, rifampin, interferon, methotrexate (high dose), vincristine, vinblastine, and corticosteroids can all cause delirium.

○ **What are the common causes of delirium, other than medications, in HIV patients?**

Substance intoxication or withdrawal, hypoxia, anemia, CNS opportunistic infections, neoplasms (primary CNS lymphoma), seizures, and metabolic disturbances may also be causes of delirium in HIV patients.

○ **What is the pharmacologic treatment of delirium in HIV-positive patients?**

Low doses of Haldol (0.5–5.0 mg/d) in combination with lorazepam (0.5–2.0 mg/d) or other benzodiazepines with short half-lives and no active metabolites is usually an effective treatment for delirium in HIV patients. Care should be taken when benzodiazepines are administered as paradoxical agitation, with exacerbation of delirium, may occur in a small percentage of patients.

○ **A patient with a CD$_4$ count of 200 has sudden changes in mental status. What is the differential diagnosis?**

The differential diagnosis should include CNS opportunistic infections, neoplasm, drug-related toxicity, anemia, substance abuse, metabolic problems, and Axis I psychiatric disorders.

○ **A patient with a CD$_4$ count of 20 presents with confusion, flu-like illness, and meningeal signs. What would be the important diagnostic tests?**

Brain imaging studies, viral titers levels, spinal tap, and a toxicology screen.

○ **What are some common causes of sudden mental status changes in a patient with human immunodeficiency virus (HIV) and herpes infection?**

HIV encephalitis, AZT treatment, and aseptic meningitis.

○ **What is the differential diagnosis of mania in an HIV patient?**

The differential diagnosis includes CNS opportunistic infection/tumors, primary psychiatric illness, concurrent substance abuse including steroids and cocaine, metabolic disturbances, seizures, and medications, such as AZT.

○ **What are some consequences of untreated mania in a patient with AIDS?**

Consequences of untreated mania in AIDS patients may result in noncompliance with medications, sexual hyperactivity with subsequent spreading of the virus, impaired judgment, and poor impulse control.

○ **Can lithium toxicity develop in HIV patients with therapeutic blood levels of lithium?**

Yes, this hypersensitivity may be associated with an HIV-related compromise of the blood–brain barrier integrity, exposing the CNS to greater levels of lithium.

○ **What are the problems of treating HIV mania with Depakote?**

Although Depakote is safe in combination with most antiretroviral medications, it is known to cause elevated levels of AZT. It also causes thrombocytopenia, increased LFTs, neurotoxicity, and interacts with aspirin.

○ **What are the problems of using carbamazepine in AIDS mania?**

Carbamazepine induces hepatic enzymes. This decreases serum levels of coadministered drugs including AZT. Also, patients are at a high risk of hematologic and dermatologic complications. Particular patients may develop suppression of bone marrow, further exacerbating the low WBC count characteristic of the illness.

○ **How common is major depression in HIV/AIDS patients?**

Major depression is diagnosed in 5% to 15% of HIV/AIDS patients who are hospitalized and seen by psychiatrists.

○ **Is major depression a "normal" consequence of HIV disease?**

No.

○ **What are common psychosocial factors related to the presence of major depression in persons with AIDS?**

Common psychosocial factors include rejection by family and friends, recent notification of AIDS, loss of autonomy, unemployment, low education level, unresolved grief, and loss of friends who may also be HIV positive. A premorbid history of mood disorders, psychoactive substance abuse, dementia, and delirium may also increase the risk for depression.

○ **What laboratory tests should be ordered in patients with depression and HIV?**

If asymptomatic or with CD_4 lymphocyte counts greater than 500/UL, few tests are required. For symptomatic HIV infection and counts <500/UL, obtain a CBC, electrolytes, fasting glucose, LFTs, TSH and free T3, vitamin B_{12}, free testosterone, Treponema serology, and possibly head CT/MRI.

○ **Is there a relationship between CD_4 lymphocyte counts and depression in patients who are HIV positive?**

Possibly, because such patients may have a more rapid decline in counts. However, this finding has not been consistently replicated in other studies.

○ **What are the common endocrinologic and metabolic disturbances contributing to depression in AIDS?**

Adrenocortical insufficiency, euthyroid sick syndrome, vitamin B_{12} deficiency, hypogonadism and hypotestosterone states, and protein/calorie malnutrition may all exacerbate depression in a person with AIDS.

○ **How does one titrate an antidepressant in an HIV-positive patient?**

Start with the lowest dose available, increasing every 5 to 7 days. The effective daily dose is usually half that of healthy adults.

○ **What are the problems of treating AIDS depression with an SSRI?**

Aside from the common side effects of gastrointestinal upset, headache, anxiety, sexual side effects, agitation, extrapyramidal side effects (which occur with greater frequency in persons with AIDS), SSRIs are heavily protein bound causing elevation of other drugs (e.g., warfarin) by displacement. Inhibition of cytochrome P-450 enzymes (3A4 and 2D6) can also lead to elevation of drug levels.

○ **What are some problems associated with the use of tricyclic antidepressants (TCAs) in HIV patients?**

Patients with HIV are more prone to the common side effects of TCAs, including hypotension, anticholinergic side effects such as urinary retention and confusion, cardiac side effects, and sedation. Of note is that the side effect of xerostomia predisposes HIV patients to oral candidiasis.

○ **What are the main concerns in treating an HIV-positive patient with maprotiline or bupropion?**

HIV-infected patients are at increased risk for seizures, and these agents lower the seizure threshold.

○ **Prior to treating an HIV-positive patient with ECT, what should be evaluated carefully?**

Contraindications to the use of ECT, especially in HIV patients, include the presence of preexisting confusion, increased intracranial pressure (CT to rule out toxoplasmosis, lymphoma), cardiac abnormalities, and electrolyte abnormalities ($\downarrow$Na).

○ **When are stimulants used in AIDS patients?**

Stimulants may be used for HIV-related major depression, as a primary agent, or as an adjuvant. Low doses are effective for anergia, apathy, and anorexia.

○ **Does a past history of substance abuse contraindicate stimulant abuse?**

No, but increased caution is required.

○　**What are the prevalent methods of suicide among AIDS patients?**

Poisoning with drugs (35%), use of firearms (25%), and suffocation (13%) are some of the means whereby AIDS patients commit suicide.

○　**What are the major risk factors for suicide in AIDS?**

Social isolation, gay youths, Caucasian race, psychoactive substance abuse, and financial/occupational problems are risk factors for suicide in the AIDS population.

○　**What aspects of AIDS increase the risk of suicide?**

The presence of coexisting psychiatric disorders, impulsivity, and psychosocial stressors can increase the risk for suicide in AIDS patients. AIDS is associated with psychiatric illnesses that are themselves linked to risk factors for suicide including depression and psychosis, as well as drug and alcohol abuse. Impulsive suicidal behaviors in AIDS can be related to cognitive disorders secondary to HIV encephalitis and opportunistic infections. Other suicide risks related to AIDS include chronic pain, marked decline in physical functioning and activities of daily living, disfigurement, unemployment, loss of financial and social supports, stigmatization, and loss of autonomy.

○　**Is HIV infection a risk factor for suicide?**

This is controversial. While a 1985 study completed in New York City showed a 36-fold increase in suicide with men who had AIDS, a later study showed that HIV-positive military service applicants did not have a significantly greater risk of suicide in the months following HIV screening. Also, another study of HIV seroprevalence among suicide victims in New York City from 1991 to 1993 showed that a positive HIV serostatus is associated with, at most, a modest elevation in suicide risk. Nonetheless, clinicians should carefully assess for suicidality in all HIV-positive patients.

○　**What factors can precipitate suicidal ideation in an HIV-positive patient?**

Suicidal ideation may be precipitated by a concomitant psychiatric syndrome (depression), medication side effects (infection, steroids), response to a specific crisis or stressor, loss of control or functioning, pain, loss of significant others, and fear of abandonment.

○　**How are anxiety disorders treated in AIDS patients?**

Buspirone may be considered in substance abusers, although it may be ineffective if there is prior exposure to benzodiazepines. Otherwise, a benzodiazepine with high potency and a short half-life can be considered. Psychotherapy (cognitive-behavioral, psychodynamic, or interpersonal) is also a valuable adjunct to pharmacotherapy.

○　**What is the percentage of HIV-positive patients who suffer from sleep problems?**

Eighty percent.

○　**What are the drawbacks of prescribing benzodiazepines to HIV-positive patients?**

The side effects of confusion, abuse, tolerance, and disinhibition, as well as accumulation with long half-life medications, and interaction with protease inhibitors limits the efficacy of benzodiazepines in HIV-positive patients.

○ **A patient with AIDS, previously stable on AZT is started on methadone. He has headaches and gets extremely restless, irritable, and agitated. What may be a possible factor?**

Methadone increases AZT levels to toxic doses, which is manifested by the above symptoms.

○ **An HIV-positive patient on methadone maintenance is hospitalized and diagnosed with tuberculosis. He is started on isoniazid, rifampin, ethambutol, and pyrazinamide. He complains of diarrhea, sweating, anxiety, and insomnia. What is the possible reason?**

The patient may be in opiate withdrawal. Treatment with rifampin increases methadone metabolism.

○ **Why should one not simultaneously prescribe different narcotic analgesics to treat pain experienced by HIV-positive patients?**

Use of multiple analgesics often results in an increased likelihood of toxicity rather than enhancement of analgesia.

○ **If an HIV-positive patient with pain becomes refractory to increasing doses of a narcotic analgesic, what may one do next?**

Switch to longer-acting agents such as methadone or controlled release morphine, or consider hydromorphone. Adjuvant use of stimulants, neuroleptics, tricyclic antidepressants (with or without depression), or anticonvulsants may enhance analgesia.

○ **What are the drawbacks to the use of meperidine in the HIV population?**

Disadvantages of meperidine use in HIV patients include meperidine's short duration of action and normeperidine toxicity manifested as CNS toxicity (normeperidine is the active metabolite of meperidine).

○ **What are the common causes of dementia in an HIV-infected patient?**

CNS infection, CNS neoplasms, and CNS responses to drugs are frequent causes of dementia in HIV patients.

○ **What are the cognitive deficits of AIDS dementia complex (ADC)?**

Cognitive deficits of ADC include loss of fine motor speed and control, decreased concentration and attention, and reduced executive function and visuospatial performance, as well as short-term memory loss, word finding difficulty, and difficulty with sequential tasks.

○ **In evaluating patients for ADC, which neuropsychological areas should be tested?**

Essentially, a complete neuropsychological evaluation is indicated with careful assessment of attention and concentration, processing speed, motor functioning, abstraction, reasoning, visuospatial skills, memory, learning, and speech and language capabilities.

○ **In screening for ADC, which neuropsychological bedside screening tests may be more helpful than the Folstein Mini-Mental Status Exam?**

Trail making tests A and B, finger tapping tests, Rey auditory verbal learning test, and verbal fluency tests may be more sensitive indicators of cognitive and motor deficits than the Folstein.

○ **In assessing neuropsychological deficits in HIV-positive patients who are asymptomatic, what must the clinician account for?**

Deficits in these patients may not be secondary to HIV but rather due to a prior history of substance abuse, preexisting psychiatric disorders (e.g., the pseudodementia of depression), prior head injuries, and medication use.

○ **Can one make the diagnosis of ADC on MRI?**

No. MRI and CT scans may often show cortical atrophy, ventricular enlargement, and/or demyelination within white matter, but these findings are not diagnostic. ADC is a clinical diagnosis.

○ **What problems are associated with the use of neuroleptics in the HIV population?**

Extreme sensitivity to extrapyramidal side effects (EPS) including akathisia, pseudoparkinsonism, and an increased risk for neuroleptic malignant syndrome limit the use of neuroleptics in the HIV-positive population.

○ **Describe the benefits of intravenous administration of haloperidol to control symptoms of delirium in patients with HIV.**

Intravenous administration of haloperidol in HIV-positive patients is advantageous because of the reduced incidence of EPS (mechanism unknown), reduced risk of abscess and pain, and avoidance of intramuscular injections, which are contraindicated when hemostasis is compromised. (These benefits also apply to the general population as well.)

○ **An HIV-infected mother delivers a baby. What are the symptoms related to HIV that may be seen in the baby?**

Pseudobulbar palsy, microcephaly, weakness, extrapyramidal rigidity, and seizures.

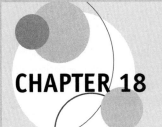

CHAPTER 18

Consultation Liaison Psychiatry

○ **What are the most common psychiatric disorders in patients who are dying?**

Anxiety disorders, depression, and delirium.

○ **What conditions might produce anxiety or restlessness?**

Hypoxia, sepsis, delirium from any cause, and any psychiatric disturbances.

○ **Why are neurovegetative symptoms such as fatigue and loss of energy not helpful in diagnosing depression in terminally ill patients?**

The illness may be producing the symptoms instead of reflecting the patient's mental status.

○ **What pharmacologic agents are used in patients whose dysphoric mood is associated with severe psychomotor slowing and cognitive impairment?**

Psychostimulants are frequently used because they have a rapid onset of action; improve attention, concentration, and overall performance on neuropsychiatric tests; improve appetite; counter feelings of weakness and fatigue; and increase the patient's sense of well-being.

○ **How significant is depression and suicide in the terminally ill patient?**

Depression is a factor in 50% of all suicides. Patients with depression are at 25 times greater risk of suicide than the general population. Hopelessness is the key variable that links depression and suicide.

○ **Why is social support important for terminally ill patients?**

The presence of a strong support system for the terminally ill patient may act as an external source of control and significantly reduce the risk of suicide, especially when family members and health care providers may withdraw prematurely from the dying patient.

○ **What is the difference between euthanasia and physician-assisted suicide?**

The intentional termination of a patient's life by an individual defines euthanasia. Physician-assisted suicide is the provision by a physician of the means by which patients can end their own lives. Passive euthanasia refers to the withholding or withdrawal of life-sustaining measures.

○ **What are the roles of the consultation-liaison psychiatrist in treating patients with terminal illnesses?**

The consultation-liaison psychiatrist has a multidimensional role in the treatment of terminal illness. In addition to recommendations regarding control of comorbid psychiatric disorders (anxiety, depression, and delirium), pain and physical symptoms, the psychiatrist often provides psychotherapy for anticipatory bereavement of the patient and the survivors, and may, at times, participate in the ethical decision-making process regarding end-of-life decisions such as resuscitation, withdrawal of life support, and evaluation of requests for physician-assisted suicide.

○ **What are significant risk factors for suicide among patients with terminal illness?**

Risk factors for suicide among patients with terminal illness include depression and hopelessness, debilitating illness, uncontrolled pain, delirium and disinhibition, previous history of depression and/or suicide attempts, a family history of depression, lack of social supports, a history of substance abuse, feelings of being a burden on others and recent loss or bereavement.

○ **What are some psychiatric complications that patients develop during the course of surgical treatment?**

Operative syndromes range from acute psychotic episodes to addiction, suicidal depression, disruptive behavior, and delirium.

○ **What psychological stressors are inherent in any surgical situation?**

Basic threat to bodily and psychic integrity, fears of the unknown, loss of identity and control, and fear of pain and death.

○ **What are some techniques known to reduce patient distress?**

Self-guided relaxation exercises, pharmacologic intervention, rehearsal, desensitization and orientation to the hospital environment.

○ **What is Munchausen syndrome?**

Categorized in the *DSM-IV* as factitious disorder with predominantly physical symptoms, Munchausen syndrome is a factitious disorder in which there is intentional feigning of physical symptoms and a need to assume the sick role. In contrast to malingering, patients with Munchausen's syndrome are not motivated in their behaviors by economic incentives. Munchausen's syndrome often occurs in people with severe character pathology, a history of mood disorders and/or childhood abuse, and an actual history of a physical disorder during childhood.

○ **What problems might arise in psychiatric patients who are abruptly withdrawn from psychotropic medications before surgery?**

Acute withdrawal of many psychotropic medications can precipitate a number of withdrawal syndromes. Malignant arrhythmias can occur upon withdrawal from heterocyclics and butyrophenones, while SSRI withdrawal can precipitate serotonergic withdrawal. Cholinergic rebound occurs upon discontinuation of conventional heterocyclics and phenothiazines, while withdrawal seizures can occur with abrupt discontinuation of clozapine. Finally, delirium and/or psychosis can occur upon abrupt discontinuation of MAOIs.

○ **What factors might complicate psychopharmacologic interventions postoperatively?**

Factors that may complicate postoperative medication management include NPO orders, compromised gastrointestinal absorption, altered hemostasis, and perioperative myocardial infarctions or stroke.

○ **What might be seen perioperatively relating to unforeseen substance withdrawal?**

Perioperative symptoms of substance withdrawal may include hyperthermia, hypertension, hypotension, seizures, hallucinations, respiratory changes, and delirium.

○ **What are some causes of preoperative cognitive disturbances?**

Microemboli from diseased valves or chronic atrial fibrillation, long-standing arrhythmias, hypotension, congestive heart failure, or asystolic arrest may all cause subtle CNS dysfunction.

○ **What characteristics of borderline personality disorder make treatment of such patients difficult?**

Characteristics of patients with borderline personality disorder that hamper medical care include the presence of intense affect, a history of impulsive behavior, superficial social adaptiveness, a history of brief psychotic episodes under stress, loose thinking in situations of too little structure, and relationships that vacillate between transient superficiality and intense dependency.

○ **What psychological side effects might be caused by β-blockers?**

Depression, anergia, suicidal ideation, hallucinations, lethargy, confusion, and impotence are reported side effects of β-blockers.

○ **What ophthalmic complications may result from psychotropic medications?**

Ophthalmic complications associated with psychotropics include anticholinergic effects and acute angle closure glaucoma from TCAs/neuroleptics, blindness with thioridazine doses >800 mg/d secondary to retinitis pigmentosa, anterior cataracts with chlorpromazine and oculogyric crisis with lithium and neuroleptics.

○ **What are some risk factors for burn injuries?**

Alcoholism, cognitive degeneration or dementia in elderly patients, chronic mental illness, and family dysfunction are common risk factors in burn patients.

○ **What percentage of burn patients develop delirium?**

Thirty to seventy percent of burn patients develop delirium within the first 24 to 72 hours after the burn, presumably from stress and burn-induced metabolic disturbances.

○ **What are some psychiatric complications from postoperative cosmetic surgery?**

Severe depression, anxiety, isolation, and withdrawal may occur after cosmetic surgery.

○ **What potential psychiatric conditions does an "insatiable" cosmetic surgery patient reveal?**

Borderline personality and/or body dysmorphic disorder.

○ **What is delirium?**

An organically caused, nonspecific, global cerebral dysfunction, characterized by concurrent disturbances of level of consciousness, attention, thinking, perception, memory, psychomotor behavior, emotion, and the sleep–wake cycle.

○ **What six groups of patients are at increased risk for delirium?**

1. Elderly patients

2. Postcardiotomy patients

3. Burn patients

4. Patients with preexisting brain damage (dementia or stroke)

5. Drug-dependent patients experiencing withdrawal

6. HIV patients

○ **What features describe the prodrome to delirium?**

Restlessness, anxiety, irritability, and disturbances in the sleep–wake cycle may precede delirium.

○ **What are the differential diagnoses for delirium?**

The pneumonic I WATCH DEATH is a helpful aid for remembering the differential diagnosis of delirium.

I—Infection	W—Withdrawal	D—Death
	A—Acute metabolic abnormalities	E—Endocrinopathies
	T—Trauma	A—Acute vascular disease
	C—CNS pathology	T—Toxins
	H—Hypoxia	H—Heavy metals

○ **What pharmacologic agents might be responsible for inducing delirium?**

Many drugs may cause delirium. In particular, narcotic analgesics such as levorphanol, morphine, and meperidine, and the chemotherapeutics methotrexate, fluorouracil, vincristine, vinblastine, bleomycin, carmustine, cisplatin, asparaginase, procarbazine, and glucocorticosteroid are notorious for induction of delirium.

○ **What is the drug of choice for treating delirium in the medically ill patient?**

Haloperidol, a potent dopamine blocker, is given 1 to 3 mg every 1 to 4 hours po, IV, subcutaneously, or IM. Commonly, lorazepam 0.5 to 1 mg every 12 hours is given along with haloperidol, which is more effective than haloperidol alone in rapidly sedating an agitated patient with delirium. However, one must be aware of the risk for additional paradoxical agitation known to occur with benzodiazepines.

○ **Describe the characteristics of AIDS dementia complex (ADC), a common neurologic complication of AIDS.**

ADC is characterized by disturbances in motor performance, cognition, and behavior. Cognitive impairment includes memory impairment, mental slowing, and impaired concentration. Motor impairment includes clumsiness, unsteady gait, tremor, and impaired handwriting. Behavioral changes include apathy, withdrawal, depression, and anxiety.

○ **How do neuropsychiatric tests distinguish ADC from major depression or adjustment disorder?**

ADC is generally referred to as subcortical dementia characterized by impaired fine and rapid motor movement, difficulty with complex sequencing, reduced verbal fluency, impaired short-term memory, diminished visual–motor and visual–spatial abilities, and impaired integrated sequential problem solving. In contrast, feelings of helplessness, passivity, and loss usually accompany the depressed state of adjustment disorders, while anhedonia, insomnia, psychomotor retardation, loss of energy, indecisiveness, decreased ability to think and/or concentrate, and suicidal ideation are associated with major depression.

○ **What are some adjuvant medications used in pain management?**

SSRIs, SNRIs, TCAs, psychostimulants, neuroleptics, and anxiolytics are all effective as adjuvant medications for the treatment of pain.

○ **What type of dosing schedule is preferred in pain management?**

Around the clock dosing is preferred over *prn* dosing, because it is thought to prevent breakthrough pain and decrease the need for higher doses of medication if breakthrough pain occurs.

○ **What group of women are at greatest risk of psychiatric illness after an induced abortion?**

Women at greatest risk for psychiatric illness after an abortion include those who are not permitted to make an autonomous choice, those aborting due to genetic defects diagnosed in the fetus, and those with prior or current psychiatric illness.

○ **What developmental period is most sensitive to teratogenic agents?**

The embryonic period from the third to eighth week of gestation.

○ **What is the prevalence of prescription use in pregnant women?**

Eighty percent of pregnant women are prescribed medication and more than a third may take psychotropics at some time during their pregnancy.

○ **What changes occur during pregnancy that may alter serum concentrations of psychotropic medications?**

There are many physiological changes of pregnancy that may alter the metabolism of psychotropic medications. Elevation of drug plasma levels may be caused by delayed gastric emptying (which increases absorption), lower levels of protein binding, and decreased renal clearance secondary to a reduced glomerular filtration rate. Conversely, the increased volume of distribution and increased rate of hepatic metabolism associated with pregnancy may lower serum concentrations of many medications.

○ **What is the mechanism of placental transport?**

Simple diffusion. It is dependent on several properties of the substance including molecular size, percent protein binding, polarity, and lipid solubility.

○ **What distinctive physiological attributes of the fetus contribute susceptibility to CNS drug exposure?**

Increased cardiac output, increased blood–brain barrier permeability, lower levels of plasma proteins and binding affinity, and lower hepatic enzyme activity, all result in a net increase in fetal CNS drug exposure and concentration.

○   **What considerations must be given concerning the neonate when treating a pregnant woman with medications?**

The glucuronidation and oxidation systems of the neonate are immature at birth and may operate at only 20% of the adult level. Also, glomerular filtration is 30% to 40% lower than adult levels and tubular secretion is 20% to 30% lower than adult levels. Therefore, the neonate may be exposed to high serum concentrations of the parent compound and/or metabolites.

○   **Fifty percent of new mothers plan to nurse. What mechanism accounts for excretion of drugs into breast milk?**

Passive diffusion of the unionized and unbound plasma fraction as well as the pH gradient between the maternal serum and breast milk are the major determinants of the quantity of drug passed to the newborn.

○   **What are the categorical risks of psychotropic medication use during pregnancy and lactation?**

Somatic teratogenicity, neurobehavioral teratogenicity, direct toxic effects, drug effects on labor and delivery, and effects on the breast feeding infant.

○   **What are the FDA use-in-pregnancy ratings?**

- A—controlled studies show no risk.
- B—no evidence of risk in humans.
- C—risk cannot be ruled out.
- D—positive evidence of risk.
- X—contraindicated in pregnancy.

○   **What relative risks to the fetus do the various classes of antidepressants pose?**

In general, TCAs are FDA category C or D, while MAOIs, SSRIs, and SNRIs are all category C. The one antidepressant with known potential for teratogenic risk is paroxetine, which has a 1.5- to 2-fold increased risk for ventricular or atrial septal defects. In addition, the neonate can be at risk for either serotonin toxicity (because of reduced hepatic metabolism) and/or serotonergic withdrawal syndrome.

○   **What relative risks to the fetus do antipsychotics pose?**

Most antipsychotics are category C, except clozapine, which is category B. All agents used to treat EPS are category C.

○   **What risks are associated with the use of antipsychotics during pregnancy?**

Risks associated with the use of antipsychotic medications during pregnancy include limited teratogenicity, neuroleptic malignant syndrome (NMS), and extrapyramidal side effects (EPS). Also, in utero exposure may produce neonatal jaundice and intestinal obstruction postnatally. If the use of antipsychotics is indicated during pregnancy, the piperazine phenothiazines are reported to have the lowest teratogenic potential.

○   **How might agents used to treat EPS be problematic for the neonate?**

Many of the medications used to treat EPS are contraindicated during pregnancy. Diphenhydramine used during the first trimester has been associated with an increased incidence of oral clefts, while amantadine is reported to be teratogenic in animal studies. Benztropine has had case reports of intestinal obstruction, and benzodiazepines have a variety of teratogenic and physiological complications.

○ **Why might the use of benzodiazepines during pregnancy be problematic?**

Benzodiazepines readily cross the placenta and have been found in fetal brain, lung, and heart tissue.

○ **What is the "benzodiazepine exposure syndrome"?**

The benzodiazepine exposure syndrome is characterized by growth retardation, dysmorphism, and mental/psychomotor retardation. Infant withdrawal syndromes have also occurred and may persist up to 3 months postnatally.

○ **Benzodiazepines are generally classified as FDA category D or X, yet may be prescribed during nursing. Why?**

Benzodiazepines have a lower milk-to-maternal serum ratio which may preclude a significant dose from reaching the nursing infant.

○ **What are some good anxiolytic/sedative choices for women during pregnancy?**

Clonazepam is the only category C benzodiazepine. Category C hypnotics include zolpidem tartrate (Ambien®) and chloral hydrate (Noctec®).

○ **Lithium is contraindicated during pregnancy. What other mood stabilizers might be used?**

All mood stabilizing medications except clonazepam carry an increased risk of fetal malformation and potential deleterious effects on cognitive development. Carbamazepine and valproate, in particular, have been linked to neural tube defects.

○ **What mood stabilizer would be preferable for use during breast feeding?**

Carbamazepine and valproic acid have low milk-to-maternal serum ratios, appear at low concentrations in breast milk, and are therefore considered to be compatible with breast feeding.

○ **Define perimenopause.**

The World Health Organization (WHO) defines perimenopause as the 10-year period prior to menopause, while the American College of Obstetrics and Gynecology (ACOG) defines perimenopause as the 5-year period occurring around menopause.

○ **What effects does estrogen have on serotonin?**

Estrogen increases the number of serotonin receptors, increases neuronal reuptake of serotonin and, overall, acts as a serotonin agonist.

○ **What is the difference between postpartum blues, postpartum depression, and postpartum psychosis?**

Approximately 20% to 40% of women report some emotional disturbance or cognitive dysfunction in the postpartum period. Postpartum blues refers to this normal state of sadness, dysphoria, frequent tearfulness, and clinging dependence. Postpartum depression is more severe in that suicidal ideation occurs with feelings of helplessness and worthlessness. In severe cases, it may reach psychotic proportions with hallucinations, delusions, and thoughts of infanticide (approximately 1–2/1000 births).

○ **Estrogen may be protective against what illnesses?**

Alzheimer's disease, cardiovascular disease, osteoporosis, and depression, although there is still controversy surrounding estrogen's protective effects in depression.

○ **List risk factors for the occurrence of depression during pregnancy.**

Marital discord, unwanted pregnancy, and a previous history or family history of depression.

○ **List systemic factors that have been shown to vary during the menstrual phase.**

Pulse, blood pressure, respirations, weight, gastrointestinal transit time, urinary excretion, and arteriolar responsiveness to hormones, catecholamines, and oxytocin.

○ **Define the premenstrual phase.**

The premenstrual phase refers to the late luteal phase of the menstrual cycle (2 weeks prior to the onset of menses).

○ **Define premenstrual syndrome (PMS).**

PMS refers to both the mood and physical symptoms that occur during the late luteal phase and is found in up to 75% of women.

○ **List some medical conditions that are exacerbated premenstrually.**

Migraines, acute porphyria, allergies and asthma, seizures, irritable bowel syndrome, systemic lupus erythematosus, and genital herpes.

○ **List some psychiatric illnesses that worsen premenstrually.**

Depression, OCD, trichotillomania, PTSD, psychosis, eating disorders, and bipolar disorder.

○ **Define premenstrual dysphoric disorder (PMDD).**

PMDD is a severe depressive disorder that occurs in 3% to 5% of women. A diagnosis of PMDD requires the presence of five or more depressive symptoms during the last week of the luteal phase. PMDD resolves after the onset of menses and is absent during the week after menses concludes. It is currently categorized in *DSM-IV* as a depressive disorder NOS.

○ **What treatments have been implicated for PMS/PMDD?**

OCPs (mixed results), SSRIs, buspirone, magnesium, vitamin B_6, exercise, and cognitive-behavioral therapy (CBT).

○ **How do oral contraceptives (OCs) affect the cytochrome P-450 system?**

In general, OCs stimulate the metabolism of conjugatively metabolized drugs and drugs metabolized by glucuronidation and impair clearance of some oxidatively metabolized drugs. Psychotropic drugs that stimulate hepatic metabolism may decrease OC efficacy.

○ **Does progesterone treat PMS?**

No, although it was thought to be effective for many years, placebo-controlled trials have demonstrated no greater efficacy when compared to placebo.

○ **What are the most common complaints of PMS?**

Fatigue, appetite changes and food cravings, depression, and irritability.

○ **What is the pathophysiology of PMS?**

Although estrogen and progesterone levels are important, attempts to find differences in ovarian steroid levels in women with PMS have been inconsistent. Dietary factors and neurotransmitter abnormalities (especially serotonin) are also implicated.

○ **What dietary factors are associated with PMS?**

High consumption of chocolate and alcohol.

○ **What is the incidence of rape?**

Estimates are as high as 15%, with more than half of the victims younger than 18 years.

○ **Why might this figure be underestimated?**

Secrecy surrounding sexual victimization and a limited understanding of rape reduces the rate of disclosure.

○ **Are more rapes perpetrated by strangers or by people that are known by the victim?**

Only 22% of rapes are perpetrated by strangers; 10% by boyfriends or former boyfriends; 29% by "friends" or acquaintances; 9% by husbands or former husbands; 11% by fathers or stepfathers; 16% by other relatives; and 3% are not identified.

○ **Define sexual assault.**

Sexual assault is any unwanted sexual contact in which an unwilling participant is coerced by physical force, violence or threats of violence, abandonment, financial, or emotional punishment.

○ **What psychological aspects are typically seen in someone who has recently been sexually assaulted?**

Helplessness, terror, isolation, feelings of degradation, and abandonment.

○ **What major tasks should a physician accomplish when examining a sexual assault victim?**

During the examination of a sexual assault victim, the physician collects evidence if consent is obtained, treats injuries, and assesses for the possibility of pregnancy and the potential for sexually transmitted diseases.

○ **What prognostic indicators exist for victims of sexual assault and how they will respond to trauma?**

Younger and married victims may be more traumatized. Victims who overcome their distress in a few months were less likely to have lost a close family in the previous year and more likely to have had intimate, loving relationships with men before the rape.

○ **What are some clues to whether you are seeing a patient with a history of sexual assault?**

Multiple physical and psychological signs may be present in a patient with a trauma history including presence of flashbacks, avoidance, hyperarousal, sexual dysfunction, evidence of self-mutilation, chronic pain, functional gastrointestinal disorders, substance abuse, suicide attempts, and eating disorders.

○ **Define domestic violence.**

Domestic violence is intentional violent behavior by a person who is currently, or has previously been, in an intimate relationship with the victim.

○ **What behaviors are included in the term domestic violence?**

Physical assault, threats of death or physical injury, sexual assault or coerced sexual activity, economic control, verbal abuse, and progressive social isolation.

○ **What are the estimates of the number of domestic violence victims in the United States?**

Between 2 and 4 million women are assaulted by intimate partners each year in the United States. It has been estimated that one in three women presenting for care in emergency departments are victims of domestic violence.

○ **Describe the typical abuser.**

Men who assault their partners often appear to be normal and the majority are not mentally ill. They also generally do not exhibit impulse control problems or violent behavior in other settings. Drugs and alcohol may be part of the general pattern of violence in up to half of the cases, but the relationship to the assaults themselves is complex. In addition, treatment of the alcohol or drug problem in most cases does not address or decrease the violence.

○ **What obstacles exist that make it difficult for a woman to leave her abuser?**

Fear for her safety and that of her children; economic constraints; social isolation; and attachment to the perpetrator are factors that prolong relationships characterized by domestic violence.

○ **What is the physician's role in domestic violence intervention?**

The physician's role is to communicate concern about the victim's welfare and provide a framework to seek out required resources. It is the victim's decision on how and when a change in her life will be made.

○ **What factors should be included in a safety plan for the victim?**

A safety plan should include phone numbers for battered women's shelters, other places she can go (friends, family), resources available for leaving (car keys, money, etc.), and access to resources needed to live (clothing, medication, important documents, own finances).

○   **What "barriers to care" exist for victims of domestic violence?**

Barriers to care include feelings of powerlessness and inadequacy by the physician, feeling uncomfortable talking about violence, fear of offending the patient and/or their partner, reluctance to acknowledge the presence of domestic violence (especially in higher socioeconomic settings), and lack of time on the part of the health care provider.

○   **What factors contribute to the etiology of child abuse/neglect?**

There are multiple factors involved but a partial list includes a history of abuse in the parents, stressful living conditions, social isolation of the abuser, lack of a support system for the abuser, and parental substance abuse. Factors that increase a child's risk of abuse include prematurity, mental retardation, physical handicap, children who cry excessively or who are unusually demanding, and hyperactive children.

CHAPTER 19 — Mental Disorders Due to a General Medical Condition

○ **What are some neurologic conditions that may cause catatonia?**

- CNS neoplasms
- Head trauma
- Cerebrovascular disease
- Encephalitis

○ **What are some neurologic conditions that may cause personality change?**

- CNS neoplasms
- Head trauma
- Cerebrovascular disease Huntington's disease
- Epilepsy
- Infections with CNS involvement (e.g., HIV)
- Autoimmune disorders with CNS involvement (e.g., SLE)

○ **A consult is obtained in a medical patient with agitated behavior, suspected to be septic. What might a neurologic examination reveal?**

In systemic illnesses, focal neurologic signs are usually not found.

○ **What is one of the most common causes of delirium?**

Medications (especially anticholinergic).

○ **What CNS structural lesions may present as dementia?**

Primary or secondary brain tumors, subdural hematomas, and normal pressure hydrocephalus.

○ **What CNS structural change associated with amnesia can be recognized on MRI?**

Damage to mediotemporal lobe structures, which may be reflected by either atrophy or an enlarged third ventricle and temporal horns.

○ **Name three nutritional deficiencies that may result in dementia.**

1. Thiamine
2. Niacin
3. Vitamin B_{12}

○ **What neurologic conditions may cause sexual dysfunction?**

Multiple sclerosis, spinal cord lesions, and temporal lobe lesions.

○ **What percentage of patients with Addison's disease develop depression?**

Approximately 40% of patients with Addison's disease develop depression that is characterized by apathy, fatigue, and occasionally psychosis.

○ **What CNS lesions site results in the highest frequency of delusions?**

Subcortical (basal ganglia, thalamus, midbrain) and limbic structures.

○ **Describe the association of motor impairment to psychiatric disorders in Parkinson's disease.**

Depression is independent of motor impairment, while cognitive impairment is frequent in late stages.

○ **Approximately what percentage of patients with dementia have at least a partially reversible condition?**
One-third (33%).

○ **Reserpine may cause depression. When does this occur typically?**

A latency period of 4 to 6 months often precedes development of depression.

○ **What is the classic triad of Huntington's disease, and on which chromosome is the gene for this disorder located?**

Transmitted on as an autosomal dominant gene on chromosome 4, Huntington's disease is characterized by dementia, chorea, and a family history of the disorder.

○ **Identify some toxins that may cause dementia.**

Alcohol, polydrug abuse, metals, industrial solvents, and iatrogenic toxins, i.e., medications, especially anticholinergic, antihypertensive, psychotropic, and anticonvulsant agents.

○ **What are some drugs that may induce anxiety upon withdrawal?**

- Benzodiazepines
- Caffeine
- Alcohol
- Sedatives
- Opiates

○ **What are some common nonspecific medical symptoms that may cause insomnia?**

- Pain
- Cough
- Pruritus
- Dyspnea
- Fever

○ **What is the most frequent metabolic cause of mania?**

Hyperthyroidism.

○ **What predominant lesion locations are associated with depression after stroke?**

Left frontal and left basal ganglia lesions.

○ **Transient amnesia is associated with which neurologic condition?**

Seizures.

○ **What types of sleep disorders may occur because of medical conditions?**

- Insomnia
- Hypersomnia
- Parasomnia
- Mixed conditions

○ **What laboratory studies are useful in the evaluation of mania?**

Glucose, electrolytes, renal/hepatic function, CBC, calcium, cortisol, thyroxine, B_{12}, folate, toxicology screen, alcohol level, pregnancy test, and levels of mood-stabilizing medications.

○ **What is the most frequent metabolic cause of anxiety?**

Thyroid abnormality.

○ **What psychiatric presentations are associated with HIV?**

- Depression
- Dementia
- Anxiety
- Delirium
- Psychosis

○ **Which psychiatric symptom may be caused by carbon monoxide poisoning or other neurotoxic exposure?**

Amnesia.

○ **What psychotic symptoms are associated with a patient presenting with a right parietal brain lesion?**

Contralateral neglect syndrome can include delusions in which the patients may disown parts of their body.

○ **Fibromyalgia is associated with nonrestorative sleep. Describe the polysomnographic pattern associated with this.**

Distinct α-EEG activity during non-REM sleep.

○ **Identify the disease recessively transmitted on chromosome 13 affecting ceruloplasmin.**

Wilson's disease, which results in abnormal deposition of copper in the CNS, liver, cornea, and kidneys.

○ **What personality changes can be seen with Wilson's disease (hepatolenticular degeneration)?**

Silliness, euphoria, and hysteria.

○ **What are some causes of degenerative subcortical dementias?**

- Parkinson's disease
- Huntington's disease
- Wilson's disease

○ **Identify comorbid psychiatric disorders in patients with physical disorders that increase suicide risk.**

Depression, delirium, dementia, and personality disorders.

○ **What is the most common cause of cortical dementia?**

Alzheimer's disease.

○ **What are some basic laboratory studies to consider in assessing patients with delirium?**

- Electrolytes
- Blood glucose
- Liver function tests
- Renal function tests
- CBC
- ABG
- Urinalysis
- Urine toxicology
- ECG
- Chest x-ray

○ **What psychiatric disorder appears to be a better predictor of the occurrence of major cardiac events than traditional cardiovascular risk factors?**

Depression.

○ **Describe the relationship between chorea and mood change in Huntington's disease.**

Depression may antedate chorea by years.

○ **What are some unique characteristics of depression due to a general medical condition compared to major depression?**

Depression due to a general medical disorder, in contrast to major depression, has a male predominance, an older age of onset, a decreased family history of alcoholism, and is associated with normal REM latency.

○ **What are the common psychiatric problems that develop in patients with multiple sclerosis?**

Three-fourths of patients will develop psychiatric disorders including mood disorders (depression or mania), cognitive disorders (dementia), and personality changes.

○ **What is the classic triad of tuberous sclerosis?**

"Mental defect," epilepsy, and adenoma sebaceum.

○ **What metabolic conditions may cause catatonia?**

- Hypercalcemia
- Hepatic encephalopathy
- Homocystinuria
- Diabetic ketoacidosis

○ **Identify some medical conditions that may cause delirium.**

- Systemic infections
- Metabolic disorders
- Head trauma
- Vitamin deficiencies
- Electrolyte imbalance
- Hypoxia
- Hypertensive encephalopathy

○ **What specific CNS lesion locations are likely to present with delirium?**

Focal lesions of the right parietal lobe and inferomedial surface of the occipital lobe.

○ **Name three endocrine abnormalities that may cause dementia.**

1. Hypothyroidism
2. Hypercalcemia
3. Hypoglycemia

○ **What infection may result in diencephalic and mediotemporal lobe damage (e.g., mammillary bodies, hippocampus, and fornix) that results in amnesia?**

Herpes simplex encephalitis.

○ **What sleep changes are caused by most general medical conditions?**

Decreased total sleep duration, increased awakenings, decreased slow-wave sleep, and decreased REM sleep or phasic REM density.

○ **What psychiatric problems are associated with pellagra (which has the classic triad of gastrointestinal disorder, skin lesions, and psychiatric disturbance)?**

Depression with suicidal behavior, acute psychosis, and delirium.

○ **What endocrine disorders cause sexual dysfunction?**

Diabetes mellitus, hypothyroidism, hyper- and hypoadrenocorticism, hyperprolactinemia, hypogonadal states, and pituitary dysfunction.

○ **Identify some medical emergencies that may present as delirium.**

- Hypoxia
- Hypertensive encephalopathy
- Wernicke's encephalopathy
- Intracranial bleeding
- Infections including encephalitis

○ **Which CNS structures are involved when psychotic disorders with delusions due to neurologic conditions are more common?**

Subcortical involvement or temporal lobe.

○ **Name two degenerative neurologic disorders that may cause mood disorders.**

1. Parkinson's disease
2. Huntington's disease

○ **What metabolic disorder which causes anxiety disorders is often referred to as the "Great Imitator"?**

Porphyria.

○ **Which medical condition results in mood disorders in a majority of patients?**

Cushing's syndrome (approximately 60% of patients develop a mood disorder).

○ **What endocrine abnormalities may cause psychosis?**

Hyper- and hypothyroidism, hyper- and hypoparathyroidism, and hypoadrenocorticism.

○ **What laboratory studies may be useful to screen for partially reversible causes of dementia?**

CBC, ESR, glucose, BUN, electrolytes, calcium, phosphorus, TSH, B_{12} and folate levels, and FTA/ABS.

○ **What hemisphere of the brain appears preferentially involved in the development of mania after CNS injury?**

Right hemisphere, especially right basitemporal.

○ **Describe how dementia due to vascular insult may appear different from other dementias.**

It is characterized by an abrupt onset, and has a stepwise progression and fluctuating course, with focal neurologic symptoms often present.

○ **Differentiate between subcortical and cortical dementia.**

Subcortical	Cortical
Depressed	Euthymic
Apathetic	Disinhibited
Slowed cognitive processing	Impaired calculation

CHAPTER 20 Geriatric Psychiatry

○ **Describe the changing age demographics of the United States.**

In 1900, 1 in 25 persons was 65 years or older; in 1990, 1 in 8 was 65 years or older. By 2030, it is estimated that the number of persons older than 65 years and younger than 18 years will be equal, each approximately 20% of the population.

○ **Who should be present at a geriatric psychiatry evaluation?**

The patient and the primary caregiver, if possible.

○ **Which medication use should be reviewed with the elderly patient?**

All, including vitamins and over-the-counter medications, which may have profound effects on elderly patients' mental status.

○ **What items are included in a functional assessment?**

ADLs—the activities of daily living including bathing, transferring, dressing, toileting, grooming, and feeding. Also IADLs—the instrumental activities of daily living including using a telephone, shopping, cooking, laundering, transportation, managing medications, and finances.

○ **What percentage of older adults will have at least one chronic disease?**

Eighty percent. The most common illnesses (in order of decreasing frequency) include arthritis, hypertension, hearing impairment, orthopedic impairments, cataracts, diabetes, and sinusitis.

○ **What is OBRA 87?**

Omnibus **B**udget **R**econciliation **A**ct of 1987. This legislation affected changes in the admission and retention of nursing home patients, and ensured patients were receiving mental health treatment when indicated. This is relevant to psychiatry in that when patients are placed from a psychiatric hospital to a nursing home, they will need an OBRA evaluation, as will patients receiving psychiatric medications. An effect of this legislation was to decrease inappropriate neuroleptic and restraint use.

○ **What percentage of Americans aged 65 years and older are residing in nursing homes at any given time?**

Five percent, but the probability of a period of long-term residence in a nursing home in late life is 25%.

○ **What are the major effects of age on pharmacokinetics?**

There is decreased metabolism from decreased hepatic blood flow, while there is an increased volume of distribution and prolonged half-lives for lipophilic compounds because of the increase in the fat/lean body ratio. Lithium and hydroxy metabolites of antidepressants have a decreased clearance due to a decrease in renal glomerular filtration. In terms of pharmacodynamics, the tissue response to a given concentration of medication is altered both peripherally and centrally with aging.

○ **What is the overall prevalence of depression among people 65 years and older?**

The overall prevalence of major depression in people older than 65 years is estimated to be 1%. A larger percentage of elderly (15%) are estimated to have subsyndromal depression.

○ **How does one account for this relatively low prevalence rate?**

Factors include methodological problems of various studies, tendency of the elderly to underreport or not recall depressive symptoms or express depressive symptoms in somatic terms, health care bias that depression is a "normal" part of aging, and cohort effect of the current geriatric population.

○ **In what geriatric populations is depression prevalence higher?**

Medically ill patients (7%–36%) including those with neurologic or chronic disease, nursing home residents (12%–16%), institutionalized populations (30%–50%), and socioeconomically deprived or disabled individuals.

○ **What is late-onset depression and how does it differ from early onset?**

Late-onset depression is defined as having a first episode of depression in old age. It is associated with a lower frequency of family history of mood disorders, higher prevalence of dementia or other cognitive disorders, and brain scan abnormalities (enlargement of lateral ventricles, or white matter hyperintensities).

○ **In what neurologic illnesses is depression frequent?**

Dementia (range of 15%–20%), stroke (up to 25%), and Parkinson's disease (up to 50%).

○ **What symptoms of depression and dementia overlap and make diagnosis difficult?**

Loss of interest, decreased energy, concentration problems, and psychomotor changes (agitation or retardation) are common to both depression and dementia, making accurate diagnosis difficult at times.

○ **What features can one use to distinguish depression in dementia from dementia alone?**

Sad mood, suicidal ideation, and other symptoms such as excessive guilt and/or hopelessness are present in major depression, but not dementia.

○ **What is "pseudodementia" and what might it tell the clinician prognostically?**

Pseudodementia is a syndrome of reversible cognitive impairment that accompanies depression in some elderly patients. Typically, the cognitive changes resolve with treatment of the mood syndrome. Some investigators have noted that patients with this syndrome may have a higher risk of developing irreversible cognitive problems (dementia, at a rate estimated to be between 9% and 25% per year), which may suggest that the depression may have unmasked a subclinical dementing process.

○ **Despite their efficacy, what side effects do tricyclic antidepressants pose for the elderly?**

Especially adverse side effects of tricyclics for the elderly include anticholinergic effects (dry mouth, constipation, urinary retention, blurred vision, tachycardia, and possibly delirium) and peripheral α-receptor blockade (leading to orthostatic hypotension which may cause falls) among others. Tricyclics appropriate for use in the elderly are nortriptyline or desipramine due to their tendency to cause fewer of these side effects. Although early concerns about proarrhythmic properties of these drugs may have been overstated and related more to toxicity with overdose, recent studies do indicate that these agents may be dangerously proarrhythmic in patients who have recently suffered a myocardial infarction, and possibly in other settings of unstable coronary artery disease.

○ **Which tricyclic should never be used in the elderly?**

Amitriptyline, as it is the tricyclic that is most likely to cause the side effects noted above. In addition, the other "tertiary amine" antidepressants (imipramine, doxepin) should generally be avoided.

○ **Describe the use of selective serotonin reuptake inhibitors (SSRIs) or other nontricyclic antidepressants in the elderly.**

SSRIs are commonly used for the treatment of depression in the elderly, as these antidepressants are well tolerated and effective in geriatric depression, though placebo-control studies in the elderly are still lacking. Also, it is not known whether they are as effective as other agents (tricyclics, MAOIs) in the treatment of severe, melancholic geriatric depression. Other medications that are used in geriatric depression include MAOIs, and atypical antidepressants like bupropion, venlafaxine, nefazodone, or duloxetine.

○ **How does one go about dosing antidepressants in the elderly?**

In general, by following the old maxim of "Start Low and Go Slow." Add to this the advice of "Don't Stop!", meaning do not undertreat or give an inadequate drug trial to an elderly patient. Generally, one should initiate a medication at less than half of the starting dose for a younger adult and titrate to efficacy slowly (paying attention to any side effects). In general, geriatric patients (because of age-related physiological changes) may require lower doses to achieve efficacy and therapeutic plasma levels as compared with younger patients.

○ **What is the use of psychostimulants (methylphenidate or dextroamphetamine) in geriatric depression?**

Although their sustained efficacy in the treatment of major depression in the elderly has not been established, they are sometimes used to target symptoms of apathy and anergy in medically ill patients. Advantages include rapid onset of action and minimal side effects when used in proper dosages.

○ **What are the indications for the use of electroconvulsive therapy (ECT) in geriatric depression?**

Indications for the use of ECT in the elderly include medical illness that precludes the use of antidepressant medication, rapid treatment response needed due to risk for suicide or to treat the medical complications of severe depression (dehydration, electrolyte disturbances, etc.), and a past history of good response to ECT. ECT can also be considered a first-line treatment for delusional/psychotic depression in the elderly, as it is often better tolerated than tricyclic-neuroleptic combinations. Geriatric patients sometimes develop prolonged confusion after ECT, especially with bilateral ECT.

○ **What about the suicide rate in older individuals?**

Suicide is more frequent in the elderly than in younger individuals, and elderly white men have the highest suicide rate (43.5/100,000). "Psychological autopsy" studies have indicated that many of these patients had late-life depressions. Many elderly people who commit suicide have seen their primary health provider in the month prior to their deaths.

○ **Describe features of mania in the elderly (in addition to those seen in younger patients).**

Symptoms of mania in the elderly include confusion, disorientation, agitation, irritability, and depressive thought content. While these symptoms can certainly occur in younger patients, they occur more frequently in the elderly.

○ **Describe the difference between early- and late-onset mania in the elderly.**

Mania in the elderly is a heterogeneous condition. Elderly patients presenting with mania may be presenting with their first mood episode (meaning they had never before been depressed or manic, consistent with late-onset mania), their first manic episode (meaning they have a history of prior depression but they have never had an episode of manic, which is consistent with a switch of "polarity" in late life), or a recurrence of mood episodes with an onset in earlier adulthood (long-standing bipolar disorder, consistent with early-onset mania). Early-onset mania is associated with a family history of bipolar disorder, while late-onset mania is associated with comorbid medical conditions, especially neurologic conditions.

○ **What is the differential diagnosis of a new-onset mania?**

The differential diagnosis of new-onset mania includes switch of polarity if there is a history of depression (occurs in 5%–18% of unipolar depressives), secondary mania (due to a medical disorder), agitated depression, dementia, delirium, or late-onset schizophrenia.

○ **What are the treatments for mania in the elderly?**

Lithium, carbamazepine, valproic acid, and ECT. Neuroleptics are also antimanic agents, but are not usually used for maintenance treatment, as tardive dyskinesia is a long-term risk.

○ **Name some of the particular concerns with lithium in the elderly.**

With lithium, one needs to make dose alterations as there is an age-associated decline in renal clearance in the elderly. There is also the potential for adverse drug interactions (with NSAIDS, thiazide diuretics, ACE inhibitors, theophylline), which can alter lithium levels. All of the drug interactions just mentioned, with the exception of theophylline (which *decreases* lithium levels), will *increase* lithium levels. Neurologic side effects including cognitive impairment and tremor are also seen more frequently, even at relatively low lithium levels.

○ **Describe causes of secondary anxiety in the elderly.**

These include underlying medical illness (hyperthyroidism, COPD, CHF, etc.), drug reaction (steroids, caffeine, thyroid supplements, etc.), depression, dementia, and substance intoxication or withdrawal (barbiturates, benzodiazepines, caffeine, etc.).

○ **What is a "masked depression"?**

"Masked depression" is a major depression that is overshadowed by prominent anxiety symptoms. Often, this type of depression goes untreated or is inappropriately treated with benzodiazepines alone.

○ **What about primary anxiety disorders in the elderly?**

The limited data available suggests that anxiety disorders tend to be chronic with remissions and exacerbations and have a lower prevalence after the age of 65 years. However, despite this decreased prevalence as compared with younger adult populations, anxiety disorders are still, as a group, the most common psychiatric conditions in the elderly. The most common anxiety disorders in the elderly are phobias and generalized anxiety disorder (GAD). While agoraphobia, posttraumatic stress disorder (PTSD), and obsessive-compulsive disorder (OCD), especially in females, may arise for the first time in old age, most other anxiety disorders arise earlier or in association with another disorder (medical illness or depression). New-onset panic disorder or OCD in an elderly patient should alert the physician to a possible underlying condition (medical illness or depression).

○ **Describe the workup for new-onset anxiety in an elderly patient.**

Completion of a comprehensive history (onset, frequency, severity of symptoms, medications the patient is taking, family history of anxiety) and physical examination, laboratory tests (including thyroid function, EKG, glucose), mental status examination, and consideration of substance abuse or withdrawal constitute a thorough workup for new-onset anxiety in the elderly.

○ **Name two classes of medications used in the management of panic disorder in the elderly.**

Antidepressants, such as SSRIs, SNRIs, or TCAs, and benzodiazepines.

○ **Name three common side effect of benzodiazepines that occur often in the elderly.**

1. Excessive sedation
2. Ataxia
3. Decreased cognition

Short half-life medications that are not metabolized by oxidation (and thus have less tendency to accumulate), such as lorazepam, are preferred to minimize toxicity.

○ **What is cognitive behavioral therapy and when should it be considered as an alternative to pharmacotherapy in the elderly?**

This therapy focuses on changing behavior and interactions in the "here and now." It is useful when specific cognitive (cognitive distortions with depression-prone individuals) or behavioral (agoraphobia in panic disorder) symptoms can be targeted. It should be considered as an alternative to psychotropic medications when there are serious concurrent medical problems, side effects, or drug interactions that preclude the use of medications. It is also a good adjunct to medications.

○ **What is the role of psychological treatments in the elderly?**

There are few studies that have looked at psychotherapy's effectiveness in the elderly, but it is widely thought to be a valuable treatment in many cases, especially as an adjunct to medication where it may aid compliance. There is no data to support that the elderly are "too old" for psychological change. As the elderly often experience multiple psychosocial losses (deaths, changing roles in society, poor health, etc.), attention to psychosocial issues is often helpful. Elderly patients who are resistant to psychiatric treatment may be more accepting of treatment presented in medical terms, so psychoeducation regarding the biologic basis of depression, anxiety, or dementia is often helpful.

○ **What are some of the goals of psychotherapy in older patients?**

Mastery of past life stresses, enhancement of current functioning, resolution of past and current conflicts, and enhancement of self-esteem may be some goals of psychotherapy with elderly patients (as well as young patients).

○ **What percentage of older adults have progressive dementias?**

Progressive dementias are seen in 7.5% of the elderly population. The breakdown of the dementias is estimated to be as follows: 50% to 60% are of the Alzheimer's type (DAT), but up to 30% of these DAT cases may be the Lewy body variant of DAT; 15%–30% are secondary to vascular dementia; and 10%–15% are secondary to a combination of DAT and vascular dementia. The remaining causes of dementia include Pick's disease (5%), Parkinson's disease, Huntington's chorea, and alcohol-related or head trauma–related dementias (1%–5%).

○ **What is the prevalence rate of dementia in patients older than 80 years of age?**

More than 20% of persons older than 80 years have dementia, the lifetime risk being 1:3 for those who survive to 85 years of age.

○ **Which chromosomes have been associated with familial Alzheimer's disease?**

Chromosome 14 and 21 are associated with early-onset familial disease, while chromosome 1 is associated with early-onset disease in Volga Germans. Chromosome 19 is associated with late-onset familial disease.

○ **Which chromosome has been associated with Huntington's disease?**

The short arm of chromosome 4.

○ **What tests should be performed to rule out reversible causes of dementia?**

The laboratory tests one should obtain to rule out reversible causes of dementia include electrolytes, glucose, renal function, hepatic function, CBC with differential, urinalysis, EKG, thyroid tests, B_{12}, folate, sedimentation rate, VDRL, brain MRI or CT, chest x-ray, and HIV screening, if any risk factors exist.

○ **How is dementia of the Alzheimer's type (DAT) diagnosed?**

DAT is a clinical diagnosis based on symptomology in the cognitive, behavioral, and functional realms. A definitive diagnosis requires histologic examination of brain tissue, usually postmortem. However, using *DSM-IV* criteria, an antemortem diagnosis of DAT is supported in 85% of cases. It is no longer considered a diagnosis of exclusion.

○ **What are clinical criteria for diagnosing dementia of the Alzheimer's type (DAT)?**

Criteria for the diagnosis of DAT include the development of multiple cognitive deficits manifested by memory impairment, and one or more of the following: aphasia, apraxia, agnosia, or executive functioning problems. These impairments must cause significant social or occupational difficulties, and represent a decline from a previous level of functioning. It is not due to any other medical condition or substance. Specifiers include early-onset, late-onset, with delirium, with delusions, with depressed mood, with behavioral disturbance, and uncomplicated.

○ **What are the classic neuropathologic findings in DAT?**

The classic neuropathologic findings in DAT are β-amyloid plaques (neuritic, senile), which are composed of a central amyloid core and the neurite (cellular debris), and neurofibrillary tangles, paired helical filaments composed primarily of a hyperphosphorylated form of the microtubule-associated phosphoprotein tau.

○   **In what other conditions can amyloid plaques and neurofibrillary tangles be found?**

Normal aging, as well as other pathologic, dementing conditions. However, there is a greater concentration of these lesions in DAT.

○   **Which type of memory is most susceptible to aging effects?**

Secondary memory, the ability to encode, store, consolidate, and retrieve new material, is the most susceptible to the effects of aging. Primary memory, such as digit span, and tertiary (remote) memory are both preserved in normal aging.

○   **What is usually the first recognizable symptom of DAT?**

Anterograde memory deficit—a rapid forgetting of information. Early in the disease course this may be confined to secondary memory, but later primary and tertiary memory may be affected.

○   **In what other areas besides memory do DAT patients have difficulties?**

Executive functioning—the ability to perform simultaneous mental operations, which is often described in terms of cognitive flexibility, concept formation, and self-monitoring. An example of this is participating in a group conversation, which requires simultaneous monitoring of each person's contribution, and formation and expression of one's own thoughts.

○   **Which lobe(s) of the brain is/are most affected by DAT?**

The cortex association areas, in particular, the parietal–temporal junction and the limbic system (including the hippocampus), show atrophy in DAT.

○   **What is the most common distinguishing feature of DAT in brain imaging by CT or MRI scans?**

There are no distinguishing features of DAT on CT or MRI. DAT patients may have cerebral atrophy, but so do many patients with normal aging. Thus, DAT cannot be diagnosed using brain imaging alone.

○   **In which lobe(s) has hypoperfusion been noted in PET and SPECT scans of DAT patients?**

The parietal and temporal lobes.

○   **In which neurotransmitter system have aberrations been most associated with DAT?**

Acetylcholine. This deficiency of acetylcholine is likely not a primary finding, but rather an expression of an underlying degenerative process of cholinergic neurons, which may contribute to the cognitive decline. Other implicated neurotransmitter systems include serotonin and norepinephrine.

○   **In which area of the brain associated with cholinergic synthesis has neuronal loss been described in DAT?**

In the nucleus basalis of Meynert (substantia innominata), which suffers extensive neuronal loss in DAT.

○   **Which apolipoprotein and subtype is associated with an increased risk for DAT?**

ApoE 4 homozygotes may have up to an eightfold risk of developing DAT.

O   **What is the Godot syndrome?**

Godot syndrome refers to anxiety about upcoming events experienced by dementia patients. It is manifested by repeated questioning about when the event will occur.

O   **What types of behavioral disturbances are seen in DAT?**

- Paranoid/delusional ideation: 40% of patients believe caregivers are hiding or stealing belongings, and 25% want to go home when already home.
- Hallucinations: Visual hallucinations are most common, but all types may occur, and can be well systematized.
- Activity: Verbal repetition, pacing, wandering, and hiding objects.
- Aggression: Verbal outbursts, anger, resistance. At most, 25% of DAT patients are always violent.
- Sleep disturbances: Fragmented.
- Affective disturbances: Depression is the most common.
- Anxiety and phobias: 40% fear being left alone, while concerns about finances, taxes, toileting, and bathing are also common. These disturbances are most prominent in moderately severe stages of DAT.

O   **Are there any psychosocial treatments for managing DAT?**

Yes, support groups for patients suffering from early dementia, and adult day care centers are very helpful in providing safe, structured activities and socialization.

O   **How common is major depression in caregivers of dementia patients?**

Thirty to fifty percent of caregivers meet criteria for major depressive disorder.

O   **What psychosocial supports are available to caregivers of a dementia patient?**

The Alzheimer's Association has local branches, and can provide guidance to community services, support groups, behavior management, and legal and financial guidance for families.

O   **What pharmacologic options are available to treat the behavioral disturbances in dementia?**

- Agitation (aggression/anxiety/activity): Trazodone, buspirone, sodium valproate, low-dose benzodiazepines, carbamazepine, and antipsychotics.
- Insomnia: Trazodone, zolpidem, low-dose benzodiazepines.
- Hallucinations: Low-dose antipsychotics.
- Mood disturbances: Antidepressants, sodium valproate, carbamazepine, lithium.

O   **List risk factors for tardive dyskinesia (TD).**

- Cumulative neuroleptic exposure
- Age
- Female gender
- Mood disorder
- Cognitive disorder

Age is an independent risk factor, with a 4% to 5% annual incidence in younger adults, compared with 30% in patients older than 45 years. Fewer instances of spontaneous remissions are noted in older patients.

○ **What types of pharmacologic treatments are available for DAT-related cognitive impairment?**

Currently, central acting cholinesterase inhibitors are the only available treatments that prolong the presence of acetylcholine in the synapse. These treatments do not cure DAT, but rather delay the deterioration in the course of the illness by approximately 1 year. Two agents are available: tacrine (Cognex®), which is associated with elevations in liver transaminases, is poorly tolerated and requires frequent lab draws for LFTs; and donepezil (Aricept®), which has not been associated with hepatotoxicity but has mild gastrointestinal distress and dizziness as potential side effects. Other newer cholinesterase inhibitors are also available: galantamine (Reminyl®), galantamine hydrobromide (Razadyne ER®), and rivastigmine (Excelon®). The newest drug to be introduced is memantine (Namenda®) which blocks glutamate-related neurotoxicity in the brain. Memantine can be used in combination with one of the cholinesterase inhibitors.

○ **How should depressive symptoms in DAT be addressed?**

Although mild-to-moderate DAT and depression may have similar symptoms, they are often difficult to distinguish. Frequently, it is best to treat suspected cases of depression, which may be a reversible cause of dementia.

○ **How may an EEG help distinguish depression from dementia?**

DAT will likely show excessive diffuse showing of background rhythm, while in depression, an EEG will likely be normal or only show mild slowing.

○ **What are two common causes of morbidity and mortality in end-stage DAT?**

Aspiration with subsequent pneumonia and decubiti.

○ **What is the primary neuropathologic finding in Pick's disease?**

Pick bodies, intracytoplasmic masses of neurofilaments and neurotubules found in the frontal lobe, not the temporal/parietal lobes as in DAT.

○ **How does early Pick's disease present?**

Pick's disease presents with personality changes including decreased impulse control, inappropriate affect, and stereotyped behaviors. Gradual progressive abnormalities in language also occur over time.

○ **What is pseudobulbar palsy, and in what conditions is it seen?**

Pseudobulbar palsy is an upper motor neuron disorder secondary to involvement of the frontal lobes. Dysarthria, dysphagia, hyperactive gag and jaw jerk reflexes, emotional lability with pathologic laughing and crying, and cognitive impairment are seen. It may occur in dementias involving the frontal lobe, multiple cerebral infarctions, head trauma, multiple sclerosis, or cerebral palsy.

○ **What is Lewy body disease?**

Lewy body disease is a progressive dementing process with mild Parkinson-like features. Lewy bodies, which are typically found in the substantia nigra in Parkinson's disease are found throughout the cerebral cortex. Up to one-third of patients with clinically and pathologically confirmed DAT were found to have Lewy bodies, and these appear to be a distinct subgroup of dementia patients.

○ **Which type of dementia is second in frequency to Alzheimer's disease?**

Vascular dementia (formerly known as multi-infarct dementia).

○   **How can vascular dementia be differentiated from DAT?**

By focal neurologic deficits. Early in the dementia, it may be difficult to distinguish, but history, risk factors, and a neurologic examination may help clarify the diagnosis. In the past, it was described as a stepwise decline, which may or may not be seen.

○   **What is the number one risk factor for vascular dementia?**

Hypertension.

○   **What are the characteristics of delirium?**

Delirium is associated with a rapid onset (hours to days), disturbance of consciousness, fluctuating course, and evidence that the condition is due to consequences of a physical illness. It is classically thought of with agitation, but a quiet delirium may be present which is not readily recognized.

○   **What EEG finding would rule out delirium?**

Usually, a normal EEG. This may be helpful in the case of a quiet delirium, where a depression is suspected due to the withdrawn nature of the patient. In depression or psychosis, the EEG background rhythm would usually be normal, but in delirium there would be a background slowing.

○   **How can delirium and dementia be differentiated?**

By the level of alertness; patients with dementia do not have a fluctuating level of consciousness. Collateral history from the caregiver is also very helpful to determine the level of prior functioning. Delirium and dementia may coexist, and preexisting dementia is a risk factor for delirium.

○   **How is delirium treated?**

The optimal treatment of delirium is to diagnose and treat the underlying medical problem. Environmental treatments that address the symptoms of delirium include providing for safety, a quiet room and orientation cues. For agitation and confusion, low-dose haloperidol may be used while the delirium is resolving. In the elderly, the delirium may persist for weeks after the medical condition has been corrected.

○   **What events may precipitate a delirium?**

Medications, drug interactions, drug and/or alcohol withdrawal, metabolic aberrations, CNS disease, cardiovascular compromise, infections, postop states, and sleep deprivation are all causes of delirium.

○   **How do psychotic symptoms seen in delirium differ from the psychosis associated with schizophrenia or mania?**

The psychotic content is generally less systematized in delirium.

○   **What is the classic triad of symptoms in normal pressure hydrocephalus?**

Dementia, gait disturbance, and urinary incontinence. Dilated ventricles are present on brain imaging, but intracranial pressure is normal.

○ **What are the distinguishing features of Creutzfeldt-Jakob disease?**

Spongiform encephalopathy, rapid onset and course of dementia, and transmission by a prion, with up to 15% of cases being familial. An EEG may show synchronous triphasic sharp wave complexes or slowing.

○ **What is the differential diagnosis of psychosis in the elderly?**

The differential diagnosis of psychosis in the elderly includes delirium, dementia, psychotic depression, mania or mixed state with psychosis, early-onset schizophrenia, late-onset schizophrenia, brief psychotic disorder, schizophreniform disorder, schizoaffective disorder, shared psychotic disorder, and psychotic disorders due to general medical conditions.

○ **What percentage of schizophrenia patients have a late onset of symptoms (older than 44 years old)?**

Up to 20%.

○ **What type of symptoms are most commonly seen in late-onset schizophrenia (after the age of 45 years)?**

Bizarre delusions, mostly of a persecutory nature. Auditory hallucinations are the second most common symptom.

○ **What is the treatment for late-onset schizophrenia?**

As with early-onset, neuroleptics are the main treatment and available data suggests that most patients show symptomatic improvement with neuroleptics. Side effects including the long-term risk of tardive dyskinesia need to be considered, and often, small doses of neuroleptics may be effective. Atypical neuroleptics are also an option, but have been associated with higher rates of cardiovascular events, stroke, and diabetes.

○ **What happens to early-onset schizophrenia patients as they age?**

Little is known about the long-term course of schizophrenia; limited data suggests that one-third of patients may undergo remission or continue with only mild symptoms over time. Often "positive" symptoms (hallucinations, delusions) become muted over time with the persistence of "negative" symptoms (affective flattening, amotivation).

○ **What factors contribute to an age-associated decline in the reported prevalence of alcoholism?**

Premature deaths in chronic alcoholics, abstinence prior to old age, underreporting due to problems with recall or embarrassment about excessive drinking, fewer external sources where problems could arise (employment, etc.), clinician underreporting or underdiagnosis, family denial due to shame, and cohort effect.

○ **What tends to happen to "cluster B" personality disorders with age?**

With age, borderline and antisocial patients tend to show less flamboyant behavior as compared with younger patients, but little is known systematically.

○ **How does sleep change with aging?**

With age, sleep continuity and the amount of slow-wave sleep decrease, REM sleep occurs earlier in the sleep period, and daytime napping increases.

CHAPTER 21 Substance Abuse

○ **What is the definition of substance dependence?**

According to the *DSM-IV*, substance dependence is a pattern of substance use over a 12-month period of time characterized by three of the following seven criteria:

1. Tolerance
2. Withdrawal
3. Use of the substance for longer periods than intended
4. Unsuccessful attempts to discontinue use
5. Continued use of a specific psychoactive substance despite known physical/psychological harm
6. Reduction of social, occupational, or recreational activities because of substance use
7. Investment of significant amounts of time to obtain the substance, use it, or recover from its effects

○ **According to the *DSM-IV*, what is the difference between substance dependence and abuse?**

Essentially, tolerance and withdrawal do not occur with substance abuse.

○ **Define tolerance.**

Tolerance is the need for markedly increased amounts of a substance to achieve intoxication or desired effects and/or a diminished effect with continued use of the same amount of a substance.

○ **Define withdrawal.**

Withdrawal is a condition whereby a characteristic syndrome for a particular substance occurs after diminished use of that substance. Withdrawal is relieved by administration of the substance, or a substance with similar pharmacologic properties.

○ **Name the principles and techniques of an intervention that addresses substance abuse/dependence.**

- Learn about the illness being confronted.
- Gather people significant to the person being confronted.
- Be specific.
- Demonstrate care and concern.
- Preparation will always help.
- Review treatment options.
- Use benevolent coercion.
- Choose an appropriate location.
- Timing is everything.
- Expect the unexpected.
- Know that an unsuccessful intervention never occurs.

○ **Name the characteristics that promote the abuse of a substance.**

Characteristics of addictive substances include rapid absorption and entry into the brain, low protein binding, high pharmacologic activity of the drug, high oral bioavailability, and a short half-life.

○ **What are some common medical problems that you should look for in a person with chemical dependency?**

- Heart disease
- Hypertension
- Diabetes
- Cancer
- Tuberculosis
- HIV infection
- Hepatitis
- Syphilis
- Intoxication syndromes
- Withdrawal syndromes

○ **Name the factors involved in the pharmacologic treatment of drug intoxication.**

Strategies used in the pharmacologic treatment of drug intoxication include increased drug clearance from the body, blockade of neuronal sites where the drug is active, and use of agents to counteract the effect of a drug.

○ **According to the *DSM-IV*, substance dependence can be applied to many substances except one. What is that substance?**

Caffeine.

○ **Which substances do not cause intoxication delirium according to the *DSM-IV*?**

Caffeine and nicotine.

○ **Which substances cause withdrawal delirium according to the *DSM-IV*?**

Alcohol and sedative-hypnotics.

○ **According to the *DSM-IV*, which substances have not had withdrawal demonstrated in humans?**

Hallucinogens, PCP, and related substances.

○ **What comorbid conditions or symptoms are often associated with substance abuse?**

Antisocial personality disorder, depression, and suicide.

○ **How long do urine drug screens remain positive?**

Depends, of course, on the substance of use/abuse. Amphetamines: 1 to 3 days, cannabis: 7 days to 4 weeks (6–11 weeks with heavy use), cocaine: 2 to 5 days (10–22 days with heavy use), opiates: 1 to 2 days, PCP: 2 to 8 days, alcohol: 3 to 10 hours, benzodiazepines: up to 6 weeks.

○ **Does a positive urine drug screen indicate the presence of a substance-related disorder?**

By itself, a positive urine drug screen does not indicate a substance-related disorder, nor does a negative drug screen by itself rule out a substance-related disorder.

○ **How do you diagnose alcohol and drug dependence?**

Although there is no gold standard, you can use the *DSM-IV* or *ICD-10*.

○ **Name some of the screening tests used to detect alcohol abuse/dependence.**

The Michigan Alcoholism Screening Test (MAST), Alcohol Use Disorders Identification Test (AUDIT—developed by the World Health Organization), Substance Abuse Subtle Screening Inventory (SASSI), Self Administered Alcoholism Screening Test (SAAST), CAGE questions (cut down, angry, guilty, eye-openers), and Adolescent Drinking Inventory (ADI) are just a few of the screening tests for alcohol abuse.

○ **What are the ASAM criteria and what are they used for?**

The American Society of Addiction Medicine (ASAM) Patient Placement Criteria (ASAM PPC-2R) are guidelines developed for determining the level of care indicated by the severity and duration of substance use, co-occurring conditions, amenability to treatment, and medical status. Separate guidelines have been developed for adolescents and adults. The levels of care range from early intervention, outpatient services, intensive outpatient services, and residential treatment to inpatient medical hospitalization. Use of the guidelines is encouraged to determine an objective level of care needs.

○ **Name some laboratory tests that are abnormal in people who abuse alcohol.**

Abnormal laboratory findings associated with alcohol abuse include increases in GGT, MCV, AST, ALT, uric acid, HDL, triglycerides, alkaline phosphatase, bilirubin, amylase, and transferrin, while levels of glucose, potassium, iron, magnesium, calcium, zinc, red and white blood cells counts, and platelet counts are decreased. These tests are nonspecific, but can alert a physician to a problem. An elevated MCV in combination with an elevated GGT corresponds to a 95% sensitivity for alcohol abuse, while an AST:ALT ratio of >2:1corresponds to a 70% sensitivity for alcohol use. The biomarker, carbohydrate-deficient transferrin (CDT), is highly specific for alcohol abuse, and relapse can be detected within a week. However, its low specificity and high cost limit its utility as a screening tool for alcohol abuse (Spiegel et al. 2008).

○ **According to the National Comorbidity Survey, what is the lifetime prevalence for alcohol dependence in men and women in the United States?**

The lifetime prevalence for alcohol dependence is 20% for men and 8% for women.

○ **How many deaths are attributed to alcohol abuse each year in the United States?**

Approximately 85,000 (Mokdad et al. 2001).

○ **How is alcohol metabolized?**

Ninety percent of alcohol is metabolized by the liver, while 10% is excreted unchanged in the lungs and kidneys.

$$\text{Alcohol} \xrightarrow{\text{Alcohol dehydrogenase}} \text{Acetaldehyde} \xrightarrow{\text{Aldehyde dehydrogenase}} \text{Acetyl Coenzyme A}$$

○ **Describe the behavioral effects of alcohol and the blood levels at which they occur.**

0.05%—thought and judgment influenced

0.1%—clumsiness, legal intoxication

0.2%—the entire motor area is depressed

0.3%—confusion and stupor

0.4% to 0.5%—coma

>0.5%—death secondary to respiratory depression or aspiration

○ **What is the most important vitamin you can give to a person with alcohol dependence and why?**

Thiamine, thiamine, and more thiamine. These people will already have low thiamine levels and this sets them up for Wernicke's and /or Korsakoff's syndrome (denoted as alcohol-induced persisting amnestic disorder in the *DSM-IV*).

○ **If an alcoholic patient comes into the ER, which should you give first, thiamine or glucose?**

You should give thiamine first because if glucose is given first, it will acutely deplete the remaining thiamine in the body, which could precipitate Wernicke's encephalopathy.

○ **If a patient has a blood alcohol level of 200 mg%, how long would it take to reach zero?**

The answer is 14.3 hours. Alcohol will decrease approximately 15 mg% per hour. As a rule of thumb, avoid treating alcohol withdrawal at a blood alcohol level greater than 150 mg%.

○ **How do males and females metabolize alcohol differently?**

Females metabolize alcohol at slower rates. Women may have lower levels of alcohol dehydrogenase, and they may have a higher blood alcohol concentration because of a higher percentage of body fat and a lower percentage of body water.

○ **Describe alcohol withdrawal.**

Symptoms of alcohol withdrawal can vary from mild anxiety, tremors, headache, reduced appetite, increased blood pressure, and insomnia to severe agitation, hallucinations, diaphoresis, tachycardia, hyperreflexia, seizures, sleep disturbance, clouded sensorium, increased temperature, and even death.

○ **What are the four syndromes associated with alcohol withdrawal?**

1. Minor withdrawal
2. Withdrawal seizures
3. Alcoholic hallucinosis
4. Delirium tremens

○ **What is delirium tremens?**

Delirium tremens (or alcohol withdrawal delirium, per the *DSM-IV*) is an acute, reversible delirium beginning approximately 72 hours after the last drink. It is associated with hallucinations, disorientation, agitation, hyperarousal, diaphoresis and seizures, may last 2 to 6 days, and has a mortality rate of up to 5%.

○ **What are the risk factors for delirium tremens?**

An extended period of heavy alcohol use, an older age, poor medical status, a prior history of alcohol withdrawal, and presentation greater than 2 days since the last use of alcohol.

○ **What class of medications do you give to prevent alcohol withdrawal?**

Benzodiazepines. Administration of benzodiazepines (usually lorazepam or oxazepam due to their shorter half-lives) in accordance with an alcohol withdrawal protocol, such as the Clinical Institute Withdrawal Assessment for Alcohol Scale (CIWA scale), allows for symptomatic treatment of alcohol withdrawal, minimizing sedation and length of stay.

○ **What receptor do benzodiazepines bind to?**

The GABA receptor.

○ **If a patient has alcoholic hepatitis and needs to be detoxified, what medication would you use?**

Lorazepam or oxazepam. Remember, chlordiazepoxide is hepatically metabolized by phase I and II, whereas lorazepam and oxazepam are metabolized by phase II only.

○ **If a person is in alcohol withdrawal and has a seizure, what would you do?**

Continue to administer benzodiazepines. The use of phenytoin may be indicated if status epileticus occurs.

○ **When the treatment of delirium tremens becomes refractory to treatment with benzodiazepines, what other options does one have?**

Refractory delirium tremens can be managed with the use of phenobarbitol or propofol. However, mechanical respiration and very close monitoring is necessary with these two pharmacotherapy approaches.

○ **What is the mechanism of action of propofol?**

Propofol potentiates the action of the GABA receptor by opening chloride channels in the absence of GABA.

○ **Name medications used in maintenance therapy for people with alcohol dependence.**

- Disulfiram (Antabuse®)
- Acamprosate (Camprel®)
- Naltrexone

○ **What is the mechanism of action for disulfiram (Antabuse®)?**

Disulfiram inhibits aldehyde dehydrogenase that results in toxic accumulations of acid aldehyde that causes the adverse symptoms of flushing, nausea, vomiting, anxiety, and hypotension.

$$\text{Alcohol} \xrightarrow{\text{Alcohol dehydrogenase}} \text{Acetaldehyde} \xrightarrow{\text{Aldehyde dehydrogenase}} \text{Acetyl Coenzyme A}$$

○ **Name the voluntary support group founded by an alcoholic stockbroker and surgeon.**

Alcoholics Anonymous (AA).

○ **Who is Dr. Bob?**

The surgeon who cofounded AA with W. Bill, a stockbroker.

○ **Why do some people of asian descent turn red when they drink alcohol?**

Because they have a variant of alcohol dehydrogenase that results in increased acetate levels, which causes the "alcohol flush."

○ **Describe findings associated with fetal alcohol syndrome (FAS).**

FAS is associated with microcephaly, low IQ, delayed growth, limb and heart defects, and craniofacial abnormalities. It is the number one known cause of mental retardation.

○ **Why is it not a good idea to drink alcohol and use cocaine?**

Besides the obvious, these two combine to form cocaethylene, which is neurotoxic.

○ **To which neurotransmitter is the action of cocaine related?**

Dopamine.

○ **Name the most common causes of death related to cocaine.**

The most common causes of cocaine-related deaths include sudden death by myocardial infarction, cerebral vascular accident, and sequelae of the Mueller's maneuver (pneumothorax caused by exhaling against a closed glottis).

○ **If someone uses cocaine and takes a neuroleptic, what should you look out for?**

Cocaine lowers the threshold for dystonic reactions.

○ **Name some "street names" for cocaine.**

Snow, Coke, Girl, and Lady to name a few.

○ **Does cocaine have any medicinal value?**

Yes, in 1880 it was used as a local anesthetic and even today is used by ENT for the same purpose.

○ **How do the effects of amphetamines differ from cocaine?**

Amphetamines, in contrast to cocaine, have no local anesthetic properties, have a longer duration of action, and may have more potent peripheral sympathomimetic effects.

○ **Name the common physical effects of stimulant use.**

Pupillary dilation, bruxism, stereotypic movement, pulmonary edema/failure, increased blood pressure, PVC, tremor, increased reflexes, seizures, nausea and vomiting, and increased temperature.

○ **Name some designer amphetamines.**

- MDMA (also known as Ecstasy or 3,4-methylenedioxymethamphetamine).
- DOM (2,5-dimethoxy-4-methylamphetamine, also known as STP).
- MMDA (5-methoxy-3,4-methylenedioxyamphetamine).

○ **Which neurotransmitter does MDMA affect?**

Serotonin, so if someone is on Prozac, they will not be able to get high if they use MDMA.

○ **Why is ammonium chloride used in stimulant intoxication?**

Ammonium chloride inhibits the absorption of amphetamines into the body by lowering the pH. This treatment modality, however, has no action on cocaine.

○ **Describe stimulant withdrawal.**

Symptoms of stimulant withdrawal include depression, anergia, anhedonia, increased drug craving, psychomotor retardation or agitation, increased appetite (hunger), somnolence, increased REM sleep, "crash," anxiety, tremulousness, dysphoria, lethargy, fatigue, nightmares (vivid unpleasant dreams), muscle cramps, profuse sweating, and insomnia or hypersomnia.

○ **Name the four types of opiate receptors.**

1. Mu
2. Kappa
3. Lambda
4. Delta

○ **What are skin poppers?**

Skin poppers are circular depressed scars sometimes complicated by underlying chronic abscesses located on the backs or thighs of people who use injectable opioids.

○ **A patient presents to the ER, and on physical examination you discover pinpoint pupils. What should you consider?**

Opioid intoxication.

○ **What drug would you give to someone with an opioid overdose?**

Naloxone.

○ **What is the most serious side effect of opioids, and how can it be treated?**

Respiratory depression, which can be treated with naloxone. Do not forget the ABCs.

○ **Describe opioid withdrawal.**

Opioid withdrawal is associated with an increased heart rate, elevated blood pressure and temperature, yawning, drug craving, insomnia, irritability, pupillary dilation, piloerection, sweating, dysphoric mood, nausea, vomiting, muscle aches, diarrhea, lacrimation, and rhinorrhea.

○ **Name medications used in maintenance therapy for opioids.**

• Methadone
• Naltrexone
• Levo alpha acetyl methadal (LAAM)
• Buprenorphine

○ **Which opioid is associated with parkinsonism?**

MPTP (1-methyl-4-phenyl-1,2,3,6-tetrahydropyridine).

○ **What nonopioid medication is also useful in decreasing the symptoms of opioid withdrawal?**

Clonidine stimulates α_2-adrenergic receptors thereby reducing the nausea, diarrhea, and sweating associated with opiate withdrawal but does not reduce muscle pain or cravings for opiates. The hypotensive effects of clonidine are poorly tolerated by some individuals, limiting its use.

○ **If opioid withdrawal is life-threatening to the fetus, what can be done?**

Low-dose methadone can be used to prevent opioid withdrawal in pregnant women dependent upon narcotics.

○ **Name the primary concern in the management of a patient with a sedative-hypnotic overdose.**

Respiratory arrest.

○ **Describe sedative-hypnotic withdrawal.**

Symptoms associated with sedative-hypnotic withdrawal include myoclonic jerks, anxiety, insomnia, psychomotor agitation, nausea and vomiting, increased temperature and pulse, tinnitus, tremor, high blood pressure, muscle fasciculations, hypersensitive areas, illusions, derealization, seizures, hallucinations, and delirium.

○ **Why can the CIWA scale be used to treat sedative-hypnotic withdrawal?**

Because sedatives and hypnotics act at the GABA receptor just like alcohol, albeit at different sites of the receptor.

○ **Describe the sedative tolerance test (pentobarbital challenge).**

Administer 200 mg of pentobarbital and check in 1 hour for intoxication. If the patient is not showing any signs of intoxication, give another 100 mg of pentobarbital every hour until signs of intoxication are evident. If <300 mg of pentobarbital was given, do nothing. But if the amount of pentobarbital is >300 mg, calculate the following: For each 100 mg of pentobarbital, give 30 mg of phenobarbital. For example, if a person required 500 mg of pentobarbital to become intoxicated, then you would give 150 mg of phenobarbital. Then decrease the dose of phenobarbital 5% to 10% per day to complete detoxification. The only problem with this protocol is that pentobarbital is not available in the United States at this time.

○ **What migraine medications can induce a severe withdrawal syndrome if overused and then abruptly discontinued?**

Those containing butalbital—Fioricet® (butalbital, acetominaphen, caffeine), Fiorinal® (butalbital, aspirin, caffeine), and Esgic® (butalbital, acetominaphen, caffeine). The withdrawal syndrome can be managed with the use of the CIWA protocol (using lorazepam or chlordiazepoxide replacement), or a phenobarbital and caffeine taper (30 mg/d phenobarbital is equivalent to 100 mg/d of butalbital).

○ **Give the names of some commonly used hallucinogens.**

- Phencyclidine (PCP)
- Lysergic acid diethylamide (LSD)
- Methylenedioxymethamphetamine (MDMA)
- Mescaline
- Peyote
- Psilocybin

○ **Name one nonpharmacologic treatment used when someone is intoxicated on hallucinogens.**

Reassurance or the "talking down" technique.

○ **If a patient describes flashbacks, what is the most likely drug used?**

PCP. In the *DSM-IV*, the term for flashbacks is hallucinogen persistent perceptual disorder.

○ **What illegal drug is highly lipid soluble and may cause recurring psychotic episodes over several months?**

Phencyclidine (PCP), because of its extreme lipid solubility, is readily deposited in fatty tissue and can produce psychotic episodes 3 to 4 months after ingestion. These psychotic episodes are frequently violent, so it may be necessary to give an antipsychotic agent until all the PCP has been released from the body. Low-potency neuroleptics are contraindicated due to autonomic dysfunction. Haloperidol is the drug of choice, while pimozide has also been used with good success.

○ **Describe the treatment of common medical problems associated with PCP.**

For tachycardia and hypertension associated with PCP, administer a β-blocker. Lorazepam is useful for agitation, while haloperidol can be used to treat psychotic symptoms. For intoxication, use ammonia chloride to acidify the urine and to increase the excretion of PCP. Lasix can be added to cause diuresis.

○ **Name substances in which acidification and alkalization of the urine is used to increase elimination from the body.**

Use acidification for barbiturates and alkalization for amphetamines and PCP.

○ **A teenager is brought to the emergency room by parents, and during the examination you discover a strange odor on the patient's breath. What do you make of it?**

You need to consider inhalant abuse, i.e., huffing. Also look for a rash near the nose and mouth.

○ **Name some common problems caused by inhalants use.**

Brain atrophy caused by heavy metals (copper and zinc), encephalopathy, seizures, TLE, and other changes on EEG, decreased IQ, ataxia, myoclonus, chorea, tremor, optic neuropathy, motor and sensory neuropathy, death by respiratory depression, cardiac arrhythmia and aspiration, hepatic and renal failure, and rhabdomyolysis.

○ **How do you treat inhalant intoxication?**

Supportive measures; remember the ABCs.

○ **A patient is noted to have conjunctival injection. What drug of abuse should you suspect?**

Cannabis.

○ **What is the most common effect of cannabis intoxication?**

Believe it or not, it is anxiety!

○ **What are the long-term effects of cannabis use?**

Cannabis interferes with formation of new memories and the ability to learn. This is why it is troublesome when adolescents use cannabis.

○ **What is the amotivational syndrome?**

Amotivational syndrome, which is associated with cannabis abuse, is characterized by an unwillingness to persist in tasks that require prolonged attention. The person may appear slothful, have increased weight, apathy, and anergia.

○ **Name some medical uses of cannabis.**

Some medicinal uses of cannabis include appetite enhancement, use as an antiemetic, reduction of intraocular pressure in glaucoma, and relief of asthma (at low doses, cannabis causes bronchial dilation, but in high doses, it can cause bronchial spasm).

○ **What are the most common cancers associated with cannabis use?**

Head and neck cancers usually occur earlier than lung cancer, but all are associated with cannabis use.

○ **What is the treatment for cannabis dependence?**

Education and support.

○ **What is tachyphylaxis?**

Tachyphylaxis is the development of tolerance after a single dose of a substance. It particularly pertains to nicotine.

○ **What is the most addicting substance of abuse?**

Nicotine.

○ **What is the lifetime prevalence of nicotine dependence in the general population?**

It is 20%.

○ **Name the two most common causes of death associated with nicotine.**

Cardiovascular disease (stroke and heart attack) and lung disease (cancer, COPD, and pneumonia).

○ **What health and cognitive problems are children of cigarette-smoking parents at risk for?**

Otitis media, pneumonia, asthma, SIDS, low birth weight, low performance on standardized tests, and poorer athletic performance.

○ **What is the most common drug that people with schizophrenia abuse?**

Nicotine.

○ **How do you determine which dose of nicotine patch to use?**

Use the Fagerstrom test for nicotine dependence (items on this scale include when the first cigarette of the day is smoked, the presence of difficulty refraining from smoking in nonsmoking areas, the number of cigarettes smoked a day, smoking more in the morning than evening, and smoking in bed when ill). If the scores falls between 7 and 10, use the 21-mg patch; if between 4 and 6, use the 14-mg patch; and if the score is <4, use the 7-mg patch.

○ **Name the approved medications indicated for smoking cessation.**

Bupropion (Zyban®) and varenicline tartrate (Chantix®).

○ **What is the most commonly used psychoactive drug in the world?**

Caffeine.

○ **Describe caffeine withdrawal.**

Fatigue, lethargy, headache, decreased activity, and irritability are all common. Mild depressive symptoms include nausea, vomiting, muscle pain and stiffness, and impaired psychomotor performance also occur.

○ **When can you expect caffeine withdrawal to begin?**

The onset is usually 12 to 24 hours after last use. It will peak in 24 to 48 hours and will resolve in approximately 1 week.

○ **How many cups of coffee would you have to drink to achieve a lethal dose of caffeine?**

One hundred cups of coffee over a 4-hour period.

○ **Name the unusual condition associated with the use of amyl nitrate.**

In susceptible persons, amyl nitrate can cause a condition called methemoglobinemia (the iron atom of the hemoglobin molecule becomes oxidized to the +3 state, thereby forming a molecule that firmly binds oxygen). In the laboratory, blood with methemoglobin will look like chocolate when placed on filter paper. Methylene blue is used to treat this condition.

○ **A body builder is brought to the emergency room because of violent behavior. What should you consider in the differential diagnosis?**

Steroid-induced psychosis (steroid rage) should be considered. Steroids can also cause euphoria, depressive symptoms, and personality change.

○ **What is the name of the drug used in some cases of date rape?**

Flunitrazepam (Rohypnol®) is a nitrobenzodiazepine no longer available commercially in the United States. Often referred to as "roofie," the hypnotic has powerful anterograde amnestic effects and has been used to impair the recall of intended victims of sexual assaults or robberies. The manufacturer, Roche, has added a dye to the formulation to make it more identifiable as a contaminant in beverages.

CHAPTER 22 Suicide

○ **Briefly describe Durkheim's theory of the etiology of suicide (1951).**

Durkeim, a French sociologist, divided suicide into three social categories:

1. Egoistic suicides occur when individuals fail to integrate into a social group, perhaps accounting for higher suicide rates in individuals who are unmarried

2. Altruistic suicidal behavior stems from excessive integration into a group, representing culturally excepted forms of suicide (such as the Japanese ritual of hari-kari) or mass suicides related to cult activity

3. Anomic suicides occur when a disturbed integration into society prevents the individual from conforming to the social norms. This would explain suicidal behavior in those individuals who have experienced a recent loss or change in status

○ **Discuss the psychological factors involved in suicidal behavior.**

There is a high association between suicidal risk and feelings of hopelessness or desperation. Feelings of shame and humiliation have also been associated with suicidal behavior. In classical psychoanalytic theory, Freud postulates that suicidal behavior is the manifestation of anger toward others turned inward toward the self. Suicidal behavior is often associated with aggression toward others.

○ **Discuss outpatient treatment of the suicidal patient.**

Patients with suicidal ideation being considered for outpatient treatment must be able to convincingly contract for safety with the treating clinician, and an appropriate intervention plan should be in place in the event that the patient feels unable to control his/her suicidal impulses. Crisis services must then be made available to the patient, and available family/social supports should be contacted and mobilized to aid the patient. Attempts should also be made to relieve or address psychosocial and environmental stressors within the home. In particular, any firearms or other potentially dangerous weapons should be removed from the home. If treatment of an underlying psychiatric disorder requires treatment with psychotropic medications, steps must be taken to ensure that the patient does not have a potentially lethal dose of medication in his/her possession. For patients who cannot make this contract or in cases where adequate social support cannot be identified, hospitalization is indicated.

○ **Discuss inpatient treatment of the suicidal patient.**

Once the suicidal patient is admitted for inpatient treatment, a thorough search of his/her belongings should occur to remove any objects which may be used for self-injury. Based on the clinical judgment of the physician and/or members of the treatment team, a schedule of regular observation of the patient should be maintained in order to ensure the patient's safety while on the unit. This observation may range from one-to-one supervision to frequent observation checks based on the intensity of the suicidal ideation. Any underlying psychiatric disorder should be treated appropriately, and supportive psychotherapy employed.

○   **What biologic findings have been associated with suicidal behaviors?**

A number of studies have found a decrease in 5-hydroxyindoleacetic acid (5-HIAA), a metabolite of serotonin, in the CSF of depressed patients, who have attempted suicide suggesting that decreased levels of serotonin may be associated with suicidal behavior. Postmortem studies of suicide victims have shown increased β-adrenergic binding in the prefrontal and temporal cortex.

○   **Discuss differences between suicide completers and attempters.**

In the general population, men are three times as likely as women to complete suicide. Women, however, attempt suicide four times more often than men do. Up to one-third of those who complete suicide have had a prior suicide attempt. Those who complete suicide generally plan the act, choose lethal means, and act in seclusion with little chance of rescue. Attempters tend to act more impulsively, notify others of their intention or carry out the attempt in the presence of others, and tend to use less lethal methods.

○   **Discuss the relationship of age to suicide risk.**

Suicide rates increase steadily with age, with the highest rates among older white males. In the United States, the suicide rate for individuals older than 65 years is 50% higher than that of the general population. While the highest rates occur among older people, it is important to note that suicide rates have been increasing among adolescents and young adults (15–24 years). Higher rates among the elderly may be associated with increased medical problems and the emotional losses common in these later years of life.

○   **Discuss the incidence of suicide among adolescents.**

Suicide is the third leading cause of death among adolescents 15 to 19 years old (gunshot wounds and motor vehicle accidents being the first and second leading cause of death). The rate of suicide among this age group has tripled in last three decades, and is attributed to an increase in alcohol abuse and greater availability of firearms.

○   **List important risk factors for suicide.**

A useful mnemonic for suicide risk factors is the phrase SAD PERSONS.

- **S**ex: Men are three times as likely as women to complete suicide; however, women are four times more likely than men to attempt.
- **A**ge: Suicide rates are higher among older persons.
- **D**epression: 10% to 15% of persons with a major affective disorder commit suicide.
- **P**revious attempts: Persons with previous suicide attempts are more likely to complete suicide.
- **E**thanol/drug abuse: Alcohol and drug use are associated with 50% of all suicides.
- **R**ational thinking loss: The risk of suicide increases with the presence of psychosis or confusion.
- **S**ocial supports: Lacking or inadequate.
- **O**rganized plan: Individuals with an organized plan are more likely to complete suicide.
- **N**o spouse: Suicide rates are higher among those who are divorced, widowed, or never married.
- **S**ickness: The presence of a chronic medical condition, particularly when there is significant loss of function or decrease in quality of life, increases the risk of suicide.

○   **What is the most consistent predictor of suicidal behavior?**

A previous suicide attempt.

○   **Discuss the impact of genetic factors on suicide risk.**

Studies among adoptees who have committed suicide have found higher suicide rates in their biological relatives when compared to their adoptive relatives. Twin studies have also found higher concordance rates for suicide as well.

○ **Name three factors that will decrease the risk of suicide.**

1. Convictions in opposition to suicide, i.e., religious beliefs.

2. Strong attachments to others, i.e., spouse and/or children.

3. Evidence of good impulse control.

○ **What percentage of those completing suicide have a psychiatric disorder?**

Ninety to ninety-five percent of individuals completing suicide have a diagnosable psychiatric disorder.

○ **What Axis I disorders are associated with an increased incidence of suicidal ideation?**

Affective disorders, substance dependence, and schizophrenia.

○ **Discuss the incidence of suicide among patients with schizophrenia.**

Ten percent of patients with schizophrenia will commit suicide, young male patients being most likely to complete suicide early in the illness. Frequent relapses and multiple hospitalizations are also associated with an increased risk of suicide in patients with schizophrenia.

○ **List two personality disorders associated with increased suicide risk.**

Antisocial personality disorder and borderline personality disorder.

○ **What CNS diseases are associated with an increased risk of suicide?**

- Epilepsy
- Huntington's chorea
- Multiple sclerosis
- Dementia
- Cerebral vascular accidents
- AIDS
- Head and spinal cord injuries

○ **What other physical illnesses are associated with an increased risk of suicide?**

- Cancer.
- End-stage renal disease requiring renal dialysis.
- Peptic ulcer disease cirrhosis.
- Endocrine disorders including Cushing's, anorexia nervosa, Klinefelter's, and porphyria.

○ **Discuss the impact of drug and alcohol dependence on suicidal risk.**

More than 50% of all suicides are associated with alcohol and/or drug dependence, and 15% to 25% of alcohol- and/or drug-dependent persons complete suicide. At least 70% of adolescent suicides are associated with alcohol and/or drug dependence.

CHAPTER 23 Forensic and Ethical Issues in Psychiatry

○ **What is the M'Naghten rule?**

Also known as the right-wrong test, the M'Naghten rule is based on the 1843 English case in which Mr. M'Naghten, a gentleman with persecutory delusions, in an attempt to kill Sir Robert Peel, mistakenly murdered Edward Drummond, Sir Peel's secretary. The rule states that a person is not guilty by reason of insanity if a defect in reasoning existed at the time of the act to the extent that the person did not know the nature, quality, and/or consequences of the act, or if that the person was incapable of recognizing that the act was wrong.

○ **What is the irresistible impulse rule?**

In 1922, a group of English jurists decided to revise the M'Naghten rule. The rule, also known as the "policeman at the elbow rule," states that a person is not criminally responsible for his acts, if he is unable to resist performing the act because of mental disease.

○ **What does the term *mens rea* mean and how does it apply?**

Mens rea literally means "evil thing" in Latin. In forensics, *mens rea* is the rational intent to do harm or "evil" to another. For a person to be legally culpable, they must be capable of forming this intent. If they are incapable of rational thought because of their mental disease or defect, they cannot be held legally responsible for their act.

○ **Who is David Bazelon and what did he say in the Durham case?**

Judge David Bazelon, in the 1954 case of *Durham v. United States*, enunciated the product rule of criminal responsibility. A person is not criminally responsible for his/her act if the act is the product of a mental disease or defect. The purpose of the decision was to obtain good, complete psychiatric testimony. In 1972, sitting as an appellate judge, he overruled his own case in *United States v. Brawner*, because confusion had developed over the definitions of "product," "disease," and "defect." Subsequently, American courts have adopted the recommendations of the American Law Institute regarding criminal responsibility.

○ **What are the recommendations of the American Law Institute regarding criminal responsibility?**

The American Law Institute, in its model penal code regarding criminal responsibility, recommends that persons are not responsible for crimes committed, if at the time of the act, because of mental disease or defect, they lacked the capacity to appreciate the criminality of their act, or could not conform their behavior to the requirement of the law. Additionally, repeated antisocial or criminal behavior is not taken to be evidence of a "mental disease or defect."

○ **In asserting the defense of mental disease or defect, at what point in time the physician must determine the patient's mental status?**

The physician must be convinced to a reasonable degree of medical certainty that at the time of commission of the act (the crime), the patient was suffering from a mental disease or defect. The occurrence of the disease or defect after the act does not absolve the patient of culpability.

○ **In what case did the United States Supreme Court state that it is against the fundamental principles of the American justice system to try someone who is mentally incompetent?**

In the case of *Dusky v. United States,* the court set forth a 13-point test to determine if a person is competent to stand trial. The test seeks to determine if the person has sufficient present ability to assist their lawyer in their defense, and to understand the charges against them.

○ **What is a determination of "general competency"?**

There is no such thing as "general competency." All determinations of competency are task specific (e.g., contracts, wills, consent to a treatment, and ability to stand trial). A person is presumed to be competent if they are of adult age, until determined otherwise by a court of competent jurisdiction. A physician may not make a determination of a patient's competency, only a court can.

○ **In determining if a patient is competent to stand trial, the psychiatrist considers what time frame does?**

In determining a patient's competency to stand trial, the psychiatrist is not interested in the patient's state at the time of the alleged crime, but their state of mind during the criminal proceedings and whether they can be treated so that they are competent (see *Dusky v. United States* for the 13-points of the examination).

○ **What are the elements of "competency to be executed"?**

A person's competence to be executed is based on his/her awareness of what is happening so that the punitive aspects of the sentence can be appreciated by the individual, so that the person can "make peace" in a religious sense if they desire, and so that a forgotten exculpatory detail, which may be exonerating, can be disclosed to the state in defense of the patient. The need to preserve competence until execution was most recently upheld by the Supreme Court case of *Ford v. Wainwright.*

○ **Can a physician participate in state-mandated executions of convicted criminals?**

Most medical societies, including the American Medical Association, state that it is unethical for physicians to participate in state-mandated executions, and the American Psychiatric Association (APA) has indicated that it is not ethical to participate in treating a mentally ill prisoner solely for the purpose of returning them to competency so they can be executed.

○ **Is it unethical to treat a patient to competency so that he may stand trial?**

No. Several medical groups including the American Medical Association oppose on ethical grounds the treating of patients to competency so that they can be executed, but such ethical consideration does not apply to treating them to competency so that they can assist in their defense and stand trial.

○ **What are the elements of testamentary capacity?**

Testamentary capacity is the ability to make a legal will disposing of or transferring the property of the said person. The person must be able at the time of execution of the will (or transfer) to know the nature and extent of the property, know that they are making the transfer or document, and know who their natural beneficiaries are (who would be entitled to their property).

○ **What are the elements of informed consent?**

The elements of informed consent include awareness of the risks and benefits of the proposed treatment/therapy, awareness of alternative therapies, awareness of the risks of no treatments, and a voluntary nature of the consent.

○ **A physician who fails to obtain informed consent from patients prior to treating them may be charged with what tort (wrongful act)?**

Battery. Judge Cardozo, in *Schloendorff v. Society of New York Hospitals,* stated, "Every human being of adult years and sound mind has a right to determine what shall be done with his own body" and that a physician who treats without consent commits a battery for which the patient may recover damages.

○ **When, if ever, is consent not required for treatment of a patient?**

There is an emergency exception to the informed consent rule that allows a physician to provide treatment that the reasonable person would want if they were able to consent to treatment. This applies only when there is an emergency situation and delaying treatment in order to obtain consent would have serious adverse consequences to the patient's life.

○ **What did the Gault decision hold?**

The Gault decision of 1967 holds that all juveniles must be represented by council, able to confront witnesses, and be given timely notice of charges. Additionally, emancipated minors have the rights of adults when they can show that they have control over their own lives and are living as adults. Otherwise, the parent or guardian is the person empowered to give consent for medical treatment. Most states have exceptions to this requirement for specific diseases or conditions (e.g., sexually transmitted disease, pregnancy, and substance abuse), in that minors can receive treatment for these conditions without the knowledge or consent of their parents.

○ **What does the term *parens patriae* mean and how does it apply to psychiatry?**

Parens patriae, translated from Latin, literally means, "*father of the country,*" and refers to the king's duty to care for his subjects as if they were his family. In current times, it is a legal principle that allows a unit of government to step in to protect a person who is a danger to himself, or to protect society from a person who is a danger to others. In psychiatry, it is the legal basis for involuntary commitment laws and emergency detainment statutes.

○ **What are a physician's duties after Tarasoff?**

The California Court in 1974 (*Tarasoff v. Regents of University of California, 1974*) held that a physician has the duty to warn third parties of possible serious harm to them by a patient if they are readily identifiable, and if the risk of harm is substantial and imminent.

○ **Which case holds that a psychiatrist has the duty to protect the public from a dangerous patient?**

The court in Tarasoff II (*Tarasoff v. Regents of University of California, 1976*) held that the psychiatrist not only has the duty to warn, but also the duty to protect not only the identified victim, but also the public, from a patient that they believe is dangerous. This may include breach of confidence and emergency detention of the patient.

○ **What did Judge Johnson rule in the 1971 case of *Wyatt v. Stickney?***

The federal district court in the 1971 class action suit, *Wyatt v. Stickney,* ruled that persons who have been civilly committed to a mental institution have a constitutional right to receive such treatment as might give them the opportunity to be cured or to have their mental condition improved.

○ **What did the U.S. Supreme Court rule in the 1976 case of *O'Connor v. Donaldson*?**

The Supreme Court, in *O'Connor v. Donaldson* (*1976*), ruled that a harmless patient could not be confined against his/her will without treatment if they could survive in a less restrictive environment.

○ **What is a writ of *habeas corpus*?**

A writ of *habeas corpus* is a petition that a person can file with the court if they believe that they have been illegally deprived of their liberty. In psychiatry, a patient, who has been hospitalized involuntarily and believes that he/she should be released, has the right to file such a writ, in which case the court must determine immediately if hospitalization was performed without due process.

○ **Does a patient being detained on an inpatient facility has the right to make telephone calls?**

Even if the patient is being involuntarily detained, they retain the right to have unmonitored communication with the outside world. This may be limited or restricted only during emergency situations.

○ **Does a patient have the right to have visitors during reasonable hours while on an inpatient unit?**

A patient, even if involuntarily admitted, has the right to have outside visitors during reasonable hospital visiting hours. Such rights may be curtailed only during emergency situations. Some visitors, i.e., the patient's attorney, physician, and members of the clergy, have the right to visit outside of ordinary hours. Noxious visitors (e.g., family members bringing contraband) may be curtailed.

○ **Does a patient have a right to refuse treatment?**

Patients of adult age and sound mind always have a right to refuse treatment (Judge Cardozo, 1914). This was more specifically addressed in the 1979 case of *Rennie v. Klein.* However, in 1981, the court allowed the appointment of a guardian to authorize treatment, if in the best interests of the patient (*Roger v. Oken*).

○ **What is the significance of the *Schloendorff v. Society of New York Hospitals* case?**

It is taken as the earliest case in which the right of the patient to not have treatment unless he consented to it was enunciated.

○ **Is a psychiatrist considered a fact witness when they testify in a court proceeding?**

Depends on what the psychiatrist testifies about. A fact witness is a person that supplies information (or facts) to the court in a proceeding. As such, a psychiatrist is entitled to no greater creditability than any other witness in a proceeding and can testify only as to facts within their own knowledge. When a psychiatrist testifies as to the psychiatric condition, diagnosis, or treatment of a patient, he/she is acting as an *expert witness,* and is allowed to draw conclusions from data in the record and render opinions within his/her field of expertise. Such opinions must be stated "to a reasonable degree of medical certainty." An expert witness must prove their credentials (education and qualifications) to the court and have them accepted by the court in each case in which they testify in such capacity.

○ **Who is your client if you are appointed by a court to examine a patient?**

The court is your client if you are appointed by the court to examine a patient and the doctor–patient privilege does not apply. You must inform the patient of that prior to doing the examination and the patient may refuse to participate in the examination, since it would amount to him being forced to testify against himself.

○ **What is testimonial privilege?**

It is the legal principle that allows a physician to keep confidential any information provided to him by a patient for use in treating the patient. The privilege is owned by the patient, that is to say that only the patient can assert it or waive it.

○ **What is confidentiality?**

Confidentiality is the long-standing, ethical/moral principle that the patient has the right to expect that information provided to a physician will be kept secret and not shared with others.

○ **To whom does the duty of confidentiality extend?**

The duty of confidentiality extends to the patient. If a physician shares this information, they may be liable for breach of that duty and may be sued by the patient. The expectation of confidentiality does not extend to other caregivers and consultants as they require information to treat the patient. The supervision of physicians in training, especially psychiatrists, presents an interesting issue about the extent of the duty.

○ **When, if ever, may you breach confidentiality?**

Confidentiality may be breached when a patient tells a physician about plans to murder or harm a specific person (does not apply to past crimes); when there is a life-threatening emergency, at which time information necessary to maintain the patient's life may be provided to another provider; when subpoenaed by a court of law to provide testimony; when given permission, preferably in writing, by the patient; and when child abuse is suspected.

○ **If you receive a call from a hospital about a patient you are treating, can you acknowledge that they are your patient and provide information about their diagnosis, medication, and treatment?**

Usually you cannot disclose or even acknowledge that you are treating a patient for a mental disease or defect without the prior consent of the patient. Most courts will carve out an exception for the provision of emergency information to treat a patient in an emergency situation (e.g., types and dosages of a patient that is unable to provide the information or may be having a drug reaction). It is a good practice to obtain the patient's consent to such disclosure as soon as possible afterwards.

○ **May you disclose the diagnosis and medications of a patient who is covered by an insurance company, so that you can be reimbursed for your services already rendered to the patient?**

You cannot disclose such information to a third party such as an insurance company or employer, even if it means you will not be paid for your services, unless you have a prior written consent from your patient for the disclosure of such information to that particular party.

○ **If your patient has instructed you that they do not wish you to disclose their treatment or diagnosis in court, may you assert that wish against a subpoena for such information?**

Although the doctor–patient privilege belongs to the patient and may only be asserted or waived by them, a court may require, by subpoena, that such information be given by the doctor to the court.

○ **What is a physician's duty if he/she suspects child abuse?**

The physician has a duty, which varies from state to state, to report all cases of suspected child abuse to the appropriate governmental entity. In some states, this has also been extended to cases of suspected elder abuse as well.

○ **Does a psychiatrist have a duty to report any case of suspected elder abuse?**

While all states have requirements that any physician report any suspected case of child abuse, and hold the physician harmless if they have a reasonable basis for their belief, the same is not true for cases of elder abuse. However, it is being expanded in a growing number of states to include elder abuse.

○ **What is the most frequent basis for malpractice claims brought against psychiatrists?**

The most common cause of lawsuits filed against psychiatrists is not for sexual involvement (<6%), but in fact, is for suicide and suicide attempts. More than 50% of suicides/attempts lead to malpractice claims against the psychiatrist.

○ **How long after discharge must a psychiatrist wait before they can have personal involvement with a patient?**

The APA, in its most recent version of the code of ethics and professional conduct, has adopted the adage "once a patient always a patient." Prior codes had allowed contact after a specified period of time, but this is no longer the case.

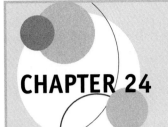

CHAPTER 24

Noncompliance with Treatment

○ **What is the essential feature of malingering?**

The essential feature of malingering is the intentional production of false or grossly exaggerated physical or psychological symptoms motivated by external incentives such as avoiding military duty, avoiding work, obtaining financial compensation, evading criminal prosecution, or obtaining drugs.

○ **When should malingering be strongly suspected?**

When a combination of the following is noted: medicolegal context of presentation; marked discrepancy between the person's claimed stress and the objective findings; lack of cooperation during the diagnostic evaluation and in complying with the prescribed treatment; and presence of antisocial personality disorder.

○ **What is the main factor that differentiates malingering from factitious disorder?**

The main difference between malingering and factitious disorder is the presence of a clearly definable goal associated with malingering.

○ **Distinguish between malingering and somatoform disorders.**

Somatoform disorders lack the volitional component of malingering. In somatoform disorder, an underlying emotional conflict is thought to be unconsciously transformed into a physical manifestation of some kind. No external or environmental outcome or reward is consciously sought.

○ **Under what category of *DSM-IV* is malingering classified?**

Additional Conditions That May Be a Focus of Clinical Attention (V Code).

○ **What factors may underlie the disinclination of professionals to label patients as malingerers?**

Clinicians may find it distasteful and a violation of the doctor–patient relationship to question a patient's intentions. Concern over legal liability also inhibits the widespread labeling of malingering. Finally, there is a concern among physicians about the anger and possible physical outbursts that might result if a patient's conscious attempt at deception is revealed to them.

○ **What is the incidence of malingering?**

Malingering is estimated to occur in 1% of mental health patients in civilian clinical practices, with the estimate rising to 5% in the military.

○ **Does the incidence of malingering increase in a litigious context?**

Yes. In a litigious context, during interviews of criminal defendants, the estimated incidence of malingering is much higher, between 10% and 20%.

○ **In what settings is malingering usually found?**

Settings with a preponderance of men, such as the military, prisons, and industrial settings.

○ **What disorders have been associated with malingering?**

Associated disorders include conduct disorder and anxiety disorders in children, and antisocial personality disorder in adults.

○ **Are there known predisposing genetic or neurophysiological factors known to be associated with malingering?**

No.

○ **The malingerer is likely hoping to achieve what ends?**

Avoidance of criminal responsibility; avoidance of military service or hazardous duties; financial gain; facilitation of transfer from prison to hospital; admission to a hospital; and/or prescription drugs.

○ **What is the clinician's best tool in the detection of malingering?**

Interviewing skills.

○ **How should the patient suspected of malingering be approached?**

A thorough evaluation should be performed, and the examiner should refrain from showing suspicion.

○ **What are the most likely psychiatric conditions to be mimicked by the malingerer?**

- Mental retardation
- Organic impairment
- Amnesia
- Psychosis
- Posttraumatic residual

○ **Should the clinical interview in suspected malingering be long or short?**

Intentional malingering is harder to maintain, as the evaluative interview becomes increasingly lengthy. In addition to basic fatigue, the pull toward reality is believed to be responsible for that phenomenon. Therefore, when malingering is suspected, the clinical interview should be as long and detailed as logistics allow.

○ **Are facial expression and eye contact good indicators of truthfulness?**

Contrary to popular myth and intuition, facial expression and eye contact are poor indicators of truthfulness.

○ **What percentage of tested persons are able to maintain a lie under sodium amobarbital or hypnotic techniques?**

Fifty percent.

○ **What symptom do criminal defendants attempting to malinger psychosis most frequently fake?**

Auditory hallucinations.

○ **What is the most widely employed psychological test for the purpose of the detection of malingering?**

The Minnesota Multiphasic Personality Inventory (MMPI) or its update, MMPI-2.

○ **Are a real psychiatric disorder and malingering mutually exclusive?**

No.

○ **What is Ganser's syndrome?**

Ganser's syndrome of approximate answers is rare and described primarily in prison populations. It involves the production of answers to questions that are relevant, but not quite correct, such as stating that the product of 7 times 4 is 29.

○ **What groups of patients are at greater risk for noncompliance?**

Patients who have chronic illness, do not feel pain or discomfort, require long-term maintenance, are hostile, and those who are on preventive regimens.

○ **What is the definition of compliance?**

Compliance is the manner in which a patient carries out his or her physician's medical and/or clinical recommendations.

○ **What percentage of hospital and nursing home admissions is due to noncompliance?**

Up to 10% of hospital and 25% of nursing home admissions can be attributed, at least in part, to poor compliance.

○ **What is the estimated percentage of patients who are noncompliant with medications?**

Approximately 50% of outpatients and 25% of inpatients.

○ **Describe the "rule of thirds" in regard to compliance.**

Around one-third of patients are compliant, one-third occasionally comply with aspects of treatment, and another third never comply with prescribed treatment.

○ **Describe the stereotypical noncompliant patient.**

There is no stereotypical noncompliant patient. Most of the studies searching for determinants of compliance have failed to show any general characteristic of a noncompliant patient.

○ **List five factors that tend to increase compliance.**

1. Patient satisfaction
2. Supervision
3. Patient insight into his/her disease
4. Family influences on the patient
5. Family stability

○ **List seven factors that tend to decrease patient compliance.**

1. Asymptomatic illness
2. Lengthy duration of therapy
3. Complex treatment regimens
4. Adverse side effects
5. Social isolation
6. Anxiety
7. Substance abuse

○ **What physician factors increase compliance?**

Enthusiasm, older age, experience, and increased time spent talking to patients. Written or visual instructions on medications and treatment plans are often more helpful than verbal ones.

○ **What patient factors are generally necessary for patient compliance?**

Patients must view their disease as a serious disorder that can affect them personally. Also, they must believe it can be controlled with a prescribed treatment.

○ **What groups are overly represented among noncompliant patients?**

Children, elderly, and the disadvantaged.

○ **What are the magic numbers for compliance with medication?**

Patients tend to be noncompliant when they must take more than two medicines a day or when they have to take their medicines more than three times per day.

○ **What are some typical countertransference reactions exhibited by physicians toward noncompliant patients?**

Many countertransference reactions can occur when patients are noncompliant with treatment regimens. Some physicians may harshly declare that their patient must find another provider. The physician may hope that deserting their patient may cause them to experience a hurt that will make them regret their lack of compliance. Physicians may also withhold useful information or help in order to see patients "learn their lesson" by experiencing a relapse of their illness. Awareness of these reactions, and hence prevention of acting out on the part of the physician, is preferred.

○ **Is the following statement more likely to increase or decrease compliance: "If you don't take your medicine every day, you'll have a heart attack"?**

This is an example of a statement that is counterproductive to compliance. Treatment directions are more likely to be followed and remembered if they are given with a pleasant demeanor followed by a positive discussion of expected outcome.

○ **What are the three stages of compliance?**

1. Comprehension
2. Supervision
3. Independence

○ **True/False: Lack of understanding instructions is generally related to patients' intellectual or cognitive deficits.**

False.

○ **What is the one certain way to determine a patient's comprehension?**

Ask the patient to describe his or her own interpretation of medication administration to instructions ascertain that it is in agreement with the actual prescription.

○ **What symptom of psychiatric patients may contribute to noncompliance?**

Psychiatric patients may have complex delusional systems and less insight into their illness, whereby compliance with a treatment regimen may be compromised.

○ **What are the two symptoms of depression that may contribute to noncompliance?**

Decreased energy/motivation and passive suicidal ideation.

○ **How does anxiety contribute to noncompliance?**

Patients with anxiety may forget directions or worry about medication side effects.

○ **List some of the traits of schizophrenic patients that are associated with higher rates of noncompliance.**

- Severe anxiety
- Paranoia
- Grandiosity
- Depression
- Hostility
- Global psychopathology
- Coexisting personality disorders
- Substance abuse hinder medication compliance in psychotic patients

○ **What are some common misconceptions that can lead to noncompliance among schizophrenic patients?**

Common misperceptions regarding medications in patients with schizophrenia include the interpretation that taking medications equates with being ill, a lack of education about medications, and paranoid beliefs about medications.

○ **Name two secondary gains associated with medication noncompliance in patients with schizophrenia.**

Sometimes schizophrenic patients may have delusions that they are very powerful or special with unique abilities (these thoughts can be a source of positive self-image that vanish with antipsychotic medications). Also, if schizophrenic patients do not take their medications, they are freed from society's usual demands on them.

○ **What are some of the ways in which schizophrenic patients can exercise autonomy over their medications?**

Allow patients to self-adjust their dose of medications within set limits and encourage patients to keep a log of their medication administration.

○   **How can family and friends help chronically mentally ill patients comply with taking medication?**

Ways in which family and friends can aid compliance include monitoring of medication schedules and medication administration, providing supportive feedback to the patient for taking medication, encouraging the patient to participate in positive activities when they demonstrate improvement, and acting as a source of information to the physician, which may help modify treatment plans to fit the patient's lifestyle.

CHAPTER 25 Cultural Psychiatry

○ **What universal behaviors are seen in children of all cultures?**

Smiling as a social greeting, separation anxiety from 6 to 12 months of age, taboo against incest and homicide, gender-specific roles, and more aggression in males than females.

○ **What is the difference between acculturation and assimilation?**

Ethnic groups that have adopted some of the characteristics of a larger society, yet retain their own ethnic identity are acculturated, while groups that have been totally absorbed into a society with loss of ethnic traditions have become assimilated.

○ **What is culture shock?**

Culture shock is a condition of anxiety or depression, accompanied at times by a sense of isolation, derealization, and depersonalization that is precipitated by an abrupt change in cultural setting. It is minimized when at least a part of the family unit accompanies an individual to another culture. While higher rates of psychiatric hospitalizations and acute psychotic episodes have been reported for immigrants than the native born, their prognosis is good.

○ **What are the findings of cross-cultural studies regarding child-rearing practices?**

Across different cultures, child-rearing practices vary considerably. However, young infants universally require indulgence and care to become healthy adults. The care can be provided by a variety of caregivers, in addition to the mother. The ability of the caregivers to negotiate issues of independence–dependence and love–hate relationships influences to some degree adult personality structure. The extent, however, is not fully known.

○ **What is a culture-bound syndrome?**

A culture-bound syndrome is a psychiatric condition specific to, and recognized by, certain societies that occurs abruptly and has a limited clinical course.

○ **Describe the culture-bound syndrome known as "ataque de nervios."**

Seen in societies of Costa Rica and Latin America, "ataque de nervios" presents as uncontrollable episodes of shouting, crying, trembling, and a sensation of heat in the chest rising to the head. Associated symptoms include headache, insomnia, anorexia, diarrhea, anger, despair, and fear.

○ **What Southeast Asian culture-bound syndrome is characterized by dissociation associated with outbursts of violence, aggression, and even homicidal behavior?**

"Amok," a condition prevalent primarily in males, is often precipitated by a perceived insult or slight, and may be accompanied by persecutory ideas, amnesia, and exhaustion.

○ **What term is used in India to describe severe anxiety and hypochondriacal concerns associated with feelings of weakness, exhaustion, and discharge of semen into the urine?**

"Dhat."

○ **In episodes of sudden, intense anxiety that the penis, vulva, or nipples will recede into the body and possibly cause death is associated with which East Asian culture-bound syndrome?**

"Koro."

○ **An excessive startle reaction associated with echopraxia, echolalia, command obedience, and dissociative or trance behavior best describes which Indonesian culture-bound syndrome?**

Primarily seen in women, "latah" is found also in Thailand, Japan, Africa, Malaysia, and the Philippines.

○ **How does the culture-bound syndrome "mal de ojo" present?**

"Mal de ojo" presents as episodes of fitful sleep and crying without an apparent cause in young children. Somatic symptoms include diarrhea, emesis, and fever. Of Spanish origin, the phase translates into English as "evil eye."

○ **Describe "piblokto."**

Also known as Arctic hysteria, "piblokto" is observed primarily in Arctic and subarctic Eskimo communities. During the dissociative episode, which lasts for 1 to 2 hours and is followed by amnesia, the patients (usually female) will scream, destroy clothing, and prostrate themselves upon the snow and ice despite subzero temperatures. Peers are reluctant to touch the patient while in such a state, as it is thought to be caused by possession of evil spirits.

○ **What are "qi gong" psychotic reactions?**

These acute, time-limited episodes of dissociation and paranoia occur after participation in the Chinese folk health-enhancing practice of "qi gong" (exercise of vital energy).

○ **What is "rootwork"?**

Also known as voodoo, "rootwork" is a set of cultural interpretations seen in African American subgroups (Haitians) that ascribe illness to hexing, witchcraft, and sorcery. A "root doctor" or healer in this tradition treats illness through the use of rites, trances, and suggestion.

○ **What are the characteristics of "Sangue D'ormido"?**

A culture-bound syndrome of Portugal, "Sangue D'ormido" is characterized by a multitude of symptoms including pain, numbness, tremor, paralysis, convulsions, stroke, blindness, cardiac arrest, infection, and miscarriage.

○ **Describe the Chinese folk label "Shenkui."**

"Shenkui" is a state of marked anxiety and panic symptoms accompanied by somatic complaints such as dizziness, backache, fatigue, insomnia, frequent dreams, premature ejaculation, and impotence. These symptoms are attributed to excessive semen loss from frequent intercourse, masturbation, nocturnal emission, or passing of white, turbid urine. It represents loss of one's vital essence and is perceived as life-threatening.

○ **What is the trance state called in which individuals communicate with deceased relatives or spirits, and which is accompanied by brief periods of personality change?**

Such a trance state is called a "spell," and is seen among African Americans and European Americans from the Southern United States.

○ **What is "Zar"?**

A general term applied to dissociative states in Ethiopia, Somalia, Egypt, Sudan, and Iran, Zar is attributed to being possessed by spirits. The dissociative episode is characterized by shouting, laughing, singing, weeping, hitting one's head against a wall, and withdrawal from daily activities.

○ **Describe "windigo."**

"Windigo" is an Algonkian Indian syndrome characterized by the fear that one will become a cannibal if possessed by the Windigo monster.

○ **What is the difference between the Japanese culture-bound syndromes of "Shinkeishitsu" and "Taijin-kyofusho"?**

"Shinkeishitsu" is a syndrome characterized by obsessiveness, somatic complaints, social withdrawal, and perfectionism, while "Taijin-kyofusho" is a state of anxiety in which one fears rejection, avoids eye contact, and is concerned about body odor.

○ **What Mohave Indian culture-bound syndrome is associated with anorexia, depression, and suicide when an unwanted separation from a loved one occurs?**

"Hi-Wa itck."

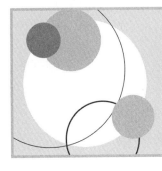

Section IV

SELECT TOPICS IN CHILD PSYCHIATRY

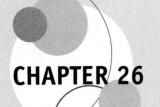

CHAPTER 26

Normal Growth and Development

○ **What are the three types of temperament described by Chess and Thomas (1986)?**

The three types of temperament described by Chess and Thomas are easy, difficult, and "slow to warm."

1. Easy temperament is characterized by easy adaptability to change without negativity, a generally positive mood, well-modulated internal regulation (sleep, hunger, etc.) and curiosity when approaching new stimuli. Approximately 40% of infants are of this type.

2. Difficult temperament characterizes approximately 10% of infants, who display irritability or intense negative reactions to change, withdrawal from new stimuli, and biologic irregularity of sleep–wake cycle, hunger, and mood.

3. The third type of temperament is the "slow-to-warm" type, exemplified by infants who tend to withdraw from new stimuli, are slow to accept change, and have frequent negative reactions of low intensity. They are sometimes described as "shy."

○ **What two hormones reach higher levels in adolescents than in adults?**

LH and testosterone peak at higher than adult baseline levels in late adolescence (by around the age of 17 years), after a steady increase throughout adolescence. Testosterone is responsible for masculinization and estradiol is responsible for feminization.

○ **A 14-year-old female presents with concern that her breasts look like "double bumps," and that her left one seems larger. She is uncomfortable that she will remain this way. On further questioning you determine that she had her first menses approximately 1 year ago, but it is sometimes irregular, and that her pubic hair has not spread to her medial thighs. What is her Tanner stage?**

She is Tanner stage 4 both in breast and pubic hair development. It is important to keep in mind that early adolescents are extremely sensitive about their physical appearance, the opinions of their peers, and fear deviating from the norm.

○ **Describe the Tanner stages of development.**

Tanner I—No pubic hair, small testicular volume, and no breast development.

Tanner II—Downy hair at base of penis or on labia majora, testicular volume increases to 1.6 to 6 mL, penis length unchanged, and breast bud forms and areola widens.

Tanner III—Hair coarsens, testicular volume increases to 6 to 12 mL, penis lengthens to 6 cm, and breast elevates.

Tanner IV—Pubic hair extends across pubis, testicular volume 12 to 20 mL, scrotum larger and darker, penis length 10 cm, breast increases in size and elevation, and areola and papilla form secondary mound.

Tanner V—Pubic hair extends to medial thighs, testicular volume >20 mL, penis 15 cm in length, and adult breast size with areola within contour of breast and papilla projecting.

○ **True/False: Infants respond to pleasant and unpleasant smells at birth.**

True. Infants have been shown to smile in response to a banana smell and to protest the odor of rotten eggs.

○ **Identify four factors that have been shown to be protective to a child having experienced a high-risk trauma (i.e., refugee, death of parent).**

Factors that have been identified as protective to children in traumatic situations include:

1. The presence of strong social supports
2. A structured upbringing
3. A high level of intelligence
4. The ability to "bounce back"

○ **A toddler has just learned to build a tower of two blocks, can say "ma-ma" and "da-da" along with several other words, walks with only an occasional tumble, and enjoys feeding himself finger foods. How old is this child?**

By 15 months, most infants are developing the beginnings of meaningful language, and have developed enough fine motor control to use a pincer grasp with some skill, and to construct a basic tower.

○ **According to Gessell (1925), at what approximate age does a child develop a "social smile" in response to the voice or face of a caretaker?**

Although infants smile spontaneously from within the first weeks of life, the "social smile" in response to a familiar person does not occur until four to eight weeks of age. Of interest is that even blind infants smile "reflexively."

○ **What is anaclitic depression?**

Severe maternal deprivation syndrome. Infants whose mother became unavailable for a long period develop a syndrome of crying, weight loss, insomnia, apathy, impaired development, and susceptibility to infection. After 3 months, the damage becomes irreversible and leads to eventual death due to marasmus—an extreme emaciation due to wasting of body tissues.

○ **What is the age of maximum risk for accidental ingestion or poisoning?**

Children between 2 and 3 years of age have the greatest incidence of accidental poisoning, because their motor activity skills are far more advanced than their judgment.

○　**A 4½-year-old child is brought to your office for nocturnal enuresis. His mother reports that he has never been completely dry for more than a week, but the frequency of his "accidents" has increased. What are the possible etiologies for this behavior?**

First reassure the mother and child that 30% to 40% of children at his age still have nocturnal enuresis, especially males. Possible causes include urologic disease or malformation, regression secondary to increased stress, immaturity of his urinary and neurologic systems necessary for absolute sphincter control, impaired stage 4 sleep, and familial genetic factors.

○　**What is the most common cause of death in adolescents?**

Accidents are the number one reason, homicide is the second, and suicide is the third. However, in some areas, homicide has become the number one cause of death among adolescents.

○　**A 9-year-old attempts to explain to his 6-year-old cousin that because 3 + 8 = 11, obviously 11 − 8 = 3. His cousin could not understand this Piagetian concept. What is it?**

Understanding reversibility is one developmental task of latency, as demonstrated in the above example. Reversibility is also the concept that ice melts into water and refreezes back into ice. Another concept acquired during the stage of concrete operations is conservation, which is best demonstrated by understanding that a tall, thin glass can contain the same amount of water as a short, wide glass.

○　**A blanket that is needed by a 2-year-old can best be described as what type of object?**

A transitional object, an item that serves to soothe a child during times of stress or during the absence of a caretaker.

○　**By what age does core gender identity become well established?**

Gender identity is generally established between the ages of 2 and 3 years in both males and females. By this time they have also recognized the anatomic differences between the genders.

○　**Describe the type of play that is characteristic of each age group as described by Piaget.**

Between 9 and 12 months the child develops object permanence, which allows the child to retain an object in mind when no longer visible. Thus, games such as peek-a-boo become enjoyable. Around 18 to 24 months symbolic thought is acquired, and the toddler begins to play symbolically. Between 2 and 7 years, symbolic play expands to rich imaginative creativity driven by magical thinking. By latency, concrete operations take hold and children use rigid rules, turn taking, and rituals to establish group games and clubs.

○　**A 5-year-old girl is devoted to a stuffed dog whom she carries everywhere and relates to as if it were human. She carries on complete conversations with this toy as if it were her close friend. How would you best describe this behavior?**

This is a fairly frequent variant on the imaginary friend, in this case a toy dog that has been anthropomorphized. The imaginary friend is quite common, some studies suggesting as high as 50%. They most often appear during preschool age and usually disappear by the age of 12 years. Their purpose appears to be to relieve loneliness and to reduce anxiety.

○　**What are the three stages in moral development according to Kohlberg?**

Kohlberg's first stage of moral development is premorality, in which obedience to the parent and avoidance of punishment are key. Morality of conventional role-conformity follows, motivated by a desire to gain approval and maintain good relations. The highest level is morality of self-accepted moral principles or compliance with voluntary rules derived from ethical principles. In this last stage, exceptions can be made to the rules in specific circumstances.

○　**Which phase of adolescence is most characterized by psychological turmoil and anxiety, difficult relationships with parents, acting out behavior, and sexual experimentation?**

Early adolescence, from 12 to 15 years, is a period of dissolution of intense ties to siblings, parents, and parental surrogates. It is a time of needing to belong to the peer group and learning to adjust to significant internal hormonal changesand their external manifestations.

○　**At what age does a child fully understand that death is permanent?**

Most children have developed this understanding by 8 to 10 years of age. At earlier ages, there is a concept of death as a separation, such as going to sleep, but not the full understanding of the permanence of death.

○　**A 6-year-old boy repeatedly awakens screaming. He does not seem to recognize familiar faces, and remains frightened, unable to be soothed, and is somewhat unarousable. What is this phenomenon called?**

Night terrors, or pavor nocturnus, occurs during non-REM sleep, usually stage 3 or 4. Children frequently remain in an "in-between state," as the dream continues even when their eyes open.

○　**What is the difference between bonding and attachment?**

Attachment, according to Bowlby, occurs when the infant has a warm, intimate, and continuous relationship with the mother and both mother and child find satisfaction and enjoyment. Bonding concerns the mother's feelings for her infant and differs from attachment because the mother does not rely on the infant as a source of security (a requirement of attachment). Research suggests bonding occurs when there is direct contact between mother and child. Attachment can be assessed by the "strange situation" test.

○　**Caretaker deprivation, or a lack of attention and interaction with the infant can result in a wide variety of pathology. Identify several potential outcomes.**

Psychosocial dwarfism, separation anxiety disorder, avoidant personality disorder, depressive disorders, delinquency, learning disorders, borderline intelligence, and failure to thrive. The outcome depends on many different factors including the severity of the deprivation, the developmental phase of the child and the attachment relationship, the availability of alternative sources for support, and the inherent resilience of the child.

○　**A 4-year-old child reprimands the dresser drawer for hitting her in the head, and inquires why it would do that. This is an example of which concept of preoperational thinking?**

Animistic thinking, which is the tendency to endow physical events and objects with lifelike psychological attributes such as feelings and intentions.

○　**During a therapy session, a business executive expressed that his wife was frustrated because he cannot "put himself in her shoes," in order to understand how she feels. Which preoperational thinking style does this demonstrate?**

Egocentrism, in which the child views themselves as the center of the universe and is unable to take on the role of another person. This can also be a feature of a narcissistic personality structure.

○　**Children who become extremely violent frequently have witnessed or experienced extreme violence. Identify other factors that also occur more frequently in violent children than in nonviolent children.**

Violent children have a higher likelihood of having a history of facial and head trauma (often inflicted by parents), increased exposure to violence in their environment (including fantasy materials such as movies, video games, and television), a severe reading disability, and repeated subjugation to frustration.

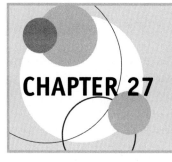

CHAPTER 27 Pervasive Developmental Disorders and Communication Disorders

○ **Why is autistic disorder also known as Kanner's autism?**

In 1943, Leo Kanner provided the first comprehensive description of the disorder in his classic paper, "Autistic Disturbances of Affective Contact."

○ **What is the gender distribution of autistic disorder?**

The male-to-female ratio of distribution is 4 to 5:1, but girls tend to be more seriously affected.

○ **Is it true that autistic disorder is found more frequently in families lacking emotional warmth (emotional refrigeration)?**

This phenomenon was noted in Kanner's initial report. However, there is no evidence that parenting deficiencies cause autism, as suggested in Kanner's initial report.

○ **What are the CT findings associated with autistic disorder?**

There are no specific anatomic abnormalities directly associated with autism. Nonspecific CT findings do include ventricular enlargement, left temporal lobe abnormalities, and asymmetry.

○ **What is the evidence of a genetic contribution to autistic disorder?**

Siblings of those with autism have a higher risk of developing autism, and the concordance rate of autistic disorder in monozygotic twins is higher that that in dizygotic twins.

○ **A boy asks, "Do you want the candy?" when he means that he wants the candy. What is this phenomenon called?**

Pronominal reversal, a feature of the impairment in communication and language skills characteristic of autism.

○ **Describe the level of intellectual functioning to be expected in patients with autistic disorder.**

Approximately 70% of autistic patients have an IQ below 70. The IQ scores tend to be low in verbal sequencing and abstraction skills, rather than in visuospatial or rote memory skills.

○ **What is meant by splinter functions and "idiot savant"?**

Even with full-scale IQ scores in the mentally retarded range, many children with autism possess unusual cognitive or visuomotor abilities. These capabilities are referred to as "splinter functions" or "islets of precocity." The most striking examples are idiot savants, who have rote memory capabilities or calculating abilities beyond those of their normal peers.

239

○   **What are the clinical differences between children with autism and those with schizophrenia?**

Hallucinations and delusions are features of childhood schizophrenia, but not autism.

○   **What are the differentiating features between autistic disorders and mental retardation?**

Unlike children with autism, mentally retarded children are able to relate to people, use language in accordance with their mental age, and have a relatively even profile of functions without splinter functions. However, the two conditions may coexist, and the clinician must be aware of the autistic individual's level of cognitive functioning in order to better recommend appropriate treatment options.

○   **In terms of nonverbal communication, how are autistic disorder and mixed receptive-expressive language disorder differentiated from each other?**

Children with autism have elementary, or totally lack nonverbal communication skills. Children with mixed receptive-expressive language disorder, although impaired in language ability, are able to communicate nonverbally, and are more interactive with people than children with autism.

○   **What laboratory tests can differentiate congenital hearing impairment from autism?**

An audiogram or auditory-evoked potentials. Significant hearing loss is generally not associated with autism.

○   **What is the difference between children with autism and deaf children in respect to their response to sound intensity?**

Deaf children respond only to loud sounds, whereas children with autism may ignore loud or normal sounds, but respond to soft or low sounds. Additionally, some children with autism are exquisitely sensitive to certain sounds, and can either become exceedingly fearful, or act out when those sounds occur.

○   **How does one differentiate psychosocial deprivation from autistic disorder?**

Children with psychosocial deprivation may improve rapidly when placed in a favorable and enriched psychosocial environment, but such an improvement does not appear in children with autism.

○   **What is the adult outcome of autistic disorder?**

Most adults with autism remain severely handicapped. Only 1% to 2% acquire an independent status with gainful employment, although 5% to 20% can achieve a borderline normal status.

○   **What are the goals of treatment in autistic disorder?**

Goals of multimodal treatment programs for children with autism include social skills training, development of verbal and nonverbal communication, maximizing independent living skills, and support of community support systems, such as family, schools, churches, assisted living organizations, and mental health facilities.

○   **What is the prevalence of seizure disorders in patients with autistic disorder?**

Approximately 35% to 50% of patients with autism will have a seizure disorder, which adversely affects prognosis.

○ **How are haloperidol and risperidone used in the treatment of autistic disorders?**

Haloperidol and risperidone have been found to both accelerate learning and reduce behavioral symptoms (hyperactivity, stereotypies, withdrawal, fidgetiness, and irritability) in individuals with autism.

○ **Why is it important to establish baseline rating of abnormal movements in children with autism before starting treatment with antipsychotics?**

Stereotypies and drug-induced dyskinesias are difficult to differentiate from each other, especially when both occur in the same body areas (e.g., orofacial area). It is also difficult to differentiate reemergence of stereotypies from dyskinesia caused by drug withdrawal.

○ **When is lithium used in the treatment of autistic disorders?**

Lithium is not a first-line drug for the treatment of autistic disorder. It may be indicated for aggressive or self-injurious behaviors when other medications fail.

○ **What is the role of psychotherapy in the treatment of autistic disorder?**

It is not appropriate in young children with autism. However, it may be helpful for emotional distress in older children with higher levels of functioning.

○ **What is the main differentiation of Landau-Kleffner's syndrome from autistic disorder?**

Children with Landau-Kleffner's syndrome have no severe impairment in social interactions. They attempt to communicate through nonverbal means. Children with autism have no interest in social interactions.

○ **What is Landau-Kleffner's syndrome?**

It is a type of acquired childhood language disorder, characterized by a progressive loss of acquired language skills concomitant with the appearance of a convulsive disorder. It is also known as acquired epileptic aphasia. Its onset usually occurs before the age of 10.

○ **What deficits in communication skills occur in Rett's disorder?**

Both receptive and expressive language development are impaired. Psychomotor retardation occurs with loss of previously acquired purposeful hand skills. Social skills plateau at levels between 6 and 12 months of age.

○ **What are the neuromuscular deficits of Rett's disorder?**

Poor muscle coordination and an unsteady, stiff gait.

○ **Does Rett's disorder have a genetic basis?**

It is likely, as Rett's disorder is observed only in girls, and has complete concordance in monozygotic twins.

○ **What respiratory abnormalities may be observed in Rett's disorder?**

Irregular respiration, episodes of hyperventilation, apnea, and breath holding.

○ **What is the prognosis of Rett's disorder?**

The prognosis for children with Rett's disorder is very poor, especially in language abilities. Most patients also develop muscle wasting and are eventually wheelchair-bound.

O   **What is childhood disintegrative disorder?**

Childhood disintegrative disorder is a developmental disorder that occurs subsequent to at least 2 years of normal development. These children lose previously acquired skills and have deficits in multiple spheres.

O   **What previously acquired skills may be lost in children with childhood disintegrative disorder?**

Expressive/receptive language, social skills, motor skills, and bowel/bladder control.

O   **What is the most important difference between Asperger's disorder and autistic disorder?**

Language development. Asperger's disorder lacks a delay in language development, while considerable delay of language skills is a core feature of autistic disorder.

O   **What are the clinical features of developmental coordination disorder?**

Clinical features of developmental coordination disorder include delays (not related to physical disorders) in achieving motor milestones such as sitting up, crawling, and walking. Patients also have deficits in other motor activities that require coordination, such as handwriting. They are often described as "clumsy" and frequently drop things.

O   **Can mental retardation be comorbid with developmental coordination disorder?**

Yes. However, to diagnose a developmental coordination disorder, motor difficulties must be in excess of those usually associated with the degree of mental retardation.

O   **Does the disturbance in developmental coordination disorder improve with age?**

No. The disturbance generally persists into adolescence and adult life.

O   **What is the Montessori technique?**

Developed by Maria Montessori, it is a technique that emphasizes the development of motor skills. It may be useful with preschool children.

O   **Why is there no *DSM-IV* diagnosis of receptive language disorder?**

When receptive skills are impaired enough to warrant a diagnosis, expressive skills should also be impaired, and the diagnosis should be mixed receptive-expressive language disorder.

O   **What behavioral problems may appear in children with expressive language disorder?**

Behavioral difficulties that may occur in children with expressive language disorder include hyperactivity and short attention span, social withdrawal, thumb-sucking, bed-wetting, temper outbursts, disobedience, accident proneness, and conduct disorder in older children.

O   **How does one differentiate expressive language disorders from mental retardation?**

Nonverbal intellectual capacity and functioning are within normal limits in children with expressive language disorder.

○ **What differentiates expressive language disorder from pervasive developmental disorders, such as autism?**

Children with expressive language disorder, though frustrated, may use nonverbal expression to form warm and meaningful social relationships. Children with autism are neither capable nor interested in verbal or nonverbal socialization.

○ **What is the prognosis for expressive language disorder?**

As many as 50% of children with mild expressive language disorder recover spontaneously without any sign of language impairment, but those with severe language disorder may have features of mild-to-moderate language impairment.

○ **What is the goal of language therapy in expressive language disorder?**

The goal of therapy is to increase the number of phrases by using block-building methods and conventional speech therapies.

○ **Can a child with mixed receptive-expressive language disorder also be deaf?**

No. The diagnosis for mixed receptive-expressive language disorder requires ruling out of speech/motor or sensory deficits. A child with mixed receptive-expressive language disorder may appear deaf, but auditory evoked potentials are within normal limits and the child does respond normally to nonlanguage sounds.

○ **What therapy is recommended for mixed receptive-expressive language disorder?**

Speech and language therapy to improve language skills is imperative, while psychotherapy for emotional and behavioral problems is often helpful.

○ **What are the differences between the causes of dysarthria and apraxia?**

Both disorders can cause difficulty in expressive language. Dysarthria is an impairment in the neural mechanisms regulating the muscular control of speech, while apraxia is an impairment in the muscle function itself.

○ **What misarticulations may appear in children with phonological disorder?**

Distortion, substitution, and omission.

○ **What is lateral slip?**

A lateral slip is the pronunciation of "s" sounds as "ssh." It is the most common type of distortion in children with phonological disorder.

○ **Do children outgrow phonological disorder and finally acquire the correct phoneme?**

Most do by the third grade. However, after the fourth grade, spontaneous recovery is unlikely.

○ **Omissions, distortions, and substitutions also occur normally in the speech of young children. How does one differentiate normal children who are learning to talk from those with phonological disorder?**

Normal children soon replace their misarticulations, but children with phonological disorder do not. Even if they learn the correct phoneme, they may use it only in newly acquired words and may not correct the words learned earlier.

○   **What is the treatment of choice for phonological disorder?**

Speech therapy.

○   **What are the indications for speech therapy in the treatment of phonological disorder?**

The indications for speech therapy include severity (when the problem is severe, such as when omissions and substitutions are involved), age (when the affected child is older than 8 years), and loss of functioning (when a speech problem causes problems with peers, learning, and self-image).

○   **What are circumlocutions?**

Circumlocutions are word substitutions one uses to avoid problematic words. It is a phenomenon seen in stuttering.

○   **Stuttering usually appears at what age?**

Stuttering usually appears before the age of 12 years, mostly from 1.5 to 9 years, with two sharp peaks of onset from the ages of 2 to 3.5 years and 5 to 7 years.

○   **What are the evolving phases in the development of stuttering?**

Phases	Ages	Features
1	Preschool period	Stuttering occurs most often when excited or upset, and under communicative pressure. High percentage of recovery.
2	The elementary school years	Chronic, with few, if any, intervals of normal speech.
3	Late childhood and early adolescence	Stuttering comes and goes in response to specific situations.
4	Late adolescence and adulthood	Stuttering comes and goes in response to specific situations.

○   **How does one differentiate spastic dysphonia from stuttering?**

Spastic dysphonia has an abnormal breathing pattern.

○   **What percentage of stutterers recover spontaneously?**

Fifty to eighty percent.

○   **Which medicine has been used to treat stuttering and how effective is it?**

Haloperidol. There is no data to accurately assess the efficacy of haloperidol.

○   **What is the theoretical basis of behavior therapy for stuttering?**

Stuttering is a learned form of behavior. It is not necessarily associated with a basic mental disorder or neurologic abnormality.

CHAPTER 28 Learning Disorders

○ **When was the field of learning disabilities as a separate entity of study/research formed?**

In the early 1960s. In 1963, Samuel Kirk first proposed the term learning disorder as a descriptive term for children with disorders in development of language, speech, reading, and associated communicative skills necessary for social interaction.

○ **The passage of which law mandated appropriate education for children with learning disabilities?**

PL 94-142: The Education for All Handicapped Children Act (EAHCA).

○ **Name the three main tenets of PL 94-142.**

PL 94-142, established in 1975, states that children with learning disabilities are entitled to a free and appropriate education that is based upon evaluation of individual needs, and occurs in the least restrictive environment possible.

○ **Special education services were extended to infants, toddlers, and preschoolers in 1986 by what law?**

PL 99-457, enacted in 1986, amended PL 94-142 to extend services to younger children.

○ **What is the Individuals with Disabilities Education Act (IDEA) of 1991?**

IDEA is a revision of PL 94-142 and PL 99-457, that defines children with disabilities as those individuals with mental retardation, autism, traumatic brain injury, learning impairments, emotional difficulties, other health impairments, and hearing, visual, language, or orthopedic impairments. These children, because of their disabilities, have special education needs that are assessed through an individualized education plan (IEP) that describes the child's current educational abilities, determines goals for improvement, and describes the specialized services the child will be given to meet these goals. The educational setting should be as close to the child's home as possible, and education should occur in the least restrictive setting possible (i.e., the child should be educated with his/her peers as much as possible).

○ **The legal definition of learning disabilities rules out what deficits as constituting a learning disability?**

Problems with self-regulatory behaviors, social perception, and social interaction. These deficits may be present but cannot be diagnosed as a learning disorder on their own.

○ **Name the two global subtypes of learning disabilities.**

1. Audiolinguistic: Language and reading learning disorder.
2. Visuospatial: Math and social learning disorder.

○ **The cognitive profiles of children and adults with learning disabilities are consistently significant for what pattern?**

Significant scatter or variability across the subtest, either within a particular domain (verbal or visual–perceptual) or between the domains.

○ **Adults with learning disabilities are more likely to have what characteristics?**

Under achievement in reading, written language, or math; grade repetition; high rate of high school dropout; failure to go on to postsecondary programs; low self-esteem; greater dependence on family systems for financial and social support; and disproportionate unemployment or underemployment.

○ **According to the *DSM-IV*, what three criteria must be met in order for a learning disorder to be diagnosed?**

In order to diagnose a learning disorder according to the *DSM-IV*, a specific academic achievement must be substantially below expectations based on age, school grade, and IQ. Additionally, the deficit in learning must significantly interfere with academic achievement or with activities of daily life involving that skill. Finally, if a sensory deficit is present, the learning disorder is in excess of that usually associated with the sensory deficit.

○ **How is a learning disorder diagnosed?**

By comparing a person's level of intelligence on a standardized test with their level of academic achievement on a standardized test.

○ **What discrepancy between IQ and academic achievement is considered significant enough to warrant a diagnosis of learning disorder?**

A discrepancy of more than two standard deviations.

○ **What test scores cannot be used to make a diagnosis of learning disorder?**

Classroom test performance, school grades, nationwide administration of standardized tests (i.e., IGAR, CAT), and group administered achievement tests.

○ **In what situation can a learning disorder be diagnosed if a sensory deficit is also present?**

When the learning difficulties are in excess of those usually associated with the deficit.

○ **What are some associated general features of a learning disorder?**

Low self-esteem, school dropout, social skill deficits, unemployment, attention, and memory deficits.

○ **What are several general medical conditions frequently associated with a learning disorder?**

Lead poisoning, fragile X syndrome, fetal alcohol syndrome, cerebral palsy, and spina bifida.

○ **What psychiatric disorders are often comorbid with a learning disorder?**

Attention-deficit/hyperactivity disorder (ADHD), conduct disorder, oppositional defiant disorder (ODD), dysthymic disorder, and major depressive disorder.

○ **How are cultural or ethnic background features adequately controlled for when diagnosing a learning disorder?**

By using tests in which the person's relevant characteristics are represented in the standardization sample of the tests.

○ **While not due to sensory deficits, what underlying impairment is assumed to be the cause of a learning disorder?**

A processing deficit resulting from underlying neurologic (CNS) impairment.

○ **A child has poor academic achievement despite a higher potential for learning. What then is considered to be the reason for that child's learning disorder?**

A specific information-processing limitation.

○ **What percentage of students in U.S. public schools are diagnosed with a learning disorder?**

Approximately 5%; prevalence rates vary from 2% to 10% depending on the nature of assessment, population, and definitions applied.

○ **What are other explanations for poor school performance that must be ruled out before diagnosing a learning disorder?**

Normal variation in academic achievement, impoverished environment, poor teaching, cultural factors, lack of opportunity, and high rates of absenteeism.

○ **In addition to the academic content area of a learning disorder (reading, math), what other deficits contribute to a child's learning disorder?**

Other deficits that can contribute to a child's learning disorder include organizational problems, problems with study skills (note taking, outlining, strategic memorization), and difficulties with memory, completion of tasks, and working in group situations.

○ **Within special education classes in public schools, what is the most frequent qualifying diagnosis?**

A learning disorder; 47% of all children in special education are diagnosed with a learning disorder.

○ **Treatment (intervention) for a learning disorder focuses on what two main processes?**

The two treatment processes are remediation (i.e., finding strategies to teach information so the child can master the skill) and compensation (i.e., to help the child identify and develop strategies for overcoming/working around his/her deficit).

○ **Name several examples of compensatory interventions for a learning disorder.**

Compensatory interventions for learning disorders include the use of books on tape for reading disorders, the use of calculators and math fact tables for math disorders, and the use of computers, typewriters, or tape recorders for disorders of written expression.

○ **Treatment for learning disabilities has been expanding rapidly. Name some treatment modalities that do not have scientific evidence of efficacy.**

Methods of treating learning disorders that do not have scientific evidence of efficacy include EEG biofeedback, optometric training, diet/nutritional treatment, chiropractic manipulation, and sensory integration treatment.

○   **What percentage of all learning disorders are reading disorders?**

Reading disorders account for 80% of all learning disabilities (or, in other words, approximately 4% of all school-age children have a reading disorder).

○   **At what grade is a reading disorder typically diagnosed?**

First or second grade, but if associated with a high IQ, it may not be diagnosed until fourth grade or later.

○   **Which learning disorder has the highest genetic predisposition?**

Reading disorder is most prevalent among first-degree relatives with a learning disorder, with heritability as high as 0.5.

○   **What is another name commonly associated with a reading disorder?**

Dyslexia.

○   **How is the term "dyslexia" different from the diagnosis of a reading disorder?**

Dyslexia describes a broader population of individuals who have deficits in phonological processing and related language abilities including reading, spelling, writing, vocabulary acquisition, general language proficiency, and the formulation of ideas.

○   **Who was the first to propose that reversals are especially symptomatic of dyslexia?**

Samuel Orton; however, subsequent research has not supported this notion.

○   **Reading disorder is due to what two primary impairments?**

Phonological deficits and deficits in working memory responsible for auditory processing.

○   **Research has identified what deficit as the most frequent cause of a reading disorder?**

The ability to accurately process phonological features of language, which in turn results in difficulty identifying words accurately and quickly.

○   **Children and adults with a reading disorder have consistently been shown to have what type of memory deficit?**

Research indicates that individuals with a reading learning disorder have deficits in short-term memory, especially memory for primarily verbal information and memorization of a sequential order. It appears likely that these memory deficits play a role in reading disorders.

○   **What are the major components of intervention for a reading learning disorder that have been successful in treating this disorder?**

Explicit and systematic instruction in phonological awareness, letter recognition and formulation, sound–symbol connections, decoding, vocabulary building, comprehension strategies, and motivation for independent reading.

○   **What percentage of children with a reading disorder also have ADHD?**

Twenty-five percent.

○ **Studies of successful adults who were diagnosed with a reading learning disorder as children reveal what chronic impairment?**

Lifelong problems using language, most notable in their difficulty with spelling, and use of written language.

○ **Math disorder and written expression disorder are rarely found in the absence of what other disorder?**

Reading disorder.

○ **How do the math skills of a child with reading and math disorders differ from children with a math disorder but no reading disorder?**

Children with both reading and math disorders have trouble memorizing math facts and understanding word problems, while children with only a math disorder have problems understanding fundamental math concepts, which is hypothesized to be related to deficits in right hemisphere spatial cognition.

○ **What is the prevalence of math disorders?**

One in every five cases of learning disorders is a math disorder. One percent of all school children are estimated to have a math learning disorder.

○ **If a child is bright (has a high IQ), at what grade level is a math learning disorder typically diagnosed?**

It may not become a problem until the fifth grade. Typically, a math learning disorder is diagnosed in second or third grade.

○ **What are some of the related skills which may be impaired in a math disorder?**

- Linguistic skills (math terms, concepts, operations, decoding word problems into math symbols).
- Perceptual skills (recognizing symbols/signs, clustering objects into groups).
- Attention skills (copying figures/numbers correctly, carrying numbers, observing correct operation sign).
- Math skills (sequencing of steps, counting objects, learning multiplication tables).

○ **What types of writing problems are not typically diagnosed as written expression disorder?**

Spelling problems or handwriting problems only, with no other written deficits (i.e., difficulties writing, organizing content, grammar, and punctuation errors).

○ **At what grade is a disorder of written expression diagnosed?**

Typically, at the end of first grade. Difficulty in tasks of copying, writing to dictation, and spontaneous writing are often necessary in order to diagnose.

○ **What diagnosis is most appropriate if a child evidences poor handwriting due to motor coordination deficits?**

Developmental coordination disorder; if delays in other fine/gross-motor skills are present (i.e., walking, tying shoes, playing ball).

○ **What diagnosis is used if a child has impairments in reading, math, and written expression that significantly interfere with academic achievement, but performance of skills in isolation on standardized tests are not significantly below expectations for age, IQ, and schooling?**

Learning disorder, NOS, can be used for a learning disorder not meeting criteria for a specific learning disorder.

○ **Name several factors (deficits) in preschool years that may develop into a learning disorder.**

Behavioral, motor, and perceptual problems as well as deficits in language skills.

○ **Name areas of learning during preschool years that are critical for later academic achievement.**

Basic sound–symbol matching; associating labels with abstract properties of objects; beginning to print letters/numbers and draw basic shapes.

○ **What learning disorders are considered right hemisphere or nonverbal learning disabilities?**

Specific problems in math and/or handwriting (separate from reading problems); problems in social cognition, attention, and conceptual skills; and poor fine-motor coordination.

○ **Describe the deficits present in children with a nonverbal learning disorder.**

Deficits associated with nonverbal learning disorders include poor affect modulation, impaired social skills, impairment of sensory perception and visuospatial skills, difficulty in the use of pragmatic language, poor adaptability to novelty, and difficulty with math concepts.

○ **Children with a nonverbal learning disorder are most similar in their cognitive profile and functioning as what psychiatric diagnosis?**

Asperger's disorder, a pervasive developmental disorder.

○ **What is the relationship between a learning disorder and attention problems?**

While learning disabilities and attention problems are two distinct deficits (i.e., learning disabilities are NOT caused by attention problems), there are a substantial number of children who have both ADHD and learning disabilities (between 19% and 26% of children with ADHD have a least one type of learning disorder).

○ **In research of learning-disabled children with and without ADHD, in what way do the groups differ?**

Children diagnosed with ADHD only often have deficits in higher level cognitive skills (i.e., organization, working memory, executive functioning), while children with learning disabilities and ADHD have more difficulties with written language problems as a result of the organizational and working memory demands of writing assignments.

○ **What percentage of children with learning disorders have social problems?**

Anywhere from 35% to 59.1%, with approximately similar rates found regardless of age.

○ **Studies show that children with learning disorders have adequate understanding of social norms. To what, then, are their social deficits attributed?**

Problems in affect (i.e., depression, anxiety), self-concept and attributions, and social skills.

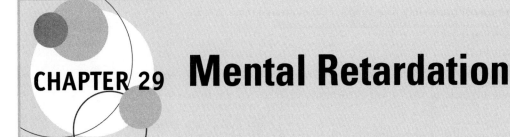

CHAPTER 29 Mental Retardation

○ **What is the prevalence of mental retardation in the general population?**

Approximately 1%. Males predominate at all levels of mental retardation.

○ **On what *DSM-IV* Axis is the diagnosis of mental retardation coded?**

Axis II. Axis II conditions in general are conceptualized as permanent conditions present by early adulthood.

○ **What are the four degrees of severity of mental retardation?**

1. Mild: IQ level 50–55 to approximately 70
2. Moderate: IQ level 35–40 to 50–55
3. Severe: IQ level 20–25 to 35–40
4. Profound: IQ level below 20 or 25.

○ **What defines mental retardation according to the *DSM-IV*?**

Significantly subaverage general intellectual functioning *and* significant limitations in adaptive functioning. The onset must occur before the age of 18 years.

○ **What percent of mentally retarded persons have *mild* mental retardation?**

Eighty percent have an IQ between 50 and 70.

○ **In the United States, what condition ranks first for chronic conditions causing major limitations in activity?**

According to the Centers for Disease Control, 1996, it is mental retardation.

○ **What age group has the highest incidence of mental retardation?**

School-age children, with a peak at 10 to 14 years. The prevalence decreases in older people due to higher mortality rates associated with severe or profound mental retardation.

○ **What generalizations can be made about the etiology of mental retardation?**

No etiology is known in 75% of borderline intellectual function cases, while the cause is known in 75% of severe mental retardation cases. Genetic, biologic, psychosocial, and environmental factors are involved.

○ **What are the three most commonly identified causes of mental retardation?**

1. Down's syndrome

2. Fragile X syndrome

3. Fetal alcohol syndrome

These three represent approximately 30% of all identified cases of mental retardation.

○ **What disorders are included in the differential diagnosis of mental retardation?**

Borderline intellectual functioning (IQ 71 to 84), dementia, pervasive developmental disorders, learning disorders, and communication disorders.

○ **When is the *DSM-IV* diagnosis of mental retardation, severity unspecified, used?**

In cases of probable mental retardation in which standardized testing cannot be done.

○ **What is the best treatment for mental retardation?**

Primary, secondary, and tertiary prevention. Primary prevention consists of genetic counseling, proper prenatal and postnatal medical care, eradication of disorders known to cause central nervous system damage, and health education to increase awareness of mental retardation. Secondary prevention develops methods to shorten the course of the illness, e.g., by treating phenylketonuria and hypothyroidism. Tertiary prevention acts to minimize sequelae and consequent disabilities, e.g., by treating comorbid psychiatric disorders, providing comprehensive education involving adaptive skills training, family education, and social interventions (such as Special Olympics International). Pharmacologic management of aggression, self-injurious behaviors, stereotypical motor movements, and attention deficit disorders may be indicated.

○ **What scale is commonly used to assess adaptive functioning in mental retardation?**

The Vineland Adaptive Scale. Deficits in adaptive functioning can also be verified through the use of reliable informants such as teachers and medical professionals.

○ **What intelligence tests are most widely used in the United States for children?**

The Wechsler Intelligence Scale for Children and the Stanford-Binet Intelligence Scale.

○ **What is the prevalence of mental disorders among mentally retarded individuals?**

It is greater than that of the general population. Approximately 50% of all mentally retarded children have an additional psychiatric diagnosis.

○ **What behavioral abnormalities are observed in males with the fragile X syndrome?**

Most males with the full fragile X mutation have mental retardation. Behavioral abnormalities include hyperactivity, short attention span, poor peer relations, and stereotypies.

○ **What is the typical phenotype of fragile X syndrome?**

Long face, prominent ears, and postpubertal macro-orchidism.

○ **Prader-Willi's Syndrome (PWS) is believed to result from a deletion involving which chromosome?**

PWS, characterized by marked obesity secondary to hyperphagia, is due to a microscopic or submicroscopic deletion on chromosome 15.

○ **What psychiatric disorder is common in Prader-Willi's syndrome?**

Obsessive-compulsive disorder.

○ **What phenotype is seen in Angelman's syndrome?**

This mental retardation syndrome is associated with severe retardation, severe speech delay, seizures, ataxia, and bouts of laughing. It is also caused by a chromosome 15 deletion.

○ **What is Williams' syndrome?**

A rare genetic disorder, Williams' syndrome is characterized by mental retardation, supravalvular aortic stenosis, infantile hypercalcemia, growth deficiency, and an elf-like facies.

○ **What distinguishes Rett's disorder?**

A degenerative neurologic disorder affecting only girls, Rett's disorder is an X-linked dominant mental retardation syndrome characterized by unusual behaviors, i.e., breath-holding, motor difficulties, and extreme deficits in expressive and receptive language. The onset of this disorder begins after a short period (5–48 months) of normal development. It is generally classified as a pervasive developmental disorder.

○ **How often does fetal alcohol syndrome occur in infants born to pregnant women with regular and extensive alcohol use?**

In 15%.

○ **What is the typical phenotype of fetal alcohol syndrome?**

Facial dysmorphism: microcephaly, short turned-up nose, inner epicanthal folds, short palpebral fissures, and hypertelorism.

○ **How does Down's syndrome differ from other mental retardation syndromes in behavioral terms?**

Individuals with Down's syndrome suffer less often from serious psychopathology compared to other groups with mental retardation. Sociability and social skills are relative strengths in Down's syndrome.

○ **How common is the coexistence of mental retardation and pervasive developmental disorders?**

Approximately 75% of persons with pervasive developmental disorders also have an IQ of 70 or below.

○ **How does a learning disorder differ from mental retardation?**

Learning disorders indicate a delay or failure of development in a specific area, e.g., mathematics, while mental retardation indicates generalized delays in development.

○   **What percentage of mentally retarded persons meet diagnostic criteria for schizophrenia?**

Approximately 2% to 3%, several times higher than that of the general population.

○   **What is the major cause of mental retardation and congenital malformations due to maternal infection?**

Rubella (German measles).

CHAPTER 30

Disruptive Behavior Disorders

○ **Describe a child with attention-deficit/hyperactivity disorder (ADHD).**

A child with ADHD has a persistent pattern of inattention and/or hyperactivity-impulsivity that is more frequent and severe than is typically observed in children at a comparable level of development.

○ **What are the *DSM-IV* criteria for ADHD?**

The *DSM-IV* criteria for ADHD are divided into two subsets, inattention and hyperactivity/impulsivity. Six or more symptoms from each subset must be present for at least 6 months to a degree that is inconsistent with the child's developmental level. Symptoms of inattention include careless mistakes in homework, short attention span, failure to listen when spoken to, failure to follow instructions, difficulty organizing tasks, avoidance of tasks that require prolonged mental effort, frequent loss of objects, easy distractibility, and forgetfulness of daily tasks. Hyperactivity-impulsivity symptoms include fidgeting, inability to remain seated in the classroom, excessive psychomotor activity, difficulty playing quietly, always "on the go," excessive talking, blurting out of answers before questions are completed, difficulty waiting for one's turn, and frequent interruption into conversions or games.

○ **According to the *DSM-IV*, what are the three subtypes of ADHD?**

1. Attention-deficit/hyperactivity disorder, combined type.

2. Attention-deficit/hyperactivity disorder predominately inattentive type.

3. Attention-deficit disorder, predominately impulsive type.

The category of attention-deficit/hyperactivity disorder not otherwise specified is reserved for disorders with prominent symptoms of inattention or hyperactivity/impulsivity, but do not meet criteria for any of the previously noted diagnoses.

○ **In how many settings must the symptoms of ADHD be present to meet criteria for a diagnosis thereof?**

Two, usually home and school, but other settings, such as day care, and church can be considered. In addition, the symptoms of ADHD must cause significant impairment in functioning to meet criteria.

○ **To meet criteria for a diagnosis of ADHD, by what age must symptoms be present?**

Age 7 years.

○ **At what age do most children with ADHD get referred for evaluation?**

The most frequent age of referral for children with ADHD is between 6 and 9 years.

○ **What is the prevalence of ADHD?**

According to the *DSM-IV*, the prevalence of ADHD is estimated to be between 3% and 5% of school-age children with a 4:1 to 9:1 male-to-female ratio. Other studies have found the prevalence to be higher, from 7% to 10%.

○ **Do the symptoms of ADHD remit during adolescence?**

Not necessarily. Approximately two-thirds (60% to 86%) of school-age children will meet criteria for ADHD during adolescence, and approximately 40% of ADHD children will have their symptoms persist into adulthood. The prevalence rate of ADHD in adults is estimated to be approximately 3% to 4% of the general population.

○ **Why is there a higher reported prevalence of ADHD in the United States?**

The higher reported prevalence of ADHD in the United States may be due to advanced technologies (such as lead-containing gasoline and paints and synthetic food additives) as well as differing diagnostic practices, cultural expectations, and/or prolonged compulsory schooling.

○ **Describe the familial risk factors for ADHD.**
- A child with an ADHD parent has a 50% risk of ADHD.
- A child with an ADHD sibling has a 20% to 25% risk of ADHD.
- A child with an ADHD identical twin has an 80% to 90% risk of ADHD.
- A child with an ADHD fraternal twin has a 30% to 40% risk of ADHD.
- A child with a second-degree ADHD relative has a 12% risk of ADHD.

○ **What prenatal factors can contribute to the development of ADHD?**

Poor maternal health and maternal use of cigarettes, alcohol, and drugs.

○ **Name two perinatal factors that contribute to the development of ADHD.**

Low birth weight and postmaturity.

○ **What inborn error of metabolism is associated with the development of ADHD?**

Phenylketonuria.

○ **Name the test used in the laboratory that measures the ability to sustain attention.**

The continuous performance test.

○ **What behavior rating scales are commonly used in the monitoring of ADHD symptoms?**

Conner's teacher or parent rating scales, the DuPaul ADHD Rating Scale-IV, the Child Behavior Checklist (CBCL), the Academic Performance Rating Scales (APRS), the Brown ADD Rating Scales for Children, Adolescents and Adults, the Home Situations Questionnaire-Revised and School Situations Questionnaire- Revised, the Swanson, Nolan and Pelham (SNAP-IV), the SKAMP and the Vanderbilt ADHA Diagnostic Parent and Teacher Scales.

○ **When is the use of medication indicated in the treatment of ADHD?**

The use of medication is indicated when a child or adolescent manifests inattention and hyperactivity symptoms that are interfering with the child's ability to learn (academic failure) or to develop satisfactory interpersonal relationships (social maladaptive behavior).

○ **What percentage of children with ADHD improve on a stimulant regimen?**

The symptoms of 70% of children with ADHD will improve with stimulant treatment.

○ **What are the patterns of regional cerebral blood flow studies in children with ADHD and what is the effect of stimulant medication on those patterns?**

Regional cerebral blood flow in children with ADHD is decreased in the striatal region and increased in primary sensory regions of the occipital and temporal cortex. Stimulant medication tends to normalize the pathologic flow distribution.

○ **What are the most common side effects of stimulant medications?**

Anorexia, insomnia, abdominal pain, headache, obsessive tendencies, and tics. A brief period of increased mood lability can be notable during initial treatment with stimulants.

○ **Explain why short-acting stimulants are given after breakfast and lunch.**

Short-acting stimulants are administered after meals to diminish problems with appetite suppression.

○ **What are the contraindications to the use of psychostimulants?**

Marked anxiety, agitation, glaucoma, motor tics, a family history or diagnosis of Tourette's syndrome, a history of psychosis or substance abuse, and concomitant MAOI use.

○ **Why is it not advisable to administer psychostimulants after 4 PM?**

Psychostimulants can cause insomnia if administered late in the day.

○ **Which of the stimulants can be used to treat children younger than 6 years?**

Dextroamphetamine (Dexedrine) is currently the only stimulant approved by the FDA for administration to children younger than 6 years (as young as 3 years of age).

○ **What is the so-called "rebound phenomenon" of stimulants?**

The "rebound phenomenon" of psychostimulants refers to a paradoxical exacerbation of hyperactivity and agitation that may occur up to 5 hours after the last dose of medication. Symptoms include excitability, insomnia, talkativeness, abdominal pain, and mild insomnia.

○ **How would you manage "rebound phenomenon"?**

Addition of a small afternoon dose of a short-acting stimulant may minimize rebound symptoms.

○ **What percentage of ADHD children do not improve with stimulant medication?**

Ten to forty percent.

○ **Are the doses for methylphenidate and dextroamphetamine equivalent?**

No. Dextroamphetamine is approximately twice as potent as methylphenidate and therefore, an equivalent dose of dextroamphetamine is half that of methylphenidate.

○ **What is the mechanism of action for methylphenidate-based stimulants?**

Methylphenidate-based stimulants block the reuptake of norepinephrine and dopamine into the presynaptic neuron.

○ **How is methylphenidate metabolized?**

By hepatic de-esterification to the inactive metabolite, α-phenyl-piperidine acetic acid.

○   **How would one initiate pharmacologic treatment of ADHD with methylphenidate?**

Treatment with methylphenidate is initiated with a 5-mg dose at 8:00 AM for 3 days, then titrated to 5 mg at 8:00 AM and 12 noon for 3 days. Dosage increases are then determined by the effect on target symptoms, with a maximum daily dose of 2 mg/kg/d, administered in two to four doses. When one uses a long-acting stimulant, it is generally advisable to start with the lowest dose available and titrate up.

○   **Describe the dosing, duration of action (DOA), and formulations of available methylphenidate products.**

Short Acting	Long Acting

Ritalin® 5-, 10-, and 20-mg tablets
  dose q 4 h 2–3 times/d
  DOA ~4 h
  cheap
  can be cut or crushed
	Ritalin LA® 10-, 20-, 30-, and 40-mg capsules
	  once-a-day dosing (AM only)
	  DOA ~8–10 h
	  bimodal release using SODAS technology (immediate release
	    beads & extended release, enteric-coated beads, 50/50 mix)
	  do NOT alter capsule

Ritalin SR® 20 mg
  old, once-a-day formulation
  DOA ~8 h
  wax matrix (inconsistent)
  do NOT alter capsule
	Metadate®**CD** 10-, 20-, and 30-mg capsules
	  once-a-day dosing (AM only)
	  DOA ~ 10–12 h
	  30% IR, 70% ER
	  may sprinkle, do not crush or chew
	
	Concerta 18-, 27-, 36-, 54-mg tablet
	  once-a-day dosing
	  DOA~12 h
	  OROS delivery system—a trilayer osmotic capsule (2 layers of
	    drug & "push layer" with laser-drilled orifice) & IR drug
	    overcoat (~50% released 1 h after administration, rest
	    continuously released for 6–7 h)
	  do NOT alter capsule
	  distant risk for GI obstruction

Focalin® 2.5-, 5-, & 10-mg
  d-enantiomer of methylphenidate
  two times as potent as IR
    methylphenidate
  requires dosing every 4 h, 2–3
    times daily
	Focalin®**XR** 5-, 10-, 20-mg
	  SODAS (spherical oral drug absorption system) technology with
	    d-enantiomer of methylphenidate in a 50/50 mixture of
	    immediate releases and extended release beads
	  twice as potent as IR methylphenidate
	  once-a-day dosing, AM only
	
	Daytrana® patch 10-, 20-, 30-, & 40-mg patches
	  apply to alternating hip areas in AM, remove 9 hours later, effect
	    continues for 3 h after patch removed
	  active ingredient—methylphenidate
	  keeping patch on can be problematic

○ **What is the mechanism of action of dextroamphetamine-based stimulants?**

The mechanism of action for dextroamphetamine-based stimulants is twofold. Dextroamphetamine blocks reuptake of norepinephrine and dopamine from the presynaptic cleft (like methylphenidate), and stimulates dopamine and norepinephrine efflux from presynaptic terminals.

○ **How is dextroamphetamine metabolized?**

Approximately half of a dose of dextroamphetamine is excreted in the urine as unchanged drug, while the rest is hepatically metabolized to primarily benzoic acid.

○ **Describe the dosing, duration of action (DOA), and formulations of available dextroamphetamine products.**

Short Acting	Long Acting

Dexedrine® 5-mg tablets (dextroamphetamine)
    d-isomer is 4–5 times more potent than the
        l-isomer in eliciting CNS excitation vs.
        peripheral excitation
    requires dosing q 4 h, two times daily
	Dexedrine®**spansules** 5-, 10-, and 15-mg capsules
	    capsule contains small particles of meds
	    once-a-day dosing, ideally
	    DOA ~ 6–8 h

Adderall®5-, 7.5-, 10-, 12.5-, 15-, 20- and 30-mg
    tablets
    mixed salts of:
        dextroamphetamine saccharate
        dextroamphtamine sulfate
        amphetamine sulfate
        dextroamphetamine sulfate
    requires dosing q 4 hr, 2–3 times daily
	Adderall®**XR** 5-, 10-, 15-, 20-, and 30-mg capsules
	    contains immediate and extended release beads
	        containing same active substances as Adderall®
	    can open capsule and sprinkle
	    do NOT chew or crush beads
	    Black Box for sudden cardiac death
	    once-a-day dosing (AM only)
	
	Vyvanse®20-, 30-, 40-, 50-, 60-, and 70-mg capsules
	    active compound—prodrug of dextroamphetamine,
	    "lisdextroamfetamine"(converted in GI tract and
	        liver to dextroamphetamine and *l*-lysine)
	    capsule can be dissolved in water
	    DOA: 12 h
	    once-a-day dosing

○ **What are some second- and third-line agents available for the treatment of ADHD?**

Tricyclic antidepressants, atomoxetine, and bupropion

○ **Describe the effect of tricyclic antidepressants on attention as compared to its effect on depression.**

The effect of tricyclic antidepressants on attention is more rapidly achieved than the effect on depression, but onset of action is still longer than that of stimulants, and the effect size is smaller than that achieved by the stimulants. Imipramine and nortriptyline are the tricyclics most commonly used for the treatment of ADHD.

○ **What is the mechanism of action for tricyclics in general?**

Blockade of norepinephrine reuptake.

○ **What serious side effect of tricyclics must one be aware of when prescribing these for ADHD (or any other condition)?**

Cardiotoxicity is a potential adverse effect of all tricyclics. Sudden cardiac death is particularly associated with desipramine. A baseline ECG is recommended before initiating treatment with any tricyclic, after dose increases and if there are any complaints suggestive of cardiac complications. Monitoring of plasma levels of tricyclics is also recommended.

○ **Describe the onset of action of bupropion (Wellbutrin®).**

Bupropion's onset of action for improvement of attention takes approximately 4 weeks to occur. The impact on attention is less robust than the effects of stimulants, but may be especially of benefit when stimulants cannot be tolerated or when depressive symptoms are also present.

○ **What is the mechanism of action for bupropion?**

The mechanism of action for bupropion is not well established, but it does appear to be involved in blockade of norepinephrine and dopamine reuptake.

○ **What populations are at increased risk for seizures when treated with bupropion?**

Patients with seizure disorders and eating disorders. All individuals are at increased risk for seizures when the dose of bupropion exceeds 450 mg/d in adults (or when the short-acting BID or TID dose exceeds 150 mg) and seizures are a frequent consequence of overdose with bupropion.

○ **Describe the onset of action of atomoxetine (Strattera®).**

Atomoxetine's onset of action for improvement of attention takes approximately 4 to 6 weeks to occur. The impact on attention is less robust than the effects of stimulants.

○ **What is the mechanism of action for atomoxetine?**

Atomoxetine is a selective norepinephrine reuptake inhibitor.

○ **What side effects of atomoxetine have warranted Black Box warnings?**

Hepatotoxicity and the risk for suicidal thinking

○ **What α_2-adrenergic agonists are used to treat symptoms of ADHD?**

Clonidine hydrochloride and guanfacine (Tenex®) can be used for treating the hyperactive and impulsive symptoms of ADHD, as well as aggression and the stimulant side effects of insomnia and tics.

○ **What serious symptom can occur with abrupt discontinuation of clonidine or guanfacine?**

Rebound hypertension.

○ **Why is pemoline no longer prescribed in the United States?**

Pemoline was pulled from the market as a result of the adverse side effect of liver dysfunction, which had been reported in 2% of cases in those children receiving pemoline.

○ **What treatment modalities were found to have superior outcome in the 1999 Multimodal Treatment of ADHD (MTA) study?**

"Algorithmic medication management of ADHD" was found to be superior to behavior therapy or behavior therapy combined with medication management.

○ **When is behavior therapy indicated for the treatment of ADHD symptoms?**

When parents are reluctant to treat ADHD symptoms with medication, when ADHD symptoms are mild, or when insufficient symptoms are present to meet criteria for a diagnosis of ADHD (i.e., the symptoms occur in only one setting).

○ **Which of the nonpharmacologic treatments of ADHD have been found to show the most promise as an alternative and/or adjunct to pharmacotherapy?**

Behavioral therapy. Behavior therapy that emphasizes psychoeducation, consistency in observation of behaviors and application of reinforcers, appropriate reinforcement of positive behaviors and appropriate consequences for negative behaviors (at home and in public), consistent communication with school personnel (homework log, daily report), and appropriate use of time-outs and token economies. Parent training may be necessary for successful use of behavioral techniques. The use of cognitive-behavioral training, dietary modification, or social skills training has not been found to be of benefit for the treatment of ADHD symptoms. However, family therapy and other interventions such as remedial education may be indicated in situations where there significant family dysfunction or learning disabilities are present.

○ **Which children with ADHD are likely to benefit from individual psychotherapy?**

Children with comorbid diagnoses of school phobia, anxiety disorder or major depression, and those who have undergone traumatic events (e.g., parental separation), are likely to benefit from individual psychotherapy. Individual psychotherapy is also a good format to address issues of low self-esteem, hopelessness, and feelings of rejection or abandonment, possibly precipitated by the difficulties associated with the disorder of ADHD.

○ **What is the Feingold diet?**

The Feingold diet, developed in the 1970s, is a diet that eliminates all food additives, salicylates, and dyes. In 1997, the American Academy of Child and Adolescent Psychiatry found insufficient evidence to support the Feingold diet as a treatment of ADHD.

○ **What is the significance of the presence of comorbid disorders in an ADHD child?**

The presence of comorbid disorders indicates that the child requires additional treatment modalities and may have a worse prognosis.

○ **What Axis I diagnoses are commonly associated with ADHD?**

Oppositional defiant disorder (54%–84%), conduct disorder, and learning or language disorders (25%–35%) primarily, but mood and anxiety disorders, and Tourette's disorder are also frequently comorbid with ADHD.

○ **Describe a child who is diagnosed with oppositional defiant disorder (ODD).**

Typically, a child with ODD is argumentative, disobedient, and defiant with adults. Often, the child will rather lose everything, than lose an argument.

○ **What are the *DSM-IV* criteria for ODD?**

Four of the eight following behaviors must be present for a period of at least 6 months to make a diagnosis of ODD: frequent temper tantrums, frequent arguments with adults, active defiance or refusal to follow rules/directions, deliberate annoyance of others, frequent blaming of others for one's own mistakes, easily annoyance by others, often angry, and spiteful. The symptoms must occur more frequently than expected for the child's developmental level, cause significant social and academic impairment, and must not occur only during the course of a mood or psychotic disorder. Additionally, a diagnosis of conduct disorder precludes a diagnosis of ODD.

○ **What is the prevalence of ODD?**

The prevalence of ODD is estimated to be from 2% to 16%, with a male-to-female ratio of 2 to 3:1 before puberty, after which the male-to-female ratio is more equal.

○ **What are some proposed mechanisms for the development of ODD?**

Inconsistent parental use of behavior modification techniques, impulsive parental behavior patterns, mismatch of temperament between parents and child, and decreased parental availability may contribute to the development of ODD.

○ **What distinguishes ODD from conduct disorder?**

The behaviors of children with a diagnosis of ODD are generally less severe and do not seriously violate the rights of others, as do the behaviors of children with a diagnosis of conduct disorder.

○ **How does one distinguish the symptoms of ODD from those of separation anxiety or panic disorder?**

While temper tantrums are common to all of these disorders, the behaviors associated with separation anxiety or panic disorder are limited to situations in which the specific fear occurs.

○ **How is ODD treated?**

The best approach to ODD is a combination of parental training in behavior modification techniques and improvement of the child's social skills, affect regulation, and problem-solving skills.

○ **What comorbid disorders occur in children with ODD?**

ADHD, learning disorders, and communication disorders are often associated with ODD.

○ **When can ODD be diagnosed in a child with mental retardation?**

When a child with mental retardation exhibits more oppositional and defiant behavior than one would expect for his/her developmental age, a diagnosis of ODD is indicated.

○ **During which developmental stages does one often observe transient oppositional behavior?**

During the preschool and adolescent years.

○ **Describe a child/adolescent with conduct disorder.**

A child/adolescent with conduct disorder exhibits a consistent pattern of behavior in which the rights of others or the rules of society are violated.

○ **How are the criteria of conduct disorder grouped by the *DSM-IV*?**

The 15 *DSM-IV* criteria for conduct disorder are grouped into four subsets: aggression to people and animals; destruction of property (fire setting, vandalism); deceitfulness or theft; and serious violations of rules (truancy and running away).

○ **What are the two different types of conduct disorder in the *DSM-IV*?**

Childhood onset (before the age of 10 years) and adolescent onset. Prognosis is worse for childhood-onset conduct disorder.

○ **What disorders should one consider in the differential diagnosis of conduct disorder?**

The externalizing symptoms of conduct disorder often mask symptoms of other psychiatric disorders. More than half of children with conduct disorder will also meet criteria for ADHD, while PTSD, dissociative disorders, learning disorders, and borderline IQ/mild mental retardation are also quite common. MDD and bipolar disorder, as well as anxiety disorders, and substance abuse should also be considered.

○ **What factors predict persistence of conduct disorder into adulthood?**

Borderline IQ/mental retardation and a family history of antisocial personality disorder.

○ **How can one establish rapport with the hostile, guarded child diagnosed with conduct disorder?**

Interviews with children diagnosed with conduct disorder can be difficult, as these children often have experiences where basic trust has been violated. Integrating mental status questions into a review of medical history can yield more information about psychiatric symptoms than direct questioning about symptoms such as hallucinations or dissociative episodes. Additionally, the child's developmental level and language skills may preclude description of their internal perceptions. Use of a concrete approach during inquiry may also be useful.

○ **What is the prevalence of conduct disorder?**

In males, 6% to 16% and in females 2% to 9%.

○ **What kinds of injuries are commonly reported in the medical histories of children diagnosed with conduct disorder?**

Head injuries, often incurred during abusive interaction with primary caregivers. Inquiry about head injuries as well as visible scars can yield information as to the nature and intensity of a child's previous traumatic experiences.

○ **What social systems often become involved in the treatment of a child with conduct disorder?**

The treatment of conduct disorder is complex and requires interaction between numerous agencies, including the juvenile court system, child protective services, psychiatric service providers, medical health providers, school systems, and the family system itself.

○ **What treatment modalities are useful in the treatment of conduct disorder?**

While problem-solving skills training, in which children/adolescents learn conflict resolution skills, can be helpful, the primary focus of treatment generally requires parental involvement, which may or may not be possible. Identification and treatment of underlying psychiatric conditions, learning disorders, and determination of intellectual capacities, is useful in stabilization of mental status, and in the tailoring of treatment strategies to the cognitive level of the child. Use of medications indicated in the treatment of the child's coexisting psychiatric disorders might help alleviate some externalizing symptoms. The use of lithium to reduce irritability and lability is particularly indicated when the family history is positive for bipolar disorder. Finally, patients may also benefit from the use of other mood stabilizers and β-blockers.

CHAPTER 31   Psychosis in Children

○ **What are the subtypes of schizophrenia with onset in childhood and adolescence?**

With questionable validity, schizophrenia in childhood and adolescence has been divided into Very Early Onset Schizophrenia (VEOS), which develops before the age of 13 years and is very rare; and Early Onset Schizophrenia (EOS), which develops after the age of 13 years. Most workers, however, consider schizophrenia developing before the age of puberty (12–13 years) as childhood-onset schizophrenia (COS).

○ **How early can schizophrenia develop in childhood?**

COS is extremely rare in children younger than 6 years, but the frequency steadily increases in those older than 11 years to a maximum around late adolescence/early adulthood.

○ **Does the age range for development of COS overlap with that for the development of autistic disorder?**

No, the age range for the development of autistic disorder is below 5 years of age while COS is very, very rare in this age group.

○ **What is the sex ratio for COS?**

In various studies, males outnumber females by up to 2.5 times. Among patients with a very early age of onset, males outnumber females even more.

○ **Is the mean age of onset different in boys and girls?**

Not before puberty. In adolescence, COS develops approximately 5 years earlier in boys.

○ **What is the relationship of social class to COS?**

COS is more common in less educated and less professionally successful families, but, as in adult-onset schizophrenia (AOS), the low social status may be the result of mental illness in the parents (downward drift theory).

○ **What is the difference in the *DSM-IV* diagnostic criteria for schizophrenia in adults and in children/adolescents?**

The criteria are essentially the same except that in adults, the criteria require that one or more major areas of functioning be markedly below the level achieved prior to the onset of illness, while in children and adolescents there should instead be a failure to reach the expected level of interpersonal, academic, or occupational achievement.

○ **How do the normal developmental stages affect the symptoms of COS?**

In the early stages of development, delusions and hallucinations are simpler, more elementary, and often involve monsters, pets, or toys. However, in older patients, they tend to be more vivid and systematized.

○ **Which is the most commonly reported symptom in COS?**

Auditory hallucinations. These are reported in approximately 80% of patients with COS.

○ **Is the presence of hallucinations alone enough to warrant a diagnosis of COS?**

No. Hallucinations should occur in a setting of identifiable delusions, disorganized thought process, and an inability to achieve or a decline in social milestones in order to warrant a diagnosis of COS.

○ **Can the presence of loose associations and illogical thinking be a part of a child's normal developmental stages?**

Yes. These are frequently found during a child's normal development, but their frequency decreases markedly by the end of Piaget's preoperational period (around 7 years of age).

○ **Name a well-known structured interview for detailed assessment of psychotic symptoms in children.**

The K-SADS (Kiddie Schedule for Affective Disorders and Schizophrenia).

○ **What is the most common mode of onset of COS?**

Insidious in approximately three-fourths of the patients, more so in the VEOS.

○ **Are there any premorbid symptoms that can precede the development of clinically recognizable COS?**

Premorbid impairments have been documented in social, motor, and language development. Premorbid developmental delays in speech are the most conspicuous and have been the most consistently documented.

○ **Are these premorbid symptoms specific to COS?**

No. All of these can also be seen in children who go on to develop schizotypal personality disorder, Asperger's disorder, or atypical pervasive developmental disorders (PDD).

○ **Can children with PDD go on to develop COS?**

Children with Asperger's disorder are at increased risk for the development of COS but not children with autistic disorder.

○ **Can COS be comorbidly diagnosed with PDD?**

DSM-IV allows autistic disorder or another PDD to be diagnosed comorbidly with schizophrenia in children if hallucinations and delusions form a prominent part of the clinical picture. However, PDD not otherwise specified (NOS) cannot be comorbidly diagnosed with schizophrenia.

○ **Which psychiatric disorders cluster more frequently in the first-degree relatives of COS?**

Higher rates of schizophrenia spectrum disorders have been reported in the families of COS probands, which may even exceed the rates of these disorders in the families of AOS probands. Bipolar affective disorder is twice as common among relatives of COS than among relatives of normal controls.

○ **Is mental retardation common in COS?**

While mental retardation can occur comorbidly with COS, mental retardation is much more common in children with autistic disorder (75%).

○ **What are the neuropsychological changes that have been documented in COS?**

On neuropsychological testing, tasks involving fine motor speed, attention, short-term, and recent long-term memory have been found to be particularly affected.

○ **What is the effect of COS on intellectual functioning?**

A decline in intellectual functioning has been demonstrated with the onset of premorbid symptoms.

○ **Is this intellectual decline progressive in nature?**

Unlike AOS, the intellectual decline in COS can progress till approximately 48 months after the onset of psychotic symptoms.

○ **Is the prevalence of schizophrenia in first-degree relatives of patients with COS more or less than in AOS?**

The prevalence is more.

○ **Are there any morphologic changes in the brain in COS?**

Significantly reduced total cerebral volume (TCV) has been demonstrated in patients of COS vis-à-vis healthy controls matched for age, sex, and handedness.

○ **What is currently known about the cause of this reduced TCV in COS?**

The reduced TCV appears to be due to a reduction in the volume of gray matter with relative sparing of the white matter.

○ **Have eye-tracking abnormalities been reported in COS?**

As in AOS, there are greater eye-tracking abnormalities in COS patients as compared to normal controls.

○ **What is known about the pattern of autonomic nervous system (ANS) abnormalities in COS?**

ANS abnormalities in COS are similar to those reported in chronic, poor prognosis AOS and include high levels of resting activity, deficient response to normal stimuli, and an inability to stop responding to familiar stimuli.

○ **What are the important causes of psychotic symptoms in children?**

Bipolar disorder, major depressive disorder, PDD, substance use, medications, seizure disorder, anxiety disorders, death of a loved one, dissociative disorders, severe abuse or neglect, obsessive-compulsive disorder, and severe language disorder are some of the common causes of psychotic symptoms in children. In most of these conditions, the symptoms are isolated, transient, and tend to occur following identifiable environmental stressors. Rates of misdiagnosis of COS, especially in children with early-onset bipolar disorder, are high.

○ **Which of the PDDs can most closely resemble COS?**

Asperger's disorder more closely resembles COS than autistic disorder. The differences are as follows: in Asperger's disorder, onset occurs before the age of 3 years, with a gradually improving course; while in COS, a better early developmental history is described, followed by gradual deterioration.

○ **Can affective symptoms appear in COS?**

Affective symptoms often appear in childhood psychosis, and if prolonged, should lead the clinician to suspect an affective disorder with psychosis, or a schizoaffective disorder as the primary diagnosis.

○ **What is the significance of affective symptoms in COS?**

COS patients with affective symptoms may show less cognitive impairment, less often have a history of neonatal complications, and have a better outcome than COS without these symptoms.

○ **Should such affective symptoms influence the choice of treatment of COS?**

Addition of a mood stabilizer to the antipsychotic regimen in this patient population may increase treatment benefits.

○ **What are the good prognostic indicators in COS?**

Presence of affective symptoms, later age of onset, acute onset, good premorbid adjustment, absence of premorbid delay in motor milestones/language acquisition, absence of premorbid attention-deficit hyperactivity disorder or learning disorder, well-differentiated symptoms, and good family support are good prognostic indicators in COS.

○ **Is the response to antipsychotics in COS influenced by the age of onset?**

COS may not respond as well to antipsychotics as AOS, particularly if the onset is before the age of 7 years.

○ **Are the typical antipsychotics effective in COS?**

Placebo-controlled trials are sparse but suggest that typical antipsychotics are effective in the treatment of COS, especially for positive symptoms, but the proportion of neuroleptic-intolerant patients at less-than-adequate doses is much higher.

○ **Has risperidone been shown to be an effective treatment for COS?**

Risperidone has been shown to be effective for both positive and negative symptoms in COS as in AOS, but there is a higher rate of extrapyramidal symptoms, dystonia, and galactorrhea than in adults.

○ **Has risperidone also been evaluated in treatment-resistant COS?**

No, risperidone has not been evaluated specifically for the management of treatment-resistant COS.

○ **What kind of intervention is appropriate for the education of patients with COS?**

Small, structured classrooms and individualized educational plans.

CHAPTER 32 Elimination Disorders

○ **Before we review anything we need to know the basics. At what age does a child typically develop bladder control?**

Between 2 and 3 years of age.

○ **Two to three years is only for daytime control; at what age does a child typically develop nocturnal (while sleeping) bladder control?**

Between 3 and 4 years of age.

○ **How does the brain control urination?**

Urination is controlled completely by an autonomic reflex at the level of the spinal cord. However, the brain can inhibit or facilitate urination through facilitory and inhibitory control centers in the brain stem. Several inhibitory centers are located in the cerebral cortex.

○ **What is the *Diagnostic and Statistical Manual-IV* (*DSM-IV*) definition of enuresis?**

The *DSM-IV* definition of enuresis is the repeated voiding of urine into inappropriate places like a bed or clothes, voluntarily or involuntarily.

○ **How often must a child urinate inappropriately, before being considered clinically significant by the *DSM IV*?**

Inappropriate urination must occur at least two times a week for at least 3 months.

○ **What diagnosis is used if a child urinates inappropriately only once a week for 4 months?**

If a child does not fit the criteria for frequency and duration, the diagnosis can still be considered as a provisional if there is significant distress or if there is impairment in social or academic functioning.

○ **Enuresis is classified into two subtypes, primary and secondary. What are the parameters for these subtypes?**

In primary enuresis, children have never achieved continence of urine, while in secondary enuresis, children have maintained continence for at least 1 year, and at some later point, have lost continence of urine.

○ **At what age would you expect the onset of secondary enuresis?**

Between the ages of 4 and 5 years.

○   **List the risk factors for developing secondary enuresis.**

Delayed onset of nocturnal continence, and exposure to four or more life stressors within a year's period.

○   **What is the risk for a child developing enuresis if either the father or mother was affected?**

It is 7.1 and 5.2 times greater, respectively.

○   **What is the probability for a child developing enuresis, if both biological parents were affected?**

The probability is 77.3%.

○   **What is the probability that a sibling of an enuretic child will be affected?**

The probability is 75%.

○   **If one twin is enuretic, what is the probability for a dizigotic and monozygotic twin developing enuresis?**

The probability is 35.7% and 67.8 %, respectively.

○   **In the Isle of Wight study by Rutter (1973), what was the prevalence of enuresis among boys and girls?**

By the age of 14 years, the prevalence of enuresis less than once a week in boys was 1.9%, and 1.2% in girls, and the prevalence of enuresis at least once a week for boys was 1.1%, and 0.5% for girls.

○   **Compared to nocturnal enuresis, diurnal enuresis requires what type of workup?**

Diurnal enuresis is more likely to be caused by a urinary tract abnormality. Depending on the history and physical, contrast studies may be required in order to determine pathology. However, this is not generally recommended for all cases of diurnal enuresis.

○   **Occasionally, we need to rule out obstructive lesions as a cause of enuresis. What is the incidence of obstructive lesions leading to enuresis in a child?**

A study by Cohan (1975) found an incidence in the primary care pediatric setting of 3.7%.

○   **After urinary tract infection and altered bladder physiology, what are the rarer causes of enuresis?**

Hyperthyroidism, constipation, and central hormonal abnormalities.

○   **Most episodes of nocturnal enuresis occur during what stage of sleep?**

Enuresis does not occur during any specific stage of sleep.

○   **A 13-year-old girl is seen in the psychiatrist's office, suffering from depression, and during the history, it is noted that she has just started to experience bed-wetting and leaking during the day. What is the most likely cause of her enuresis?**

Infection of the urogenital tract is the most common biologic cause of enuresis, especially in girls.

○   **You decide to treat a 7-year-old boy for enuresis with desmopressin acetate (DDAVP). Your objective is to treat the patient to prevent bed-wetting beginning that night. Of the two preparations, nasal spray or injection, which will have a quicker onset?**

The nasal preparation of DDAVP has an onset that is 10 times faster than the injection.

○ **Successful treatment with a medication, such as imipramine, should continue for how long?**

After 3 months, it is recommended that the medication be tapered and discontinued, and if symptoms recur, restart and titrate to the previous dose.

○ **How soon after starting imipramine can one expect to see improvement?**

Within 3 days at relatively low doses (25–75 mg).

○ **After starting a child on imipramine, the child decides to "cure" himself by taking all of the medication at once. After arriving in the emergency room, you tell the doctor to give what antidotal medication?**

Physostigmine.

○ **What is the most common side effect of DDAVP?**

Nasal stuffiness, headache, epistaxis, and abdominal pain.

○ **A 4-year-old patient is seen in the emergency room for hyponatremia and polydipsia. You hear from his mother that he is taking a pill "to stop his peeing." What is the most likely medication?**

Water intoxication and resultant hyponatremia are a rare but serious side effects found in the very young and elderly being treated with DDAVP.

○ **What is the initial clinical approach to the patient with nocturnal enuresis?**

Typically nonpunitive behavioral techniques (e.g., bell and pad) should be used, followed by pharmacologic interventions if behavioral techniques are unsuccessful.

○ **You decide to use the bell and pad method to treat a patient for enuresis. How would you describe to the parent how it works?**

A pad with two unconnected wires is placed under the child at night. When the child wets, a connection is made between the wires. When this connection is made between the two wires, an electric circuit is created and a bell sounds (annoying stimulus) and the child awakens. The child learns to either awaken prior to wetting or to retain the urine until they wake, avoiding the noxious stimulus.

○ **What is the success rate of psychotherapy alone versus the behavioral bell and pad method?**

Psychotherapy has a success rate of 20%. Bell and pad has a success rate of 75%.

○ **What are the main predictors of a poor outcome with the use of the bell and pad method?**

Childhood psychiatric disorders and family stress.

○ **There is one more behavioral method that is not commonly used called retention control. How is it taught?**

The child, while urinating, is told to stop in mid stream. This strengthens the sphincter control.

○ **Knowing how successful the bell and pad method can be, you know to recommend it before medication. What is the percentage of your colleagues who recommend the bell and pad method to parents?**

Three percent.

○   **What is the percentage of children who will spontaneously remit from enuresis?**

Twenty percent.

○   **Do children suffering from autism show the same delayed onset of toilet training as children with mental retardation?**

Children suffering from autism do not show any particular delay in the onset of toilet training.

○   **What is the *most common* mistake that occurs with toilet training?**

Beginning training too early, most often within the first year. Inconsistent reinforcement and punitive methods are also significant contributors to failure.

○   **List the different normal intestinal transit times seen at different stages in development.**

Age	Time
3 months	8.5 hours
4 to 14 months	16 hours
3 to 13 years	26 hours

○   **How long on average does it take for total intestinal transit time?**

Thirty-three hours.

○   **What does a child gain control of first, bladder or bowel control?**

Bowel control occurs slightly before bladder, between the ages of 2 and 2.5 years.

○   **At what age in the United States do a majority of children reach bowel continence?**

Age 5 years.

○   **Can social and academic impairment factor into the diagnosis of encopresis similar to that of enuresis?**

No. In the *DSM-IV*, there is no consideration of impairment; the frequency and duration are lenient enough, allowing for just one episode of inappropriate stooling per month for 3 months.

○   **Is the intentional passage of stool considered as a part of the *DSM-IV* definition of encopresis?**

Yes. The *DSM-IV* defines encopresis as repeated passage of stool into inappropriate places (e.g., in clothes or the bathtub), whether involuntarily or intentionally.

○   **A 7-year-old child with mental retardation functioning at a 3-year-old developmental level has been having "accidents" in his pants his whole life. Can this patient be considered as having encopresis?**

No. According to the *DSM-IV*, a child must have reached the chronological and/or developmental age of 4 years.

○ **A 5-year-old child has developed tropical sprue, and as a result, he has been having bowel movements in his pants during gym class and on the bus. Can this child be considered as having encopresis?**

Any child having inappropriate stooling caused by a medical condition or from medications such as laxatives is excluded from the diagnosis.

○ **What differentiates primary encopresis from secondary encopresis?**

Primary encopresis is defined as not having reached a period of sustained continence for at least 1 year. Secondary encopresis is defined as when a child has had a period of continence for 1 year or more, before the current episode of encopresis began.

○ **A 7-year-old child's mother complains that her child "doesn't go poop" and has diarrhea when sitting in class. She asks you for a diagnosis. What is your answer?**

There are two subtypes of encopresis in the *DSM-IV*. "With constipation and overflow incontinence," as demonstrated in this patient, and "Without constipation and overflow incontinence."

○ **What unique clinical descriptor is not shared between encopresis and enuresis?**

Encopresis does not have a nocturnal and a diurnal descriptor.

○ **Several conditions in psychiatry have known predictive or predisposing factors. What factors predispose a child to encopresis?**

Fecal retention and abnormal frequency of bowel movements, in children between the ages of 1 and 2 years, have been shown to predict encopresis in the later years.

○ **How common is encopresis caused by constipation?**

It is the cause of encopresis in 75% of cases.

○ **List the two main physiological factors that result from constipation.**

A poorly functioning, weak internal anal sphincter and poor or weak peristaltic contractures of the lower colon.

○ **What is the prevalence rate for encopresis?**

According to Bellman (1966), the prevalence of encopresis between ages of 7 and 8 years is 1.5%, while Rutter (1970) found a prevalence rate of encopresis between the ages of 10 and 12 years of 1.0%.

○ **What is the male-to-female ratio for encopresis?**

According to Bellman (1966) in children aging 7 to 8 years, the male-to-female ratio was 3.4:1; while Rutter (1970) found that in ages 10 to 12 years, the male-to-female ratio was 5:1.

○ **What is a common result of persistent constipation?**

Hirschsprung's disease, also called megacolon, results when constipation is so severe that bowel movements occur only one to two times a week. This causes distention of the colon to a diameter as great as 3 to 4 in.

○ **List the neurologic conditions that are most commonly associated with encopresis.**

- Cerebral palsy
- Spina bifida
- Mental retardation

○ **How do the family structure, function, and economic status play in the causation of encopresis?**

There has been no evidence that family structure, function, or economic status are risk factors for encopresis. However, it has been found that stressful life events such as divorce, illness, and family relocation were associated with the onset of encopresis in 25% of cases.

○ **List two comorbid conditions most commonly found with encopresis.**

Enuresis and behavioral problems.

○ **What is the differential diagnosis for encopresis?**

Hirshprung's disease, stenosis of the rectum or anus, smooth muscle disease, endocrine abnormalities especially hyperthyroidism or hypothyroidism, infections such as giardiasis, and exogenous causes such as laxatives and antibiotics.

○ **When concerned about a medical cause for encopresis, what is the standard workup you would use?**

Complete blood count, electrolytes, thyroid function tests, and tests for endocrine disorders.

○ **What is the only mood stabilizer currently recommended for the use in encopresis?**

Lithium.

○ **Under what conditions do you use laxatives for treating encopresis?**

Laxative use and bowel clean out is recommended only for retentive encopresis.

○ **What is the only psychopharmacologic treatment that can be used for both encopresis and enuresis?**

Imipramine.

○ **List the three main modes of the behavioral modification approach to treating encopresis.**

Education about the disorder itself and about bowel movements has been helpful in decreasing the anxiety associated with defecation. Scheduling a consistent time for bowel movements (e.g., after breakfast each day) is advisable, while positive reinforcement should be used to encourage proper bowel movements.

○ **Why is it so important for children to schedule their bowel movements after breakfast?**

Because that is when the intestinal tract has the most peristaltic movement.

○ **When negative reinforcement is used with behavioral modification, what has been shown to be an effective consequence for episodes of encopresis?**

After a child has had an inappropriate bowel movement, requiring the child to wash their soiled clothes for at least 15 minutes and sit in a cool tub of water for 15 minutes.

○ **How is biofeedback used in the treatment of encopresis?**

A three-balloon rectal tube is placed in the rectum, one in the rectum, one at the internal anal sphincter (involuntarily controlled), and one at the external anal sphincter (voluntarily controlled). Each balloon is connected to a monometric recorder to allow the patient to visualize the pressure variations. The child is then taught to contract the external anal sphincter when they visualize the decrease in pressure at the internal anal sphincter. The child is then rewarded with positive reinforcement for being able to increase the pressure of the external anal sphincter.

○ **What is the response rate to the treatment approach involving the educational–behavioral-medical model for encopresis?**

Seventy-eight percent remission for up to 6 months.

○ **By what age do almost all children either respond to treatment or experience spontaneous resolution of encopresis?**

By the age of 16 years.

○ **What is the second leading cause of work absenteeism behind the common cold?**

Irritable bowel syndrome (IBS).

○ **What is the prevalence of IBS?**

Eleven percent.

○ **What age population accounts for the majority of cases of irritable bowel syndrome?**

Forty-five to sixty-four years of age.

○ **List the three main criteria generally agreed upon by most physicians for the diagnosis of IBS.**

Abdominal pain relieved by defecation and disturbed defecation involving two or more of the following: altered stool frequency, altered stool form, altered stool passage (straining or urgency), passage of mucus, bloating, or a feeling of abdominal distention.

CHAPTER 33   Tic Disorders

○ **What is a tic?**

According to the *DSM-IV*, a tic is defined as an involuntary, sudden, rapid, recurrent, nonrhythmic, stereotyped motor movement or vocalization. It rarely lasts more than a second. It is experienced as irresistible but can often be suppressed for varying lengths of time.

○ **How are tic disorders classified?**

Motor and vocal tics can be classified as either simple or complex. **Simple motor tics** are composed of repetitive, rapid contractions of functionally similar muscle groups (e.g., eye blinking, neck jerking, shoulder shrugging, and facial grimacing). **Complex motor tics** appear to be more purposeful and ritualistic (e.g., grooming behavior, smelling of objects, jumping, touching behaviors, echopraxia, and copropraxia). **Simple vocal tics** consist of meaningless sounds and noises (e.g., coughing, throat clearing, grunting, sniffing, snorting, and barking). **Complex vocal tics** include repeating words or phrases that are out of context. They include coprolalia (the use of obscene words or phrases), palilalia (repeating one's own words), and echolalia (repetition of last heard word of others).

○ **Describe the *DSM-IV* classification of tic disorders.**

The *DSM-IV* classifies tic disorders into four diagnostic categories:

1. **Tourette's disorder** is characterized by multiple motor tics and one or more vocal tics occurring concurrently or separately for a period of more than 1 year, and during this period there was never a tic-free interval of more than three consecutive months. The onset is before the age of 18 years and is not caused by a substance or by a general medical condition.

2. **Chronic motor or vocal tic disorder** is the diagnosis given when either a motor tic or a vocal tic is present, but not both. Additionally, criteria have never been met for Tourette's disorder. Other criterion of age of onset, minimum duration, and exclusion of organic factors are same as Tourette's disorder.

3. **Transient tic disorder** is the presence of a single or multiple motor and/or vocal tics lasting for more than 4 weeks but for no longer than 12 months. Criteria have never been met for Tourette's disorder or chronic motor or vocal tic disorder. Other criterion of age of onset and exclusion of organic factors are same as Tourette's disorder.

4. **Tic disorder not otherwise specified** is the category of tic disorder that does not meet the criteria for a specific tic disorder, i.e., tics lasting less than four weeks or tics with an onset after the age of 18 years.

○ **What *DSM-IV* diagnostic criteria are common for Tourette's disorder, chronic motor or vocal, and transient tic disorder?**

In all of these subcategories of tic disorder, the age of onset of the tic disorder is before 18 years, and the tic disorder is not caused by a substance or by a general medical condition.

○ **What is the differentiating *DSM-IV* diagnostic criteria between chronic motor or vocal tic disorder and transient tic disorder?**

Both the tic disorders share similar diagnostic criterion except that transient tic disorder lasts no longer than 12 months and criteria for chronic motor or vocal tic disorder have not been met in the past.

○ **What is the differential diagnosis for tic disorders?**

Tics must be differentiated from movement disorders, (for example dystonic, choreiform, athetoid, myoclonic, and hemiballismic movements), tremors, mannerisms, and sterotypic movement disorders. Neurologic diseases in which movement disorders are a symptom include Huntington's disease, Parkinsonism, Sydenham's chorea, and Wilson's disease.

○ **What are the comorbid conditions associated with tic disorders?**

ADHD occurs in 50% to 60% of children with Tourette's disorder, while OCD symptoms occur in approximately one-half of Tourette's disorder patients. Attention difficulties often precede the onset of tics, whereas OCD symptoms often follow the onset of tic symptoms.

○ **What are the associated behavioral difficulties with tic disorders?**

Behavioral difficulties associated with tic disorder include distractibility, impulsivity, disinhibition, restlessness, and obsessive-compulsive symptoms.

○ **What conditions exacerbate tics?**

Stress, anxiety, fatigue, boredom, or an exciting event exacerbates tics.

○ **What conditions attenuate tics?**

Tics are attenuated by alcohol, orgasm, fever, relaxation, or involvement in an absorbing activity. They are markedly diminished during sleep.

○ **Which tic disorder is the most common?**

Transient tic disorder is the most common and mildest of the tic disorders.

○ **What is the lifetime prevalence of Tourette's disorder?**

The lifetime prevalence of Tourette's disorder is around 4 to 5/10,000.

○ **What is the gender difference in prevalence of Tourette's disorder?**

Tourette's disorder occurs approximately three times more often in boys than in girls.

○ **Describe the prevalence of tic behaviors (other than Tourette's disorder).**

The rate of tic behavior has been estimated to be from 100 to 1000 times greater than that of Tourette's disorder. The prevalence of tics, twitches, mannerisms, and nervous movements range from 1% to 13% in boys and 1% to 11% in girls. Children between the ages of 7 and 11 years appear to have the highest rate.

○ **What is the age of onset of tic disorders?**

The median age of onset of Tourette's disorder and motor tics is 7 years. The median age of onset of vocal tics is 11 years, while the onset of transient tic disorder occurs between 3 and 10 years of age.

○ **Describe the course of tic disorders.**

Tourette's disorder is a usually chronic, lifelong disease with relative remissions and exacerbations. New tics may replace old ones. Severely afflicted people may have serious emotional problems, including major depressive disorder and suicidal attempts. **Chronic motor or vocal tic disorder** usually lasts four to six years and stops in early adolescence. **Transient tic disorder** disappears permanently or recurs during periods of stress. Only a small percentage (usually after a partial remission) develop chronic motor or vocal tic disorder or Tourette's disorder.

○ **What is the suggested mode of genetic transmission of Tourette's disorder?**

Family pedigree studies suggest that Tourette's disorder appears to be inherited through an autosomal pattern intermediate between dominant and recessive (also called bilinear transmission).

○ **What is the most compelling evidence of genetic inheritance of Tourette's disorder?**

The most compelling evidence of genetic inheritance is provided by twin studies of Tourette's disorders and chronic motor tic disorder that show significantly greater concordance in monozygotic (>50%) than in dizygotic twins (10%).

○ **What is the neurochemical etiology of tic disorders?**

Evidence for **dopamine system** involvement comes from the fact that tics are suppressed by dopamine antagonists (haloperidol, pimozide, fluphenazine) and exacerbated by agents that increase central dopaminergic activity (methylphenidate, amphetamine, pemoline, and cocaine). **Endogenous opiates** may be involved in tic disorder, as some evidence indicates that endogenous opiate antagonists (i.e., naltrexone) reduce tics. Abnormalities of the **noradrenergic system** have been implicated in some cases by the reduction of tics with clonidine.

○ **What is the neuroanatomic etiology of tic disorders?**

Abnormalities in the **basal ganglia** are implicated as possible sites of disturbance in Tourette's disorder.

○ **State the immunologic factors associated with the etiology of tic disorder.**

A poststreptococcal syndrome caused by autoimmune processes secondary to streptococcal infection has been identified as a potential mechanism causing Tourette's disorder.

○ **Describe diagnostic laboratory tests of Tourette's disorder.**

There is no specific laboratory test for any tic disorder. Tourette's disorder has nonspecific abnormal EEG findings. CT and MRI studies have not revealed any specific structural lesions.

○ **What is the goal of the drug therapy of tic disorders?**

The goal of therapy is to reduce tics to a tolerable level while minimizing side effects. Pharmacotherapy of tic disorders is strictly symptomatic and not curative.

○   **What are the guidelines for the use of medications in the treatment of tic disorders?**

Pharmacotherapy is reserved for the treatment of severe tic disorders only. Motor or vocal tic disorder or transient tic disorder patients generally do not require pharmacotherapy until tics are severe and impairing. Pharmacotherapy is most effective for Tourette's disorder, though a patient with mild symptoms may not require medications.

○   **What drugs are used for the treatment of tic disorders?**

- **Haloperidol** has been the mainstay in the drug therapy. Up to 80% of patients have a favorable response with haloperidol, the usual dose being 0.5 to 6 mg/d. However, only 20% to 30% of patients continue long-term maintenance therapy due to the side effects of haloperidol (or any pharmacotherapeutic agent).
- **Pimozide** is useful for patients who cannot tolerate or fail to respond to haloperidol. Usual dose is 1 to 10 mg/d. The use of atypical neuroleptics, such as risperidone, may also be of benefit.
- **Clonidine** seems to be most effective in reducing motor tics. It is somewhat more effective in patients with both tic disorder and ADHD than in patients with ADHD alone. Usual dose is 0.15 to 0.30 mg/d in divided doses of 0.05 mg.

○   **What is the role of behavioral therapy in tic disorders?**

Several behavioral techniques are reported to reduce tic frequency, particularly the habit reversal treatment, in which a competing response paired with a tic or urge to tic. Behavioral treatments are most effective in treating transient and chronic motor or vocal tic disorders. Tourette's disorder responds less favorably to behavioral therapy.

○   **What is the role of psychotherapy in treating tic disorders?**

Psychotherapy appears to have no effect on tics and is not recommended as a primary treatment for chronic tic disorder, although it may help a patient to cope with symptoms of the disorder.

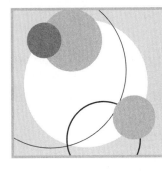

Section V

TREATMENT MODALITIES

CHAPTER 34 Psychopharmacology I

○ **What are the phases of drug development in the United States?**

Investigational New Drug application granted by the Food and Drug Administration (FDA).

↓

Phase I: Given to normal persons. Pharmacokinetics and adverse effects (safety and tolerability) studied.

↓

Phase II: Given to patients. Efficacy in specific disorders studied.

↓

Phase III: Larger trials in patients to confirm the findings, determine optimum dosage, and use in special populations (e.g., young, elderly, renal impairment, hepatic impairment).

↓

Phase IV: Postmarketing surveillance.

○ **What are the FDA categories for rating the safety of a drug's use in pregnancy?**

- Category A: controlled studies in humans show no risk
- Category B: animal studies show risk but this is not substantiated in human studies

OR

animal studies do not show risk and human studies have not been done

- Category C: animal studies show risk or have not been done

AND

human studies have not been done
    (*Implication*: use in pregnancy only if the potential benefit outweighs the risk)

- Category D: human studies show risk but the benefit may outweigh the risk
- Category X: use of the drug in pregnancy is contraindicated because the risks outweigh the benefits

○ **What is the difference between pharmacokinetic and pharmacodynamic interactions?**

Pharmacokinetic interactions occur when one drug affects the metabolism of another drug or the protein binding of another drug. An example of a pharmacokinetic interaction is the inhibition of the cytochrome P-450 2D6-isoenzyme system by paroxetine, which increases the blood levels of tricyclic antidepressants (TCAs), which are metabolized by the 2D6-isoenzyme system. Pharmacodynamic interactions occur when the mechanism of action of one drug affects the mechanism of action of another drug. These interactions occur most often at the synaptic level.

○   **What does the duration of action of a drug depend on most?**

The duration of action of a drug depends more on the volume of the distribution than the half-life of a drug. The volume of distribution is dependent on how lipophilic the drug is. The more lipophilic an agent, the faster it crosses the blood–brain barrier and the faster it is stored in peripheral fat tissues. Obesity increases the volume of distribution and elimination half-life, all of which will decrease the duration of action.

○   **What are the main processes whereby most drugs are metabolized?**

Oxidation, reduction, hydrolysis, and conjugation.

○   **What is meant by the term "therapeutic index"?**

It is the ratio of the median toxic dose (TD_{50}, the dose that tends to cause toxic effects in 50% of patients) to the median effective dose (ED_{50}, the dose that tends to be effective in 50% of patients).

○   **In what way does the dosing of psychotropic drugs in children differ from that in adults?**

Despite a lower body weight, children tend to require a higher ratio of milligrams of drug to the body weight due to higher rate of metabolism.

○   **How does the mechanism of action of the atypical antipsychotic agents differ from that of traditional neuroleptics?**

The biggest difference between atypical and traditional antipsychotics is serotonin antagonism, which is most likely the means by which atypicals improve negative symptoms. The atypical neuroleptics bind much more avidly to the serotonin receptor than the D2 receptor, but nonetheless, dystonia and EPS are still reported with the use of atypicals.

○   **What is the most effective dose range of risperidone, and what are the clinical problems associated with giving higher doses?**

The most effective dose range of risperidone is 4 to 8 mg/d. Higher doses are associated with a higher frequency of EPS without the advantage of increased efficacy.

○   **Although clozapine has significant anticholinergic activity, what very annoying side effect does it paradoxically produce?**

Clozapine, an atypical neuroleptic with a high level of anticholinergic activity, can paradoxically cause significant hypersalivation that increases the risk of aspiration in some patients.

○   **What are the dose-limiting side effects of clozapine?**

The dose-limiting side effects of clozapine are hypotension, sedation, and seizures. The side effect of agranulocytosis is not dose related.

○   **What factors increase the risk of agranulocytosis in patients treated with clozapine?**

The factors that increase the risk for agranulocytosis in patients treated with clozapine are Jewish descent, female gender (male-to-female ratio of 1:2), increasing age, first 6 months of treatment, and a low white blood count at baseline.

○ **What are the advantages and disadvantages of clozapine? Which classical neuroleptic has a similar side-effect profile?**

Clozapine is almost void of any extrapyramidal effects and has a lower risk of tardive dyskinesia. In some cases, symptoms of tardive dyskinesia have actually improved when clozapine was introduced. Clozapine has also been shown to be extremely useful in the treatment of refractory psychosis. However, its disadvantages include a greater incidence of agranulocytosis, requiring absolute compliance with regular monitoring of blood counts. Clozapine also lowers the seizure threshold, has a high level of anticholinergic side effects, can cause significant hypotension and sedation, and has low potency, that is, properties which are very similar to those of chlorpromazine.

○ **What severe, but rare, adverse effect can occur when benzodiazepines are given to a patient on clozapine?**

Circulatory collapse and respiratory arrest. A condition similar to this occurs occasionally when benzodiazepines are given with low-potency neuroleptics producing deep sedation, hypotension, and decreased respirations. The elderly and patients with chronic obstructive pulmonary disease are at increased risk.

○ **What are the most common side effects of olanzapine (Zyprexa®)?**

The most common side effects of olanzapine are the anticholinergic symptoms of constipation and dry mouth, and orthostatic hypotension secondary to α-adrenergic blockade. Doses higher than 10 mg may produce tremor and sedation. Olanzapine also has antihistaminic effects, which may be responsible for the associated weight gain. There appear to be no serious hematologic side effects.

○ **How are psychotic symptoms of cerebral vascular accidents treated?**

Anticonvulsants and neuroleptics can be used to treat psychotic symptoms secondary to an organic lesion.

○ **What are the effects of blocking α-adrenergic receptors? What neuroleptics have a high degree of α-blocker activity, and which neuroleptics have a low degree of α-blockade?**

α-Adrenergic receptor blockade results in peripheral vasodilation and thus a fall in total peripheral resistance occurs, resulting in hypotension. The low-potency neuroleptics such as chlorpromazine, thioridazine, mesoridazine, and clozapine have a high degree of α-blockade. The higher potency agents, fluphenazine, haloperidol, loxapine, trifluoperazine, and thiothixene have a much lower degree of α-adrenergic blockade.

○ **Treatment of agitation and psychosis in the elderly with antipsychotic agents can be limited by what factors?**

The use of antipsychotic agents for the treatment of agitation and psychosis in the elderly can be limited due to the increased sensitivity of the elderly the anticholinergic, antihistaminic, and antiadrenergic side effects of neuroleptics. Hypotension, in particular, can lead to falls, fractures, subdural hematomas, and myocardial infarctions. Atypical neuroleptics are also associated with increased risk for death in the elderly (1.6–1.7 times greater than placebo), usually due to cardiovascular or infectious etiologies. Finally, the elderly have a higher risk of tardive dyskinesia. The use of high-potency antipsychotics such as haloperidol or fluphenazine in low doses can minimize side effects.

○ **Why is pimozide not recommended as a first-line drug in schizophrenia?**

Because pimozide is associated with significantly more cardiac conduction abnormalities than other antipsychotics. It is recommended that a baseline ECG and periodic follow-up ECGs be obtained when pimozide is prescribed. There is usually no problem with doses of 20 mg or less in patients with normal ECGs. Ziprazidone and less commonly risperidone are also associated with prolonged Qtc intervals and should be used cautiously in individuals with a history of heart disease.

○ **What are the diagnostic criteria for neuroleptic malignant syndrome (NMS)?**

The diagnostic criteria for NMS include treatment with a neuroleptic medication within the last 7 days (or 2–4 weeks for depot neuroleptics), hyperthermia (≥38°C), muscle rigidity, and three of the following seven sets of symptoms: mental status changes, tachycardia, hypertension or hypotension, tachypnea or hypoxia, elevation of CPK or myoglobinuria, leukocytosis, and metabolic acidosis. Finally, the presence of a drug-induced, systemic, or neuropsychiatric illness should be excluded.

○ **What other agents can cause a syndrome similar to NMS?**

Lithium (especially in combination with neuroleptics), tricyclic antidepressants, monoamine oxidase inhibitors, sympathomimetics (amphetamines, cocaine, and fenfluramine), psychedelics (PCP, LSD), anticholinergics, dopamine depleting agents (such as tetrabenazine and reserpine), and dopamine antagonists (such as metoclopramide) can cause NMS-like syndromes. In addition, patients with Parkinson's disease and other basal ganglia disorders can exhibit an NMS-like syndrome when abruptly withdrawn from dopamine agonists like levodopa.

○ **Low serum iron is associated with what side effects related to neuroleptic medication treatment?**

Low serum iron is associated with neuroleptic malignant syndrome and extrapyramidal reactions. Correcting with supplemental iron may reduce the risk for these conditions.

○ **Fatal hyperthermia is associated with what medication group?**

Fatal hyperthermia is associated with neuroleptics, especially those with high anticholinergic side effects. Hot weather, alcohol ingestion, and CNS disorders are also risk factors for this condition.

○ **What neuroleptics lower the seizure threshold?**

Chlorpromazine and clozapine significantly reduce the seizure threshold.

○ **Why should low-potency neuroleptics and ACE inhibitors not be coadministered?**

The mixture of low-potency neuroleptics and ACE inhibitors can cause serious hypotension leading to possible falls, fractures, and cardiac or cerebral infarcts.

○ **What percentage of patients stabilized on antipsychotic medication will relapse if a placebo medication is substituted for the neuroleptic?**

The relapse rate is 70% on placebo.

○ **How does the treatment of psychosis in delusional disorder differ from the treatment of psychosis in schizophrenia?**

The psychotic symptoms of delusional disorder tend to be much more resistant to treatment with neuroleptics than the psychotic symptoms of schizophrenia.

○ **How long should anticholingeric medication for dystonia be continued?**

Tolerance to dystonia develops in approximately 1 month. The need for prophylaxis of extrapyramidal side effects (EPS) should be re-evaluated at that time.

○ **In what population is the use of anticholinergics as prophylaxis against EPS contraindicated?**

The use of anticholinergics as prophylaxis against EPS is contraindicated in the elderly secondary to the risk of memory dysfunction, susceptibility to anticholinergic delirium, and urinary retention.

○ **What is "rabbit syndrome"?**

Rabbit syndrome is a focal, perioral, Parkinsonian tremor that is a side effect of antipsychotic agents. It usually has a late onset of presentation and responds to drug dosage decrease or antiparkinsonian agents.

○ **What drugs, although useful for akathisia, are not useful for dystonia?**

β-Blockers and benzodiazepines are useful for the treatment of akathisia but not dystonia.

○ **What is the pharmacokinetic difference between benztropine and trihexyphenidyl?**

Benztropine has a half-life of greater than 24 hours and can be given in a once-a-day dose to adults. Trihexyphenidyl has a short half-life of 3 to 10 hours and must be given three times a day.

○ **How long does it take for Parkinsonian symptoms secondary to neuroleptic use to resolve once the drug is discontinued?**

It usually takes 7 to 10 days for Parkinsonian symptoms to resolve once the neuroleptic is discontinued. However, it may, in some cases, take several weeks to months to resolve completely.

○ **Besides benzodiazepines, what other drugs are used in the treatment of antipsychotic-induced akathisia?**

β-Blockers are very useful in treating antipsychotic-induced akathisia. Propranolol appears to be more effective than pindolol and metoprolol.

○ **Contrast the difference between risperidone and clozapine in regard to their effects on mania or depression.**

Risperidone appears to have higher efficacy in patients with psychosis and depression, but is more likely to cause mania than clozapine. Clozapine appears to control manic states much better than depressive states.

○ **What is considered the best mood stabilizer to begin a patient on and why?**

Research supports the use of valproic acid over lithium and carbamazepine because valproic acid is better tolerated than lithium or carbamazepine. Valproic acid is also easier to dose, causes less cognitive impairment, has fewer drug interactions, and can be administered in loading doses.

○ **What medications are useful in the treatment of bipolar disorder with rapid cycling?**

Valproic acid and possibly carbamazepine have been shown to be the most effective pharmacologic agents for the treatment of bipolar disorder with rapid cycling.

○ **What are the gastrointestinal side effects of valproate and how can these be mitigated?**

Gastrointestinal effects are the most common side effects in patients on valproate, and include nausea, vomiting, anorexia, heartburn, and indigestion. Diarrhea may also occur. Use of the enteric-coated formulation (Divalproex sodium) or addition of a histamine-2 blocker may successfully reduce these side effects. Of note is the fact that gastrointestinal side effects are common with all three major mood stabilizers.

○ **What blood level should a patient have when treated with valproic acid?**

A therapeutic blood level of 45 to 100 μg/mL is required for valproic acid. If there is insufficient response, increase up to 125 μg/mL. Adverse effects are much more prominent and frequent above serum levels greater than 125 μg/mL.

○ **What are the three forms of valproic acid available in the United States?**

1. Valproic acid (Depakene®)
2. Sodium valproate (Depakene® syrup)
3. Divalproex sodium (Depakote®)

All these preparations may be referred to as valproate, and they all convert to valproic acid in the serum. Please note: Divalproex sodium is available as sprinkles, immediate release, and extended release formulations.

○ **Tremor is common with which of the mood stabilizers?**

Valproic acid and lithium can produce a tremor, and are even more likely to do so if combined.

○ **What liver function tests become elevated in patients taking valproic acid?**

The prothrombin time, fibrinogen levels, and serum transaminase are frequently elevated during the course of treatment with valproic acid. These changes are usually dose related and self-limited. Reports of fatal hepatotoxicity are very rare, occurring primarily in children younger than 2 years.

○ **What hematologic parameters require monitoring during treatment with valproic acid?**

The platelet count and white blood cell count require monitoring during treatment with valproate. If thrombocytopenia or leukopenia develops, it is usually dose related and will respond to dosage decrease. If dosage reduction does not result in return of the platelet count or white blood count to normal levels, the use valproic acid may need to be discontinued.

○ **What hematologic parameters require monitoring during treatment with carbamazepine?**

During treatment with carbamazepine, a complete blood count and platelet count should be checked at baseline (before treatment begins), then every 2 weeks for 2 months, and then every 3 months thereafter. In addition, the patient and family should be instructed to contact the physician if petechiae, weakness, pallor, fever, sore throat, or infection occur. A complete blood count should then be done immediately to rule out reduced white blood cell, red blood cell, and platelet counts.

○ **What effect does carbamazepine have on cardiac conduction?**

Carbamazepine slows atrioventricular cardiac conduction and should not be used in patients with heart block and used cautiously with other drugs that can increase heart block, such as tricyclic antidepressants and β-blockers.

○ **What is the overall effect of carbamazepine on levels of other drugs and how does this differ from valproate?**

Carbamazepine is a strong enzyme inducer, so blood levels of drugs, and carbamazepine itself, may fall. Valproate, on the other hand, is an enzyme inhibitor and causes the levels of various drugs to rise.

O **Carbamazepine is a potent autoinducer and heteroinducer of what isoenzyme subsystem and what are its effects?**

Carbamazepine induces the cytochrome P-450 3A4-isoenzyme system, which is also the system that metabolizes it. Consequently, carbamazepine lowers its own levels in 2 to 12 weeks. The levels of other agents metabolized by this isoenzyme system are also reduced, and include triazolam, nefazodone, alprazolam, terfenadine, ketoconazole, astemizole, and birth control pills. It is very important to discuss birth control with the patient before initiating carbamazepine, since patients have become pregnant because of the decreased effectiveness of birth control pills when coadministered with carbamazepine.

O **What hepatic and hematologic parameters require close monitoring, but not drug discontinuation, in a healthy patient taking carbamazepine?**

If the white cell count does not drop below $3000/mm^3$ or if the γ-glutamyltransferase, alanine transferase, or aspartate transaminase are not greater than three times the normal level, then carbamazepine may be continued with close monitoring.

O **What rashes are seen in carbamazepine therapy, and what is the treatment?**

Ten to twenty percent of all people taking carbamazepine will develop rashes, which may be associated with fever and myalgia. Most require discontinuation of the drug. Erythema multiform and Steven's-Johnson syndrome are the most severe dermatologic rashes associated with carbamazepine use and can result in fatal reactions.

O **Describe the interaction of valproic acid and carbamazepine.**

Valproic acid causes an accumulation of the epoxide metabolite of carbamazepine (which is not measured by laboratory assays of carbamazepine) by inhibiting its metabolism. Carbamazepine, on the other hand, causes a decrease in valproic acid levels by induction of the cytochrome P-450 3A4-isoenzyme system.

O **What is the best patient profile for the use of lithium?**

The best clinical profile for lithium is a patient having an uncomplicated episode of mania, with no history of substance abuse, a history of good interepisode functioning, and a history of cycling where the index episode is one of mania. Negative predictors of response to lithium include a history of rapid cycling, mixed states, substance abuse, incongruent psychotic features, and an index episode of depression.

O **Is the effectiveness of lithium the same in the treatment of acute mania and in prophylaxis of recurrent episodes?**

Yes. Lithium is very effective in preventing recurrent cycles, more so manic, than depressive phases. However, only 50% of patients will have full remission of manic episodes when treated with only lithium.

O **What are the clinical indications for once-a-day dosing of lithium?**

Prescribing lithium in once-a-day doses assists in compliance and can decrease polyuria.

O **What is the long-term clinical significance of abruptly discontinuing lithium in a patient whose mood disorder has been stabilized?**

Abrupt discontinuation of lithium may lead to lithium refractoriness, as well as an increased risk for development of a manic episode. A gradual taper will prevent these unsatisfactory outcomes.

○ **What is discontinuation-induced refractoriness?**

Discontinuation-induced refractoriness refers to the loss of treatment response after discontinuing lithium in a patient who was lithium responsive until discontinuing it. This is more likely to occur if lithium is suddenly stopped and not gradually tapered. This may be true for other medications, especially valproic acid and carbamazepine.

○ **What effect does lithium have on calcium metabolism?**

Lithium can cause dysregulation of calcium metabolism that results in hypercalcemia and hyperparathyroidism. This may ultimately cause osteopenia, osteoporosis, and hypermagnesemia. Increased calcium levels can also cause weakness and fatigue, which may appear as depression. Treatment is lithium discontinuation.

○ **What is considered appropriate renal monitoring in a patient on lithium?**

Renal monitoring of patients on lithium consists of periodic measurement of serum creatinine and blood urea nitrogen. If these parameters begin to rise or serum lithium levels begin to rise on a constant dose, consultation with a nephrologist is recommended.

○ **What medications increase lithium levels?**

Diuretics (amiloride, spironolactone, triamterene), tetracycline, carbamazepine, and nonsteroidal anti-inflammatory drugs. Aspirin has little effect on lithium levels. Hypokalemia increases the toxic effects of lithium, while sodium depletion increases serum lithium levels.

○ **What effect does lithium have on the ECG?**

An ECG of a patient on lithium may show T-wave flattening or inversion that is benign and disappears after discontinuation of the drug. Lithium also interferes with atrioventricular conduction and the pacemaking activity of the sinus node, and hence, is contraindicated in the sick sinus syndrome.

○ **What is the treatment of choice in a first trimester patient with acute mania?**

The treatment of choice for mania in the first trimester is electroconvulsive therapy (ECT) or neuroleptics. Mood stabilizers may be given after the first trimester. Neural tube malformations and Epstein's anomaly are teratogenic side effects of anticonvulsants and lithium, respectively.

○ **How would you evaluate the fetus of a woman who was treated with lithium during her first trimester and what would you be looking for?**

Epstein's anomaly is a serious cardiac birth defect that occurs in 0.1% to 0.7% of fetuses exposed to lithium during the first trimester (20 times higher than the occurrence of this anomaly in the general population). Echocardiography after the 16th week of pregnancy can be done to evaluate the fetus for this defect. Overall, the risk of major birth defects following exposure to lithium is two to three times that of the normal population.

○ **What fetal defects can be seen if the mother is taking valproate during her first trimester and what substance can be given to help prevent this?**

Various neural tube defects such as spina bifida and anencephaly can occur if the fetus is exposed to valproate during the first trimester. Administration of folate, 1 mg/d, may help diminish the risk. Ultrasound at 18 to 20 weeks will detect the neural tube abnormalities.

○ **When should the dose of an antidepressant be tapered or terminated in the treatment of depressive episodes of bipolar disorder?**

Once euthymia is established, an antidepressant should be slowly tapered. If mania or hypomania occurs, the antidepressant should be immediately discontinued.

○ **How are monoamine oxidase inhibitors (MAOIs) used in the treatment of bipolar disorder?**

MAOIs can be very effective in the treatment of depressive episodes associated with rapid cycling, as well as the depressive episodes of bipolar I and II disorders. Phenelzine, in particular, has been shown to be effective at low doses when combined with a mood stabilizer.

○ **Which other agents are useful in the treatment of bipolar disorder?**

Used in conjunction with mood stabilizers, bupropion and triiodothyronine (T3) are considered the first-line agents for the treatment of depressive episodes associated with bipolar disorder. Selective serotonin reuptake inhibitors (SSRIs), serotonin norepinephrine reuptake inhibitors (SNRIs), and tricyclics may be used at low starting doses and with careful titration, but must be promptly discontinued if signs of mania appear.

○ **What is the indication for the use of lamotrigine (Lamictal®) in bipolar disorder?**

Lamotrigine is an anticonvulsant that can be useful in the treatment of the depressive symptoms of bipolar disorder. Lamotrigine inhibits the presynaptic secretion of glutamate, an excitatory amino acid, and may have significant antidepressant activities, unlike the other anticonvulsants used in the treatment of bipolar disorder.

○ **What complications does one encounter when using lithium to treat elderly individuals with mania?**

The use of lithium in elderly patients is complicated because of the increased incidence of concurrent neurologic disorders and a higher frequency of secondary mania, conditions that respond poorly to lithium. Additionally, increasing age is associated with poor response to lithium. The adverse effects of lithium are also more common, and occur at lower lithium levels than in younger populations. Finally, older patients are likely to be taking other drugs that may interact adversely with lithium.

○ **What side effect of carbamazepine is more likely to cause more difficulties in elderly individuals than in young adults?**

Hyponatremia associated with carbamazepine use is more likely to cause problems in the elderly.

○ **What comorbid conditions associated with bipolar disorder also respond to valproic acid?**

Migraine headaches and panic disorder are comorbid conditions that occur with bipolar disorder and respond to valproic acid.

○ **Patients who respond to antidepressant medications do so by what week of treatment?**

Patients who are going to respond to a given antidepressant do so by the 6th week of treatment. The full response to an antidepressant, euthymia, is most often achieved by the 12th week of treatment.

○ **What percentage of depressed patients fail to respond to an initial trial of antidepressant medication?**

Thirty percent of depressed patients fail initial treatment with antidepressants.

○   **What antidepressants are available in parenteral or liquid form?**

Amitriptyline and imipramine are the only antidepressants available in parenteral form. Doxepin, nortriptyline, fluoxetine, paroxetine, and citalopram are available in liquid formulations.

○   **What antidepressant should be avoided in Parkinson's disease?**

Amoxapine should be avoided in patients with Parkinson's disease, as it has significant dopamine-blocking activity. Consequently, it should also be avoided in patients who have a history of tardive dyskinesia.

○   **What are the advantages and disadvantages of selective serotonin reuptake inhibitors (SSRIs) as compared to TCAs?**

The advantages of SSRIs as compared to TCAs include minimal anticholinergic activity, no α-adrenergic antagonism, no antihistamine activity, very low effects on the cardiovascular system (pulse, blood pressure, and cardiac conduction), and low levels of sedation. The disadvantages of the SSRIs, not associated as frequently with TCAs, include a higher incidence of sexual dysfunctional, diarrhea, nausea, insomnia, headache, tremor, and nervousness.

○   **Fluvoxamine (Luvox®) and nefazodone (Serzone®) inhibit the cytochrome P-450 3A4-isoenzyme system that metabolizes terfenadine (Seldane®) and astemizole (Hismanal®). Why is this important clinically?**

This is clinically important because inhibition of the metabolism of these antihistamines leads to elevated serum levels of these drugs, which can cause fatal arrhythmias. Ketoconazole and erythromycin also inhibit the cytochrome P-450 3A4-isoenzyme system and should not be used with these antihistamines.

○   **Why is the combination of fluoxetine and metoprolol problematic?**

Because fluoxetine inhibits the hepatic isoenzyme, CYP 2D6 (which metabolizes metoprolol), resulting in elevated levels of metoprolol and corresponding symptoms of adrenergic toxicity. Blood levels of other CYP 2D6 substrates, such as amphetamines, flecainamide, vinblastine (to name a few) can also become elevated when administered with SSRIs in general.

○   **What are the symptoms of the central serotonin syndrome?**

The symptoms of the central serotonin syndrome include mental status changes, agitation, myoclonus, hyperreflexia, tremor, incoordination, headache, diaphoresis, hyperthermia, nausea, diarrhea, tachycardia, autonomic instability, cardiovascular collapse, and rarely, death. It is thought to be caused by excessive secretion of serotonin from 5-HT$_{1A}$ receptors in the brain stem and spinal cord. It is commonly precipitated by drug–drug interactions between MAOIs and SSRIs/TCAs, but can occur between SSRIs and heterocyclic antidepressants and meperidine (Demerol®), triptans or dextromethophan (OTC cough medications). Specifically, the combination of any SSRI, SNRI, or clomipramine (serotonergic medications) with any MAOI can cause this syndrome, and is the reason for a mandatory 1 week washout when changing from an SSRI (5 weeks for fluoxetine) to an MAOI.

○   **Of the four SSRIs, fluoxetine, sertraline, paroxetine, and fluvoxamine, which can cause clinically significant muscarinic receptor blockage (although not nearly as severe as the TCAs)?**

Paroxetine has a relatively high affinity for the muscarinic receptor, thereby causing some antimuscarinic effects such as dry mouth and constipation.

○ **Blockade of what two receptors can cause hypotension?**

Blockade of both histamine and α-adrenergic receptors can result in hypotension.

○ **What antidepressants can be safely administered to a patient with narrow-angle glaucoma?**

Venlafaxine, nefazodone, trazodone, and bupropion are first-line agents for the treatment of depression in patients with closed-angle glaucoma because other antidepressants have significant anticholinergic activity that can exacerbate this condition. These agents would also be a good choice in patients with chronic constipation.

○ **In a patient with a seizure disorder, what antidepressants should be avoided, if possible?**

Amoxapine, maprotiline, bupropion, and trimipramine would be the least desirable antidepressants to use in a patient with a seizure disorder because they all lower the seizure threshold. Clomipramine also lowers the seizure threshold.

○ **What are three deleterious side effects of amoxapine that often preclude its use?**

1. The high risk of seizure.

2. High rate of mortality in overdose.

3. Risk of tardive dyskinesia (its demethylated metabolite is loxapine) are serious side effects of amoxapine.

○ **What is the recommended starting dose of heterocyclic antidepressants such as imipramine or nortriptyline when used in the treatment of panic disorder?**

The recommended starting dose of imipramine or nortriptyline in panic disorder is much lower than in the treatment of depression. This is because an amphetamine-like side effect commonly occurs that can increase anxiety in individuals with panic disorder, leading to discontinuation of the medication. The recommended starting dose is 10 mg/d, with slow titration until a therapeutic response is achieved. Addition of benzodiazepines and/or β-blockers may decrease the overstimulative effect. A therapeutic response may take up to 12 weeks.

○ **What properties of venlafaxine (Effexor®) make it different from other antidepressants?**

Venlafaxine causes downregulation of β-adrenergic receptors faster than any other antidepressant, possibly explaining its faster onset of action. It is also more weakly protein bound (27%) than other antidepressants, thereby decreasing the risk of displacing tightly bound drugs from protein binding and causing drug–drug interactions.

○ **The side-effect profile of venlafaxine is most consistent with what other class of drugs?**

The side effects of venlafaxine are most like those of the SSRIs.

○ **What is one adverse side effect of venlafaxine that is different from all other antidepressants?**

Venlafaxine can cause an elevation of diastolic blood pressure in 5% of patients at doses less than 200 mg/d and in 13% of patients at doses greater than 300 mg/d.

○ **If venlafaxine is to be discontinued, what is the recommended approach?**

If a patient has been on venlafaxine for 7 or more days, it should be tapered over 2 to 3 days. If treatment has been for more than 2 weeks, a gradual taper over a 2-week period is recommended.

○ **What is the unique mechanism of action of the antidepressant mirtazepine (Remeron®)?**

Mirtazepine is a central presynaptic α-receptor antagonist. Its action is that of an indirect agonist of norepinephrine, although it also blockades $5HT_2$ and $5HT_3$ receptors.

○ **What antidepressants are $5HT_2$ antagonists?**

Trazodone and nefazodone are $5HT_2$ antagonists. Nefazodone is the more potent of the two.

○ **What effect does nefazodone (Serzone) have on sleep?**

Nefazodone increases REM sleep.

○ **Why is there a serious risk for cardiac arrhythmias when nefazodone is used in combination with what two drugs?**

Nefazodone may pose a risk for arrhythmias when given to a patient on terfenadine (Seldane) or astemizole (Hismanal) as a result of toxic accumulation of the latter two drugs caused by nefazadone's inhibition of the cytochrome P-450 3A3/4-isoenzyme system. Loratadine (Claritin) appears to be the safest allergy medication to give to patients on nefazodone, although it too is metabolized by the 3A3/4-isoenzyme system (but is less toxic).

○ **What electrocardiogram finding is a contraindication to increasing the dose of a heterocyclic antidepressant, no matter what the blood level is? And what is the clinical relevance?**

A widening QRS interval. An increasing QRS interval reflects prolonged electrical conduction, and if it exceeds 100 ms, heart block, ventricular arrhythmias, and sudden death can occur. The ECG is of solid clinical value in monitoring direct cardiotoxicity, more so than blood levels.

○ **In what order can an MAOI and a TCA be safely added together?**

Both an MAOI and TCA can be started at the same time, at a low dosage, and the MAOI can be added to an established TCA regimen. Adding a TCA to a MAOI is contraindicated, because of the risk of precipitating the serotonin syndrome.

○ **What two TCAs combine best with MAOIs?**

Amitriptyline and trimipramine are the best TCAs to use in combination with MAOIs.

○ **Describe the action of selegiline (Eldepryl®) and what patient population it is used in.**

Selegiline is a MAO-reversible inhibitor that preferentially inhibits MAO-B. It has a low incidence of hypertensive crisis and is used in the treatment of Parkinson's disease. If the usual dose of 5 to 10 mg/d is increased, antidepressant activity is noted, but the drug loses its MAO-B specificity and becomes a MAO-A and MAO-B inhibitor, and the risk of hypertensive crisis returns.

○ **What class of drugs is beneficial in the treatment of premenstrual dysphoria?**

The SSRIs have shown effectiveness in premenstrual dysphoria and irritability.

○ **What problem is associated with the use of SSRIs in the treatment of post-LSD depression?**

SSRIs can produce recurrent flashbacks.

○ **What are the guidelines and recommendations for use of methylphenidate in the elderly?**

Apathetic, isolated, resigned to death, and disinterested elderly who are not having a major depressive episode, may respond to methylphenidate. Effects include improved energy, motivation, and a desire to again participate in life. Psychostimulants, in general, should not be used for the treatment of major depression, since they do not have antidepressant effects.

○ **What are the four components of bright light therapy?**

1. Intensity
2. Timing
3. Duration
4. Wavelength

○ **What light intensity is necessary for melatonin suppression?**

Light intensity greater than 2000 lux is necessary for melatonin suppression in most people.

○ **What is the recommended use of a bright light box in seasonal affective disorder (SAD)?**

Exposure to the eyes of diffuse visible light with an intensity of at least 2500 lux daily, preferably in the morning, for at least 2 hours, is the recommended use of bright light for the treatment of SAD. Most bright light boxes produce 2500 lux at a distance of 3 ft, and as light intensity is inversely related to the square root of the distance of the eyes to the light source, using the 2500 lux box at 1.5 ft from the eyes produces 10,000 lux, and the duration of treatment can be reduced, as 30 minutes at 10,000 Lux is equivalent to 2 hours at 2500 lux. Standard cool fluorescent tubes with minimal UV are effective and, in fact, avoiding UV is much preferred.

○ **How long it takes before a response to bright light is effective?**

Response to bright light therapy usually begins within 3 to 4 days, with full response in 1 to 2 weeks. When light therapy is stopped, relapse can occur in 3 to 4 days. In susceptible individuals, the use of bright light therapy has been associated with induction of mania.

○ **Which benzodiazepines are metabolized by glucuronidation?**

Lorazepam, oxazepam, and temazepam are metabolized by glucuronidation. The other benzodiazepines are metabolized by oxidation and, therefore, are more dependent on adequate hepatic function and have more drug–drug interactions.

○ **What effect do the benzodiazepines have on sleep?**

The overall effect of benzodiazepines is to increase total sleep time. Sleep latency and the number of nighttime awakenings are decreased. The effect on sleep architecture is to decrease the duration of stages 1, 3, and 4, and REM sleep, while increasing the duration of stage 2 sleep. The number of REM cycles increase, but the time in REM is actually decreased.

○ **What advantages does zolpidem (Ambien®) have over benzodiazepines?**

The advantages of zolpidem when compared to the benzodiazepines are a lack of tolerance, the absence of a withdrawal syndrome, and no REM rebound upon discontinuation. Conversely, the amnestic effect of zolpidem has been associated with adverse outcomes, such as driving a car while "under the influence" and being unable to recall getting into the vehicle.

○   **When is diphenhydramine used for sleep, and what is the recommended dose?**

Diphenhydramine, at a dose of 50 mg improves sleep in 60% to 70% of psychiatric patients. Doses greater than 50 mg do not increase sleep, but may increase delirium through anticholinergic action, especially in the elderly.

○   **What is yohimbine and what use it has in psychiatric medicine?**

Yohimbine is an $\alpha_2\alpha$-adrenergic presynaptic antagonist. It is most frequently used to counteract the sexual dysfunction caused by psychotropic medications, especially SSRIs. It is available in 5.4-mg doses, and one to two tablets are administered 2 hours before intercourse or on a regular schedule of one to four tablets daily. Severe side effects however limit its use, and the phosphodiesterase type 5 inhibitors have largely replaced it as treatment for sexual dysfunction.

CHAPTER 35 Psychopharmacology II

○ **What is the prevalence of poor 2D6 isoenzyme metabolizers?**

Approximately 7% to 10% of Caucasians are considered poor 2D6 metabolizers, compared to 1% to 2% of Asians and blacks, depending on the reference. The rate of substrate metabolism is related to the type and number of cytochrome P-450 2D6 alleles that have been inherited.

○ **Which drugs can be used to augment the antidepressant effect of selective serotonin reuptake inhibitors (SSRIs)?**

Buspirone, clomipramine, lithium, anxiolytics, antipsychotics, and stimulants.

○ **Which SSRIs are least likely to cause drug interactions through their effect on the P-450 system?**

Citalopram and sertraline.

○ **Name the main active metabolites of the following SSRIs and give their half-lives.**

SSRI	Active Metabolite/Parent Half-Life	Half-Life of Metabolite
Citalopram	<10% parent compound/35 h	—
Fluoxetine	Norfluoxetine/48–72 h	4–16 d
Fluvoxamine	None/15 h	—
Paroxetine	None/21 h	—
Sertraline	desmethyl-sertraline/26 h	2–4 d

○   **List common drugs and other substances that are inhibitors, substrates, and inducers for each of the main P-450 isoenzyme systems**

P-450 System	Inhibitors	Substrates Psychotropic Drugs	Other Drugs	Inducers
1A2	fluvoxamine theophylline grapefruit juice	clozapine TCAs tacrine duloxetine	propranolol theophylline warfarin caffeine	phenytoin
2C	fluoxetine fluvoxamine Sertraline	diazepam	phenytoin warfarin tolbutamide NSAIDs	
2C19	fluoxetine sertraline fluvoxamine omeprazole	citalopram diazepam clomipramine	propranolol omeprazole	phenytoin
2D6	fluoxetine paroxetine fluvoxamine sertraline duloxetine secondary TCAs moclobemide antipsychotics quinidine diltiazem vincristine labetalol (fluoxetine and paroxetine are more potent)	tricyclics antipsychotics opiates SSRIs venlafaxine duloxetine donepezil	type 1C antiarrhythmics (e.g., encainide) beta blockers	piperidines
3A3/4	fluoxetine paroxetine fluvoxamine sertraline nefazodone cisapride cimetidine ketoconazole astemizole erythromycin grapefruit juice (fluoxetine and nefazodone are the most potent)	carbamazepine benzodiazepines (especially alprazolam, midazolam, triazolam) zolpidem nefazodone sertraline venlafaxine donepezil	terfenadine astemizole loratadine, cisapride antiarrhythmics calcium channel blockers steroids carbamazepine (elevated levels of terfenadine, astemizole, or cisapride can cause QT prolongation and cardiac arrhythmias) erythromycin	carbamazepine phenytoin St. John's Wort

○ **What are the adverse effects associated with the SSRIs?**

Commonly reported side effects include anxiety, insomnia, gastrointestinal symptoms (nausea, diarrhea), headache, decreased appetite, and sexual dysfunction. Less commonly reported side effects include tremor, other extrapyramidal symptoms, lethargy, sweating, and fatigue. An increased incidence of suicidal ideation after initiation and/or increase in dose has warranted a black box warning for SSRIs as well as for all other antidepressants. Induction of manic symptoms is a risk for all antidepressants, including SSRIs. The SSRIs also have a significant risk for serotonin syndrome when combined with other SSRIs, SNRIs, triptans (5-hydroxytryptamine receptors agonists), tryptophan, MAOIs, and dextromethorphan. Laboratory findings associated with SSRI use include hyponatremia (particularly in the elderly), increased cholesterol, and a prolonged bleeding time (especially when coadministered with warfarin). SSRIs should be used with caution in individuals with a history of narrow angle glaucoma. Finally, abrupt discontinuation of SSRIs can result in a discontinuation syndrome characterized by increased irritability, insomnia, anxiety, gastrointestinal symptoms, paresthesias, headache, and dizziness.

○ **Which of the SSRIs has significant anticholinergic effects?**

Paroxetine (which is also the most potent 2D6 isoenzyme inhibitor).

○ **Use of which psychotropic drugs requires regular monitoring of LFTs?**

Tacrine (Cognex®), valproate, disulfiram, naltrexone, carbamazepine, pemoline, and monoamine oxidase inhibitors (MAOIs). Mnemonic: **T**hese **V**ery **D**rugs **N**eed **C**areful **P**eriodic **M**onitoring.

○ **What is the mechanism of action of venlafaxine (Effexor®)?**

It is an inhibitor of the reuptake of both serotonin and norepinephrine.

○ **What are the adverse effects associated with venlafaxine?**

In addition to the aforementioned side effects of SSRIs, venlafaxine is also associated with an increased risk for hypertension and seizures.

○ **How are Effexor® and Pristiq® related?**

Pristiq® (or desvenlafaxine) is the active metabolite of Effexor® (or venlafaxine), which is packaged in an "inert matrix" to achieve an extended release pattern for once-a-day dosing. The shell is excreted unchanged and may occasionally be noted by patients in the stool after toileting.

○ **What are the pharmacodynamic effects of mirtazapine (Remeron®)?**

Mirtazapine is an alpha-2 blocker that is relatively selective for central and presynaptic alpha-2 receptors. On the noradrenergic neurons, this blockade potentiates norepinephrine release. Mirtazapine does <u>not</u> inhibit the reuptake of norepinephrine. On serotonergic neurons, the alpha-2 blockade potentiates 5-HT neurotransmission. Other effects include those of 5-HT$_{1A}$ agonist, 5-HT$_2$ and 5-HT$_3$ blockade, and H$_1$ blockade (may explain the sedation, increased appetite, or weight gain that may be associated with it).

Moderate peripheral alpha-1 blockade may explain the orthostatic hypotension associated with its use, while moderate muscarinic blockade may explain the dry mouth/constipation that is an associated side effect.

○ **What are the clinically significant active metabolites of mirtazapine?**

None.

○   **What are the clinically significant effects of mirtazapine on the P-450 system?**

None.

○   **What is a potential serious adverse effect of mirtazapine?**

Severe neutropenia/agranulocytosis in 1 of 1,000 patients treated.

○   **What are the other potential adverse effects of mirtazapine?**

Elevated cholesterol/triglycerides and elevated liver enzymes.

○   **What are the pharmacodynamic effects of nefazodone (Serzone®)?**

Nefazodone is a $5\text{-}HT_2$ blocker that weakly inhibits serotonin reuptake. Together, these effects probably lead to sensitization of $5\text{-}HT_{1A}$ receptors. Its metabolite, m-chlorophenylpiperazine (mCPP), is a $5\text{-}HT_{2c}$ agonist.

○   **What are the advantages of nefazodone over trazodone?**

Lack of alpha (orthostatic hypotension) or histamine (sedation) receptor blockade.

○   **What is the mechanism of action of bupropion (Wellbutrin®)?**

Not clearly known, probably due to its noradrenergic effects. Bupropion does have dopaminergic activity, but contrary to prior belief, this probably does not account for the antidepressant effect.

○   **What are the contraindications to the use of bupropion?**

A history of seizure disorder, head trauma, CNS tumors, or other brain diseases; EEG abnormalities; recent withdrawal from benzodiazepines/alcohol; eating disorders; and current use of other medications which may lower the seizure threshold (e.g., antipsychotics, lithium).

○   **What is the incidence of seizures in patients taking bupropion?**

At doses less than 450 mg/d, 0.4%. At doses 450 to 600 mg/d, 2%. The risk for seizures in bupropion overdoses is particularly high.

○   **Which antidepressants have a relatively higher incidence of seizures associated with them?**

Bupropion, clomipramine, venlafaxine, imipramine, and maprotiline.

○   **Which antidepressant has a well-established therapeutic window?**

Nortriptyline: 50 to 150 ng/mL.

○   **What is the role of EKG monitoring in tricyclic/tetracyclic use?**

An EKG should be monitored periodically due to risk of cardiac conduction slowing. Consider decreasing the dose or stopping the drug if the PR interval is greater than 0.2 seconds or the QRS interval is greater than 0.12 seconds.

○   **What is the incidence of seizures in patients taking imipramine?**

It is 0.1% to 1% depending on the dose.

○ **Which of the tricyclics/tetracyclics is the most selective for inhibition of serotonin reuptake?**

Clomipramine.

○ **Which antidepressant is the most selective for the inhibition of norepinephrine reuptake?**

Maprotiline, while desipramine is second.

○ **Which tricyclic is the most antihistaminergic?**

Doxepin, which is quite sedating and can also be used for treatment of peptic ulcers (blockade of H_2 receptors).

○ **Which adverse effect is especially common with maprotiline?**

Seizures.

○ **Name the specific inhibitors of MAO-A and MAO-B.**

MAO-A: clorgyline. MAO-B: selegiline (Eldepryl®; used for parkinsonism).

○ **What are the common adverse effects associated with MAOIs?**

Mnemonic: **O**(h), **B**(e) **WISE**.
Orthostatic hypotension, Behavioral activation, Weight gain, Insomnia, Sexual dysfunction, and Edema.

○ **Which drugs can be used to treat a hypertensive crisis associated with MAOIs?**

Mnemonic: **No Cheese P**lease. Nifedipine, chlorpromazine, phentolamine. Note that all three lower blood pressure.

○ **Name the foods that have a very high tyramine content.**

Mnemonic: A-B-C-D-E-F and 4Ps.
Alcohol (especially beer and wine), Beef or chicken liver, Cheese (aged), Dry sausage, Extracts of meat, Fava or broad beans, Pickled or smoked fish/poultry/meats, Packaged soups, Pulp of oranges, and Pills (yeast-based vitamin pills).

○ **Which medications should never be used along with MAOIs?**

Anesthetics containing epinephrine, antiasthmatics, antihypertensives, diuretics, L-dopa, L-tryptophan, SSRIs, SNRIs, clomipramine, narcotics (especially meperidine and fentanyl, which have had fatal interactions with MAOIs), OTC cold/hay fever/sinus medications (especially those containing dextromethorphan), and sympathomimetics.

○ **What are the indications for amantadine in psychiatry?**

Neuroleptic-induced movement disorders and SSRI-induced sexual dysfunction.

○ **What are the contraindications to the use of amantadine?**

Renal disease, cardiovascular disease, epilepsy, and concurrent use of stimulants or anticholinergics.

○ **How should serious anticholinergic toxicity be treated?**

With intravenous physostigmine—a cholinergic drug that acts by inhibiting cholinesterase, which breaks down acetylcholine.

○ **What is the mechanism of action of clonidine?**

Alpha-2 adrenergic receptor agonist. Agonist effects at these receptors, which are located presynaptically, on adrenergic neurons, reduce the release of epinephrine from these neurons.

○ **What are the first-line indications for clonidine in psychiatry?**

Opioid withdrawal and Tourette's disorder (there are several other second-line uses).

○ **Why is it particularly important to taper clonidine carefully?**

Severe rebound hypertension can occur.

○ **What are the pharmacological effects of trazodone?**

Selective inhibition of serotonin reuptake, blockade of alpha-1 and alpha-2 receptors, blockade of histamine receptors, and (through its active metabolite, *m*-chlorophenylpiperazine) agonism at postsynaptic 5-HT$_{2c}$ receptors.

○ **What are the effects of trazodone on sleep?**

Trazodone increases total sleep time, decreases the number/duration of awakenings, and decreases the amount of REM sleep.

○ **Which benzodiazepine is metabolized in the gut prior to absorption?**

Clorazepate is metabolized to desmethyldiazepam in the gut and then absorbed.

○ **Which benzodiazepines are highly lipid soluble and therefore have quick absorption, quick transport into the brain, and thus, a quick onset of action?**

Diazepam, lorazepam, alprazolam, triazolam, and estazolam.

○ **Which benzodiazepines have no active metabolites?**

Lorazepam, oxazepam, temazepam. These belong to the same chemical subclass (mnemonic: L.O.T.) and are directly metabolized by glucuronidation.

○ **Which benzodiazepine has the shortest half-life?**

Overall, midazolam. Of the benzodiazepines administered by mouth, triazolam (2–3 hours).

○ **Which symptoms tend to denote a true benzodiazepine withdrawal rather than a return/exacerbation of the original anxiety?**

Observable depression, nausea, loss of appetite, depersonalization, derealization and increased sensory perception, abnormal perception or sensation of movement, and autonomic instability. Overall benzodiazepine withdrawal is essentially the same as alcohol withdrawal and is treated in the same way.

○ **What are the pharmacodynamic effects of zolpidem?**

Zolpidem acts on benzodiazepine receptors (affinity is higher for BZ_1 receptors than for BZ_2 and also higher for CNS receptors than for peripheral).

○ **What are the potential adverse effects of zolpidem?**

Mnemonic: 3D's. **D**rowsiness, **D**iarrhea, **D**izziness. Zolpidem is also known for its amnestic effects.

○ **What are the advantages and disadvantages of chloral hydrate as a hypnotic?**

Advantages—lack of rebound of REM sleep.

Disadvantages—high lethality (lethal dose is only about 5–20 times the therapeutic dose), tolerance to the hypnotic effects within 2 to 3 weeks, and significant gastrointestinal irritation.

○ **Name two potential drug interactions when using chloral hydrate.**

- With furosemide: autonomic instability.
- With anticoagulants: ↑ effect of warfarin, ↓ effect of dicumarol.

○ **What is the mechanism of action of buspirone (Buspar®)?**

Agonist/partial agonist at the serotonin type -1_A receptors.

○ **What are the indications for buspirone?**

Anxiety disorders (especially generalized anxiety disorder), anxiety/aggression in developmentally disabled persons, emotional/behavioral problems in brain-injured persons, emotional/behavioral problems in elderly patients, and augmentation of fluoxetine treatment of depression/OCD.

○ **What are the major indications for beta blockers in psychiatry?**

Neuroleptic-induced akathisia, social phobia, aggression in schizophrenia or mental disorders due to general medical conditions, adjuvant to benzodiazepines for alcohol withdrawal, and lithium-induced tremors.

○ **What are the first-line indications for bromocriptine in psychiatry?**

Neuroleptic malignant syndrome, antipsychotic-induced galactorrhea, and cocaine withdrawal (controversial).

○ **Name the most important metabolite of carbamazepine and describe its therapeutic activity.**

The 10-, 11-epoxide metabolite has antiepileptic effects but its effect in bipolar disorder is not known.

○ **What are the relatively well-established indications for use of carbamazepine in psychiatry?**

Bipolar disorder, depressive disorders, impulse-control disorders, nonacute agitation/aggressive behavior in schizophrenia (though lorazepam is more effective for acute agitation), schizoaffective disorder, and alcohol withdrawal (prevents seizures, but not withdrawal).

○ **What laboratory tests should be performed before starting treatment with carbamazepine?**

CBC with platelet count, LFTs, serum sodium, EKG (in patients over 40 years of age or with preexisting cardiac disease).

○ **What are the serious adverse effects that may occur with carbamazepine?**

Blood dyscrasias (aplastic anemia, agranulocytosis), hepatitis, hyponatremia, cardiac conduction defects, toxic epidermal necrolysis, and Stevens-Johnson syndrome.

○ **What is the risk for developing toxic epidermal necrolysis or Stevens Johnson Syndrome in patients treated with carbamazepine?**

The risk for toxic epidermal necrolysis or Stevens Johnson Syndrome is dependent on ethnicity and associated with the presence of the HLA-B allele, HLA-B* 1502. In Caucasian, the risk runs from 1 to 6 per 10,000, but in Asians the risk is much higher at approximately 10 to 60 per 10,000.

○ **What is the incidence of severe blood dyscrasias (aplastic anemia, agranulocytosis) with carbamazepine treatment?**

Aplastic anemia occurs in approximately 1 out of 125,000 patients treated with carbamazepine, while agranulocytosis occurs at a rate of 3 to 4 per 100,000 patients. Mild thrombocytopenia and leukopenia are much more common, and while these need to be monitored, generally, are not life-threatening and do not require discontinuation of carbamazepine.

○ **What is the teratogenicity of carbamazepine?**

Neural tube defects (e.g., spina bifida) in 0.5% to 1% of babies exposed to carbamazepine.

○ **How do the side effect profiles of lithium and carbamazepine compare?**

In regard to adverse effects, the action of one drug tends to be opposite of the other (e.g., carbamazepine causes leukopenia while lithium causes leucocytosis; lithium causes diabetes insipidus while carbamazepine causes SIADH). However, both drugs tend to cause hypothyroidism and can be teratogenic.

○ **What is the mechanism of action of lithium?**

Unknown. Possible mechanisms of action include alteration of cation transport, inhibition of the enzyme inositol monophosphatase (one of the enzymes involved in second messenger systems), alteration of gene expression, and modulation of cytoskeletal structure to name a few.

○ **What are the psychiatric indications for the use of lithium?**

Bipolar disorder, depressive disorders (alone or to augment other antidepressants), schizophrenia, and schizoaffective disorder. Other disorders with intermittent-type of behaviors such as impulse-control disorders, premenstrual dysphoric disorder, binge drinking, bulimia nervosa, borderline personality, and aggressive/self-injurious behavior in children with other disorders may also respond to therapeutic doses of lithium.

○ **What laboratory tests should be done prior to starting lithium?**

Serum creatinine, serum electrolytes, thyroid function tests, CBC, EKG, and a pregnancy test (if there is any possibility of pregnancy).

○ **What is the incidence of hypothyroidism with long term use of lithium?**

Abnormal TRH response 50%, elevated TSH 30%, clinical hypothyroidism 5%, and goiter 3%.

○ **What is the treatment of lithium-induced tremors?**

Administer the lithium in smaller, more frequent doses. Propranolol, 30 to 160 mg/d, may also be helpful.

○ **How should lithium-induced diabetes insipidus be treated?**

Thiazide diuretics or amilorides are used to ameliorate lithium-induced diabetes insipidus. Remember that diuretics increase lithium levels and so significant dose reduction is necessary to prevent lithium toxicity. Vasopressin (ADH) has no benefit since diabetes insipidus is caused by resistance of the kidney to the effects of vasopressin.

○ **Which fetal malformation may be caused by the use of lithium during pregnancy?**

Ebstein's anomaly (congenital displacement of the tricuspid valve into the right ventricle leading to tricuspid regurgitation). The risk is about 0.1% (lower than was previously thought) of babies exposed to lithium in the first trimester.

○ **What drug interactions are possible with lithium?**

Increased lithium levels occur in combination with:

- Thiazides, loop diuretics (mnemonic: FEB = **F**urosemide, **E**thacrynic acid, **B**umetanide)
- Potassium-sparing diuretics (mnemonic: SAT = **S**pironolactone, **A**miloride, **T**riamterene)
- NSAIDs, ACE inhibitors, and metronidazole

Decreased lithium levels occur in combination with:

- Osmotic diuretics (mannitol, urea)
- Carbonic anhydrase inhibitors (acetazolamide)
- Xanthines (theophylline, coffee)

Increased adverse effects occur when coadministered with:

- Antipsychotics (neurotoxicity)
- Anticonvulsants (neurotoxicity)
- ECT (delirium)
- SSRIs (serotonin syndrome)

○ **How should lithium overdose be treated?**

1. Discontinue lithium.
2. Remove the unabsorbed lithium from the gastrointestinal tract through emesis and/or gastric lavage (*note*: activated charcoal may **not** help).
3. Aid the excretion of lithium by the kidney by vigorous hydration, osmotic diuretics, and IV sodium bicarbonate (in alkaline urine, lithium will ionize and will not be reabsorbed in the renal tubules).
4. Remove lithium from the blood directly through peritoneal dialysis, hemodialysis (for serious symptoms of toxicity or serum lithium >4 mEq/L within 6 hours of the overdose).

○ **What is the recommended dosage of lamotrigine for the treatment of bipolar disorder?**

It is 50 to 400 mg/d.

○ **What are the potential adverse effects associated with lamotrigine?**

Headache, nausea, dizziness, ataxia, diplopia, blurred vision, and skin rash. Toxic epidermal necrolysis is the most serious adverse effect.

○ **What potential drug interactions may occur if lamotrigine is administered together with other anticonvulsants?**

Combination of lamotrigine with valproate results in markedly elevated levels of lamotrigine, while combination with carbamazepine results in elevated levels of the carbamazepine 10, 11-epoxide metabolite.

○ **What is the mechanism of action of valproate?**

In seizure disorder, it probably acts by decreasing the breakdown of GABA, the major inhibitory neurotransmitter. Mechanism of action in bipolar disorder is unknown.

○ **What are the *most* common adverse effects of valproate?**

Nausea, vomiting, diarrhea, sedation, tremor, weight gain, tremor, transiently elevated liver enzymes, and hair loss.

○ **What are the risk factors for valproate-induced hepatotoxicity?**

Risk factors for hepatotoxicity include young age (less than 10 years old), sensitivity during the first few months of treatment, severe epilepsy, and use of multiple drugs.

○ **What is the incidence of fatal hepatotoxicity with valproate?**

In those taking valproate alone, 1 in 100,000 patients.

○ **What is the teratogenicity of valproate?**

Neural tube defects, including spina bifida, occur in 3% to 5% of babies of mothers who took valproate in the first trimester.

○ **What are the drug interactions associated with valproate?**

- With other anticonvulsants: complex and variable.
- With CNS depressants: increased CNS depression.
- With antipsychotics: increased sedation and increased severity of extrapyramidal adverse effects.
- With aspirin/warfarin: increased anticoagulation.
- With fluoxetine: increased valproate levels.

  Results of laboratory studies: false positive results for urine ketones and abnormal TFTs.

○ **What are the pharmacodynamic effects of clozapine?**

1. Antidopaminergic activity: anti-D_1 effect much greater than anti-D_2; also blocks D_4; more effective in blocking dopaminergic activity in the cortical and limbic dopamine neurons than those in the basal ganglia.

2. Effects other than the antidopaminergic activity include antiserotonergic (anti-$5HT_2$), anticholinergic (antimuscarinic), antihistaminergic (anti H_1), and antiadrenergic (anti-alpha$_1$, anti-alpha$_2$) effects.

○ **What are the indications for clozapine?**

Indications for the use of clozapine in the treatment of schizophrenia and other psychotic disorders include treatment resistance, inability to tolerate extrapyramidal side effects of conventional antipsychotics, and the predominance of negative symptoms. Clozapine is also indicated for the treatment of L-dopa–induced psychosis in patients with Parkinson's disease and treatment-resistant bipolar disorder.

○ **What laboratory tests should be done prior to starting clozapine?**

Multiple CBCs (the WBC counts should be averaged), LFTs, renal function tests, and an EKG.

○ **What are the potential adverse effects associated with clozapine?**

- *H_1 receptor blockade*: sedation, weight gain.
- *Anticholinergic effects*: constipation.
- *Alpha-1 blockade*: orthostatic hypotension.
- *Others*: agranulocytosis, elevated liver enzymes, seizures, sialorrhea.

   Note: Hyperprolactinemia is notably <u>absent</u>.

○ **What is the incidence of agranulocytosis with clozapine?**

It is 1% to 2%.

○ **What are the guidelines for the management of leukopenia due to clozapine?**

If the WBC count is less than 3,500/cmm or the granulocyte count is less than 1,500/cmm, clozapine should be stopped and consultation with a hematologist should be requested. If the WBC count is less than 1,000/cmm, the patient should be placed in reverse isolation.

○ **What is the therapeutic blood level of clozapine?**

Blood levels above 350 ng/mL are believed to be correlated with therapeutic response.

○ **What is the incidence of seizures with clozapine?**

- Dose less than 300 mg/d: 1% to 2%.
- Dose 300 to 600 mg/d: 3% to 4%.
- Dose more than 600 mg/d: 5%.

○ **How should seizures induced by clozapine be treated?**

Stop clozapine, start phenobarbital or valproate, and then restart clozapine at about half the previous dose and titrate up cautiously.

○ **What are some drug interactions that can occur with clozapine?**

- With fluoxetine: ↑ clozapine levels.
- With lithium: ↑ movement disorders, ↑ neuroleptic syndrome, ↑ confusion, ↑ seizures.
- With benzodiazepines: ↑ orthostasis, syncope, respiratory suppression.
- With carbamazepine (and other drugs that may suppress the bone marrow): ↑ agranulocytosis.

○ **What is the receptor binding profile for olanzapine (Zyprexa®)?**

Blockade of 5-HT$_2$, and D$_1$ to D$_4$ receptors. Antagonism of alpha-1, histamine-1, and muscarinic receptors likely account for observed side effects.

○ **What are the adverse effects associated with olanzapine?**

- *H_1 receptors*: sedation is the most common adverse effect (30% of patients); weight gain.
- *Muscarinic receptors*: constipation.
- *Alpha-1 receptors*: orthostatic hypotension, dizziness.
- *Dopamine receptors*: akathisia, EPS, increased prolactin level seizures (less than 1%), and elevated ALT/AST.

○ **What is the receptor binding profile of quetiapine (Seroquel®)?**

Blockade of 5-HT$_2$ and D$_3$, D2, and D$_1$ receptors. Side effects are likely due to blockade at alpha-1, alpha-2, and histamine-1 receptors.

○ **What is the half-life of quetiapine?**

About 6 hours.

○ **What are the potential adverse effects associated with quetiapine?**

Sedation, dizziness, orthostatic hypotension, weight gain, metabolic syndrome, and elevation of AST/ALT.

○ **Name two drugs that can reduce quetiapine levels.**

Thioridazine or phenytoin may significantly decrease the levels of quetiapine.

○ **What is the receptor binding profile of risperidone (Risperdal®)?**

Blockade of 5-HT$_2$ and D$_4$, D$_3$, and D$_2$ receptors. Side effects are likely due to antagonism at alpha-1 and alpha-2 adrenergic receptors and H$_1$ histamine receptors.

○ **What is the half-life of risperidone?**

The half-life of risperidone and of its active metabolite is about 24 hours.

○ **What are the more common adverse effects of risperidone?**

Sedation, extrapyramidal symptoms, nausea, weight gain, metabolic syndrome, hyperprolactinemia, agitation, and orthostatic hypotension.

○ **How is paliperidone (Invega®) related to risperidone?**

It is the major metabolite of risperidone packaged in a capsule with an "osmotically active trilayer core surrounded by a subcoat and semipermeable membrane ... with two precision laser-drilled orifices on the drug layer dome," similar to the capsule that Concerta® is packaged in. The exact degree to which it offers improvements over the efficacy and side effects of risperidone is hard to find in available prescribing information.

○ **What is the receptor binding profile of aripiprazole (Abilify®)?**

Partial agonist activity at D$_2$ and D$_3$ and 5-HT$_{2A}$ receptors. Side effects are likely due to antagonist activity at 5-HT$_{1A}$ receptors as well as due to antagonist activity at alpha-1 receptors.

○ **What is the half-life of aripiprazole?**

The half-life of aripiprazole is 75 hours, and 94 hours for its major metabolite, dehydroaripiprazole.

○ **What are the more common adverse effects of aripiprazole?**

Sedation, extrapyramidal symptoms, nausea, metabolic syndrome, insomnia, and akathisia.

○ **What is the receptor binding profile for ziprasidone (Geodon®)?**

Antagonist activity at D_4, D_3, and D_2 receptors and 5-HT_2 receptors. Side effects are likely mediated through antagonist activity at alpha-1 receptors and histamine H_1 receptors.

○ **What is the half-life of ziprasidone?**

The half-life of ziprasidone is 7 hours (it has no active metabolites).

○ **What are the more common adverse effects of ziprasidone?**

Sedation, extrapyramidal symptoms, weight gain, metabolic syndrome, cough, and prolongation of the QTc interval (9–14 msec longer than risperidone, olanzapine, quetiapine, and haloperidol).

○ **In which patients should ziprasidone be used with care, if at all?**

Patients with a history of cardiac disease or those at increased thereof, such as patients with a history of anorexia. Obtaining a baseline ECG and magnesium and potassium levels may be of benefit to identify at risk patients who do not have known cardiac disease and it is highly recommended in the elderly and those on diuretic therapy.

○ **What are the risk factors for neuroleptic-induced parkinsonism?**

Female gender, older age, use of conventional antipsychotics, and use of high potency antipsychotics.

○ **What are the risk factors for neuroleptic-induced acute dystonia?**

Male gender, young age, use of conventional antipsychotics, high potency antipsychotics, and intramuscular route of administration.

○ **What are the risk factors for neuroleptic-induced akathisia?**

Female gender and older age.

○ **What are the risk factors for neuroleptic-induced tardive dyskinesia?**

Female gender, older age, long duration of treatment with antipsychotics, history of brain damage, and mood disorders.

○ **According to the DSM-IV research criteria for neuroleptic-induced tardive dyskinesia, what is the minimum duration of exposure to neuroleptics to make the diagnosis?**

Three months (1 month if age is 60 years and above).

○ **What is the incidence of neuroleptic-induced tardive dyskinesia?**

Incidence increases by 3% to 4% a year after 4 to 5 years of treatment with neuroleptics.

○ **How should neuroleptic-induced acute akathisia be treated?**

Akathisia can be treated by reducing the antipsychotic dosage or by addition of propranolol, benzodiazepines, or clonidine. Anticholinergics, amantadine, or clonidine can also be tried.

○ **How should neuroleptic-induced tardive dyskinesia be treated?**

Reduce or stop the antipsychotic if possible. Switching to clozapine may be indicated. One could also try vitamin E, or high dose buspirone. For treatment of both the psychosis and tardive dyskinesia, use of lithium, carbamazepine, or benzodiazepines is possible.

○ **What are the risk factors for neuroleptic malignant syndrome?**

Young males; use of high potency, conventional antipsychotics; use of high doses of antipsychotics; and rapid increases in the dose.

○ **What is the mortality rate with neuroleptic malignant syndrome (NMS)?**

It is 0% to 30%, depending on the reported series. It is believed that greater awareness of the syndrome has reduced fatalities. Complications of NMS include renal failure, respiratory failure, cardiac arrest, and neuromuscular abnormalities.

○ **How should neuroleptic malignant syndrome be treated?**

Discontinue the antipsychotic, cool the patient, provide supportive therapy, and monitor carefully (including vitals, urine output). Use of bromocriptine (dopamine receptor agonist) and dantrolene (direct acting skeletal muscle relaxant) to reduce muscle spasms may be indicated.

○ **What are the indications for use of dantrolene in psychiatric syndromes?**

Dantrolene is used to treat muscle rigidity in neuroleptic malignant syndrome, catatonia, or serotonin syndrome.

○ **What is the mechanism of action of dantrolene?**

Dantrolene is a skeletal muscle relaxant that acts directly on the muscles (rather than through CNS effects).

○ **What are the potential cardiac effects of the dopamine receptor blockers (especially low potency)?**

Prolongation of the PR and QT intervals, depression of the ST segment, and blunting of the T waves, which predispose patients to cardiac arrhythmias.

○ **What are the potential ophthalmic adverse effects of neuroleptics?**

Irreversible pigmentation (similar to retinitis pigmentosa) with thioridazine, whitish-brown granular deposits in the cornea and lens with chlorpromazine, and rarely glaucoma (and other eye changes) with quetiapine.

○ **Use of which conventional neuroleptics is preferred in the first trimester of pregnancy?**

If neuroleptics are unavoidable, high potency neuroleptics should be used because of the increased risk of fetal malformations and hypotension with the low potency neuroleptics. No specific malformation has, however, been associated with the low potency neuroleptics.

○ **What are the possible drug interactions with the sympathomimetics?**

Sympathomimetics increase the concentration of phenytoin, phenobarbital, primidone, phenylbutazone, tricyclics/tetracyclics, and warfarin (mnemonic: 4 Ps plus TCAs and warfarin). Sympathomimetics also decrease the effects of antihypertensives and cannot be used within two weeks of treatment with MAOIs.

○ **What are the potential adverse effects associated with the stimulants?**

Anorexia, weight loss, growth retardation, insomnia, psychotic symptoms, and tics.

○ **What is the mechanism of action of disulfiram?**

It is a competitive aldehyde dehydrogenase inhibitor. Alcohol is metabolized as follows:

$$\text{Alcohol} \xrightarrow{\text{Alcohol dehydrogenase}} \text{Acetaldehyde} \xrightarrow{\text{Aldehyde dehydrogenase}} \text{Acetyl Coenzyme A}$$

The inhibition of aldehyde dehydrogenase leads to the accumulation of acetaldehyde when alcohol is ingested. This produces a variety of unpleasant symptoms known as the disulfiram reaction, which acts as a form of aversive conditioning.

○ **What are the adverse effects of disulfiram?**

Other than the disulfiram reaction that occurs on exposure to alcohol, disulfiram can cause hepatitis, blood dyscrasias, psychosis, dermatitis, optic neuritis, or sexual dysfunction.

○ **What laboratory tests should be monitored for a patient prescribed disulfiram?**

As can be anticipated from the list of adverse effects, CBCs and LFTs should be done periodically.

○ **What medication besides benzodiazepines is helpful in alcohol withdrawal?**

Carbamazepine can be very useful in the treatment of alcohol withdrawal. This is especially true if there is a history of seizures in the past as carbamazepine has an antikindling effect, which can help prevent the occurrence of additional seizures. However, use of carbamazepine alone will not prevent alcohol withdrawal.

○ **What is the biological basis for the use of naltrexone in alcohol dependency?**

Alcohol causes release of beta-endorphins by stimulating the opioid receptor, thereby increasing the rewarding effects of alcohol. Naltrexone blocks the opiate receptors, therefore reducing much of the alcohol reinforcement.

○ **What is levo alpha acetyl methadal (LAAM) and how is it used?**

LAAM is a synthetic mu-opioid agonist and it is used in the same context as methadone. LAAM, however, appears to be superior to methadone, as LAAM can be given at a clinic three times a week with no need for take-home doses because of its half-life of 46 hours. The two active metabolites of LAAM, NOR-LAAM and DINOR-LAAM, also have long half-lives of 62 hours and 175 hours, respectively. The LAAM dose is 1.2 to 1.3 times the daily methadone dose, and the starting dose should not exceed 40 mg.

○ **What is the pharmacological effect of methadone?**

Agonist at the mu-opioid receptor.

○ **Can naltrexone be used to treat opiate withdrawal?**

No. Naltrexone is an opiate antagonist and in fact precipitates withdrawal in patients who are opiate dependent, unless a patient has withdrawn from opiates and is free of short acting opiates (heroin) for at least 5 days or long acting opiates (methadone, LAAM, buprenorphine) for at least 7 days.

○ **What is the mechanism of action for buprenorphine?**

Buprenorphine is a partial opioid agonist.

○ **What is the distinction between short-term detoxification, long-term detoxification, and methadone maintenance?**

Detoxification for up to 30 days, up to 180 days (6 months), and more than 180 days, respectively.

○ **What is the half-life of donepezil (Aricept®?**

About 70 hours in the elderly patients.

○ **Which P-450 isoenzymes metabolize donepezil?**

2D6, 3A3/4.

○ **What is the advantage of donepezil over tacrine (Cognex®)?**

Donepezil is specific for cholinesterase inhibition in the CNS while tacrine is not. Donepezil therefore has less peripheral adverse effects. Also, donepezil is not associated with hepatotoxicity while tacrine is.

○ **What are the potential adverse effects associated with donepezil?**

Nausea, bradyarrhythmias, and syncope.

○ **What are the adverse effects associated with tacrine?**

Elevated liver enzymes (potentially serious), anorexia, nausea, rash, myalgia, loss of weight, and increased sweating.

○ **Is memantine (Namenda®) also a cholinesterase inhibitor like donepezil?**

No. Memantine is an antagonist of glutamatergic NMDA receptors. It is also a 5-HT$_3$ receptor antagonist and a nicotinic acetylcholine receptor antagonist. It appears to have some benefit in slowing the rate of deterioration in moderate to severe Alzheimer's disease, but is not curative.

CHAPTER 36 Psychotherapy

○ **What is psychoanalysis?**

Psychoanalysis is a system of psychotherapy, originally developed by Freud, which through the analysis of the patient's dreams, associations, transference, and behaviors leads to a better understanding of unconscious drives and the defenses used to modify the drives.

○ **What are the three components of psychic functioning defined in Freud's structural theory?**

The id, ego, and superego.

○ **What is a parapraxis?**

A parapraxis is a lapse of memory or "a slip of the tongue." Usually these "Freudian slips" have significant unconscious meaning and are evidence of the unconscious in Freud's structural theory.

○ **Define transference.**

Transference refers to the feelings and behaviors of the patient toward his/her therapist that are based on previous experiences with significant people in their lives, particularly parental figures.

○ **What therapeutic techniques are used in psychoanalysis?**

Free association, neutrality, defense analysis, and interpretation of transference.

○ **Why is establishment of an empathic therapeutic relationship essential prior to interpretation of transference?**

Interpretation of transference events is often met with disbelief by the patients, as they are often unaware that the way in which they interact with people can be based on their previous interpersonal interactions. While interpreting such interactions, the clinician must maintain the empathic rapport and continue to validate the individual, so as to not cause the patient to experience excessive anxiety.

○ **What is the definition of "neurosis"?**

Neurosis is a psychiatric disorder, the etiology of which is presumed to be unconscious conflicts between opposing wishes or between wishes and prohibitions. As a result, one feels foreign to the self (ego dystonic), anxiety becomes a major symptom, but reality testing remains intact. The disturbance is relatively enduring or recurrent without treatment and is not limited to stressful situations.

○ **What is a defense mechanism?**

A defense mechanism is an unconscious, intrapsychic process that regulates basic biological drives, maintains psychological homeostasis, and provides relief from emotional conflict and anxiety.

○ **List four mature defense mechanisms defined by Vaillant.**

Humor, sublimation, altruism, and suppression.

○ **What is the definition of resistance?**

Resistance is a phenomenon that occurs when a patient, consciously or unconsciously, avoids speaking about various thoughts during therapy.

○ **What is the difference between defense mechanisms and resistance?**

Defense mechanisms are internal processes, while resistance is an interpersonal process.

○ **How does "primary process" differ from "secondary process."**

Primary process is found in unconscious functioning and is characterized by a disregard for order, time, or other barriers of the real world. Immediate gratification is sought. Secondary process is a preconscious, logical, sequential thought process with good judgment. It takes into account the frustrations and limits that exist in reality.

○ **What process occurs when a repressed memory and its associated affect is brought into consciousness?**
Abreaction.

○ **What disorders are characterized by intrapsychic conflicts that are given external expression such as blindness or paralysis?**
Conversion disorders.

○ **Differentiate the "pleasure principle" from the "reality principle".**

In psychoanalytic theory, the pleasure principle is the concept that people seek to avoid pain and discomfort and strive for gratification and pleasure. It precedes the reality principle and comes into conflict with the reality principle as development proceeds. The reality principle reflects compromises made to postpone gratification and is normally brought about by the demands of the outside world.

○ **What is the "ego ideal"?**

The "ego ideal" is the part of the superego that aspires to be and do, rather than the part that restricts or prohibits.

○ **What behavior is characterized by a partial return to earlier patterns of behavior or thinking?**

Regression is a process that normally occurs during sleep, play, and physical illness. The ability to regress in the service of the ego is a sign of healthy psychosexual development. Many psychiatric illnesses, however, are characterized by inappropriate regression.

○ **Which psychoanalytic term refers to the impulse to reenact earlier emotional experiences?**
Repetition compulsion.

○ **What are the autonomous ego functions as described by Heinz Hartmann?**

The autonomous ego functions defined by Heinz Hartmann include perception, intuition, comprehension, learning, thinking, motor skills, language, and intelligence. They basically represent brain functions that develop in the absence of significant conflict.

○ **Which Swiss psychiatrist coined the term "collective unconscious"?**

Carl Jung. The term refers to symbols and other mental content outside of our awareness that are perceived cross-culturally. An example of this is the "hero" concept.

○ **What are the first two stages of psychosexual development outlined by Sigmund Freud?**

The first two stages of psychosexual development proposed by Freud are the oral and anal phases, followed by the phallic, oedipal, latency, and genital phases of development.

○ **What is the Oedipus complex?**

The Oedipus complex is an intrapsychic and interpersonal event whereby the 3- to 5-year-old male child develops rivalry with the parent of the same sex and attraction to the parent of the opposite sex. The parallel process in the female child is called the Electra complex.

○ **What are the three stages of development proposed by Margaret Mahler?**

The three stages of Margaret Mahler's developmental theory are the autistic phase (0–4 weeks), the symbiotic phase (4 weeks to 5 months), and the separation-individuation phase (5 months to 3 years).

○ **Describe the four subphases of Margaret Mahler's developmental stage of separation/individuation.**

The four subphases of Mahler's separation-individuation stage include differentiation, practicing, rapprochement, and consolidation/object constancy. Differentiation occurs between 5 and 10 months of age and is characterized by the occurrence of stranger anxiety, which most often begins in the eighth month. Practicing occurs between 10 and 16 months and is significant for separation anxiety and locomotion. During the rapprochement phase, between 16 and 24 months, the child experiences the rapprochement crisis, where he/she simultaneously desires the mother's help, yet is struggling to achieve independence. Temper tantrums are common during the phase. During the last stage of Mahler's theory of development, consolidation/object constancy, which occurs between 24 and 36 months of age, the child internalizes the construct of the mother thereby achieving object constancy.

○ **Define "object constancy."**

Object constancy is the ability to have a consistent internal mental representation of another person despite one's emotional state. It becomes possible after the age of three. The term is attributed to Margaret Mahler.

○ **Define "object permanence."**

Object permanence is the concept developed by Piaget whereby a child learns that an object (or person) continues to exist even if it cannot be detected by the senses. Object permanence occurs by the age of 2 years.

○ **What is another term for Piaget's concept of "phenomenalistic causality"?**

Magical thinking. This normally occurs between 2 and 7 years of age, when thinking is less logical and the events are linked by their close temporal proximity. For instance, children often believe that a bad thought can cause someone to get ill.

○ **List some general characteristics of brief psychotherapy.**

Brief psychotherapy has a defined endpoint, such as number of sessions (usually less than twenty) or specified objectives. It is usually goal-oriented, active for both the patient and therapist, and directed toward a particular symptom or problem.

○ **What is the definition of insight?**

Insight is the conscious understanding by an individual as to why he/she has a particular thought, feeling, or behavior.

○ **Describe the difference between expressive, insight-oriented psychotherapy, and supportive psychotherapy.**

Expressive psychotherapy is a treatment method whose goal is to effect behavioral change through increased awareness of one's internal conflicts and defense mechanisms. In supportive psychotherapy, the goal is to strengthen healthy defense mechanisms and support persons through difficult phases of life (i.e., maintain functioning).

○ **Define the therapy intervention of "reflection."**

Reflection refers to the therapeutic technique whereby the physician repeats to the patient something that the patient has already said, assuring the patient that he/she has been heard.

○ **Dialectical behavior therapy is a combination of what therapeutic strategies and philosophies?**

Dialectical behavior therapy, developed by Marsha Linehan, combines the aspects of cognitive and behavioral therapy with Zen Buddhism to treat a variety of disorders, including borderline personality disorder, eating disorders, and substance abuse.

○ **How are sessions structured in a typical DBT course?**

DBT usually consists of two sets of sessions a week, one individual session dedicated to identifying maladaptive behaviors and increasing motivation for change, while the group session is didactic, teaching the patient a number of new interpersonal and affect regulation strategies. In addition, the individual therapists and group leader also meet weekly to review progress, resistance, and adverse events.

○ **What type of skills are taught in the DBT group sessions?**

DBT group sessions teach patients a variety of skills whereby they become more aware of their feelings and behaviors (mindfulness), are able to tolerate a variety of stressors (distress tolerance), can learn how to respond to situations in an appropriate manner (emotion regulation), and interact with others in a more effective manner (interpersonal effectiveness).

○ **Define "alexithymia."**

Alexithymia is the inability to verbalize or become aware of one's mood or feelings. It is a poor prognostic indicator for many psychotherapies.

○ **What is one of the most significant predictors of outcome in any type of psychotherapy?**

Therapeutic alliance (physician–patient relationship).

○ **What psychological tests are designed to describe the way the mind functions using a psychodynamic model?**

Projective tests, such as the thematic apperception test (TAT) or the Rorschach test are relatively unstructured tests designed to evaluate personality traits, defense mechanisms, and feelings toward other people.

○ **Which mental disorder is characterized by a heightened sense of self-importance or entitlement, lack of empathy, grandiose feelings of uniqueness, and taking advantage of others?**

Narcissistic personality disorder.

○ **Projection is a defense mechanism most often associated with which personality disorder?**

Paranoid personality disorder.

○ **How does an obsession differ from a compulsion?**

An obsession is a persistent, unwanted, and intrusive idea or impulse that is not seen as part of the person's character and cannot be eliminated by logic or reasoning. It is recognized as a product of the patient's mind. A compulsion is an excessive, driven urge to perform a behavior repetitively, usually in an attempt to neutralize anxiety.

○ **In the cognitive therapy model, what is the definition of the "cognitive triad"?**

As proposed by Aaron Beck, the cognitive triad that exists in depression consists of negative cognitions of oneself, the world, and one's future.

○ **What are the goals of cognitive therapy?**

The goals of cognitive therapy are to identify negative cognitions, test the validity of those cognitions, develop alternative behaviors, and revise cognitive assumptions.

○ **Define the cognitive therapy term "schema."**

Schema is a repetitive, cognitive pattern through which a person interprets his or her environment and self. For example, through a schema, an anxious person may interpret excessive sweating as an impending heart attack.

○ **Cognitive therapy has demonstrated efficacy in which types of psychiatric disorders?**

Depression, panic disorder, obsessive-compulsive disorder, personality disorders, phobias (including social phobia), and eating disorders.

○ **What is the definition of interpersonal psychotherapy (IPT)?**

Interpersonal psychotherapy is a type of short-term therapy designed to treat depression. It approaches the patient's depressed mood as a problem of grief, role transition, relationship disputes, or relationship deficit.

○ **Who developed the concept of operant conditioning?**

B.F. Skinner.

○ **Describe the difference between classical and operant conditioning.**

In classical conditioning, a neutral stimulus (bell tone) is repeatedly paired with an unconditioned stimulus (food powder) that elicits an unconditioned, autonomic, instinctual response (salivation). Over time, the neutral, conditioned stimulus (bell tone) alone will elicit a conditioned response (salivation). In other words, a neutral stimulus that had no capacity to elicit a particular response before training, will do so after repeated association of the neutral stimulus with the unconditioned stimulus. The subject is passive in this process and does not actively participate in the learning process. In contrast, in operant conditioning, the subject actively operates on the environment (the pigeon presses a lever) to receive a reward (food pellet). The association between the action and reward is discovered randomly.

○ **A fear of spiders extending itself to a fear of other insects is an example of what behavioral phenomenon?**

Stimulus generalization.

○ **Define positive and negative reinforcement.**

In positive reinforcement, an event is introduced after a subject displays a desired behavior, which increases (or strengthens) the probability of that behavior recurring (like a paycheck encouraging us to return to work). In negative reinforcement, the likelihood of a desired behavior occurring is increased by removing or avoiding an aversive stimulus (an example of which is taking out the garbage to avoid being yelled at again).

○ **What is another term for the weakening of a reinforced operant response as a result of ceasing reinforcement?**

Extinction.

○ **What term describes the process whereby addition of an adversive stimulus decreases the likelihood of a specific behavior recurring?**

Punishment.

○ **Describe the use of "token economy" in the management of social settings like psychiatric wards.**

The "token economy" works by rewarding patients with tokens when specific behaviors are demonstrated. These tokens can then be exchanged for goods or privileges. (This is not too different from how money works in our society.)

○ **What term describes an animal behavior in which an animal will follow the first moving object that it sees shortly after birth?**

Imprinting, which was described by Konrad Lorenz.

○ **For which psychiatric disorder the model of learned helplessness is used as a paradigm?**

Depression.

○ **Describe the treatment of systematic desensitization.**

Originally described by Joseph Wolpe, systemic desensitization requires the patient to be exposed to increasingly more anxiety provoking cues (stimuli) from the least frightening to most. This occurs while the patient attempts relaxation techniques thereby becoming desensitized to each stimulus in the hierarchy.

○ **How does fear differ from anxiety?**

Fear is typically an alerting signal in response to a known threat that is external and not conflict based. Anxiety, in contrast, usually results from a lesser known, internal source and is usually conflictual in origin. Physiologically and emotionally, however, the two states are indistinguishable, both manifesting as times of hyperarousal with somatic symptoms of tachycardia, tachypnea, and sweating.

○ **Describe the technique "flooding."**

Flooding, or implosion, is a behavior modification technique whereby a patient is exposed to the most anxiety provoking stimulus, either in imagination or reality, until it no longer produces anxiety.

○ **What is the definition of counterphobic behavior?**

Counterphobic behavior is any behavior that seeks out experiences that are consciously or unconsciously feared in an attempt to master those fears. An example would be parachute jumping for a person with a fear of heights.

○ **Incorporating "applied tension" is necessary when doing exposure therapy with what particular group of phobias?**

Blood/illness/injury phobias. This group of phobias is unique in that a paradoxical drop in blood pressure occurs during exposure to a particular stimulus, leading to fainting. Applied tension involves contraction of large muscle groups to maintain a normal blood pressure during exposure.

○ **The "eye-roll sign" is a test for which procedure?**

Hypnosis.

○ **In what type of therapy is an undesired behavior paired with a painful or unpleasant stimulus (punishment) in order to extinguish the undesired behavior?**

Aversion therapy, an example of which is the use of Antabuse in the treatment of alcoholism.

○ **What type of therapy is useful in the treatment of patients with alcohol dependence, gambling disorder, or narcotic abuse?**

Group therapy, usually in the form of self-help groups such as Alcoholics Anonymous.

○ **What factors can facilitate a therapeutic change in group psychotherapy?**

Transferences to group members, recognizing that the patient is not alone, a sense of belonging, and group cohesion.

○ **In what type of therapy is a device used to monitor muscle tension in an attempt to decrease the frequency of migraine headaches?**

Biofeedback.

○ **What type of supportive therapy teaches patients a more direct expression of their feelings and is useful in the treatment of social phobia or avoidant personality disorder?**

Assertiveness training.

○   **What is an anniversary reaction?**

An anniversary reaction is an emotional response to a previous event occurring at the same time of the year. Usually the event involves a loss and the reaction is depressive in nature.

○   **What symptoms differentiate depression from grief?**

While both depression and grief may follow a loss, depression is accompanied by a greater sense of guilt and worthlessness, psychotic symptoms, marked functional impairment, psychomotor retardation, and suicidal thoughts and/or actions.

BIBLIOGRAPHY

Abrams R. *Electroconvulsive Therapy.* 3rd ed. New York, NY: Oxford University Press; 2002.

Alexopoulos GS, Chester JG. Outcomes of geriatric depression. *Clin Geriatr Med.* 1992;8:363.

Altshuler LL, Cohen L, Szuba MP, Burt VK, Gitlin M, Mintz J. Pharmacologic management of psychiatric illness during pregnancy: dilemmas and guidelines. *Am J Psychiatry.* 1996;153(5):592.

American Psychiatric Association. Practice guideline for the treatment of patients with substance use disorders: alcohol, cocaine, opioids. *Am J Psychiatry.* 1995;152(11)(Nov suppl).

American Psychiatric Association. *Diagnostic and Statistical Manual of Mental Disorders.* 4th ed, Text Revision. DSM-IV-TR. Washington, DC: American Psychiatric Association; 2000.

American Psychiatric Association. Practice guideline for the treatment of patients with bipolar disorder (revision). *Am J Psychiatry.* 2002;159(4)(Apr suppl).

American Psychiatric Association. Psychiatric evaluation of adults, 2nd ed. *Am J. Psychiatry.* 2006;163(6)(June suppl).

American Psychiatric Association. Treatment of patients with eating disorders, 3rd ed. *Am J Psychiatry.* 2006;163(7)(July suppl).

American Psychiatric Association. Treatment of patients with Alzheimer's disease and other dementias, 2nd ed. *Am J Psychiatry.* 2007;164(12)(Dec suppl).

American Psychiatric Association. Treatment of patients with obsessive-compulsive disorder. *Am J Psychiatry.* 2007;164(suppl).

Andreasen NC, Black DW. *Introductory Textbook of Psychiatry.* 3rd ed. Washington, DC: American Psychiatric Press; 2001.

Bellman M. Studies on encopresis. *Acta Paediatr Scand Suppl.* 1966:170.

Bighami A, Dahl D. *Glia Cells in the Central Nervous System and Their Reaction to Injury.* Austin, TX: RG Landes Co; 1994.

Black JE, Brooks SN. Narcolepsy and syndrome of central nervous system-mediated sleepiness. In: Oldham JM, Riba MB, series ed. *Review of Psychiatry Series: Sleep Disorders and Psychiatry.* Vol 24. Washington, DC: American Psychiatric Publishing; 2005:107.

Bruck H. *Eating Disorders: Obesity and Anorexia Nervosa.* New York: Basic Books; 1973.

Busse EW, Blazer DG, eds. *Textbook of Geriatric Psychiatry.* 2nd ed. Washington, DC: American Psychiatric Press; 1996.

Buysse DJ, Germain A, Moul D, et al. Insomnia. *FocusJ Lifelong Learn Psychiatry.* 2005;3(4):568.

Calne RB. *Neurodegenerative Diseases.* Philadelphia, PA: WB Saunders; 1994.

Carr PL, Freund KM, Somani S, eds. *The Medical Care of Women.* Philadelphia, PA: WB Saunders; 1995.

Casey JE, Rourke BP, Picard EM. Syndrome of nonverbal learning disabilities: age differences in neuropsychological, academic, and socioemotional functioning. *Dev Psychopathol.* 1991;3:329.

Chess S, Thomas A. *Temperament in Clinical Practice.* New York: Brunner/Mazel; 1986.

Ciraulo DA, Creelman WL, Shader RI, O'Sullivan RL. Antidepressants. In: Ciraulo DA, Shader RI, Greenblat DJ, Creelman W, eds. *Drug Interactions in Psychiatry.* 2nd ed. Baltimore, MD: Williams & Wilkins; 1995.

Cjou JCY. Targeting novel therapies in schizophrenia: consideration for physicians and patients. Paper presented at: 20th Annual US Psychiatric and Mental Health Congress; October 10, 2007; Orlando, FL.

Cohen M. Enuresis. *Pediatr Clin North Am.* 1975;22:545.

Consensus Development Conference on Antipsychotic Drugs and Obesity and Diabetes. *Diabetes Care.* 2004;27:596.

Copeland JR, Abou-Saleh MT, Blazer DG. *Principles and Practice of Geriatric Psychiatry.* West Sussex, UK: Wiley; 1994.

de Boer T. The pharmacological profile of mirtazapine. *J Clin Psychiatry.* 1996;57(4):19.

Dixon L, Weiden P, Delahanty J, et al. Prevalence and correlates of diabetes in national schizophrenia samples. *Schizophr Bull.* 2000;26:903.

Dulcan MK, Martini DR, Lake M. *Concise Guide to Child and Adolescent Psychiatry.* 3rd ed. Washington, DC: American Psychiatric Press; 2003.

Dulcan MK, Popper CW. *Concise Guide to Child and Adolescent Psychiatry.* 1st ed. Washington, DC: American Psychiatric Press; 1991.

Duman RS. Depression: a case of neuronal life and death? *Biol Psychiatry.* 2004;56:140.

Durkheim E. *Suicide.* Glencove, IL: Free Press; 1951.

Fernandez F. Ten myths about HIV infection and AIDS. *Focus J Lifelong Learn Psychiatry.* 2005;3(2):184.

Folks D, Fuller W. Anxiety disorders and insomnia in geriatric patients. *Psychiatr Clin North Am.* 1997;20:137.

Ford ES, Giles WH, Dietz WH. Prevalence of the metabolic syndrome among US adults: findings from the third National Health and Nutrition Examination Survey. *JAMA.* 2002;287:356.

Fuster JM. *The Prefrontal Cortex: Anatomy, Physiology, and Neuropsychology of the Frontal Lobe.* 3rd ed. Philadelphia, PA: Lippincott-Raven; 1997.

Fuster JM. *Cortex and Mind: Unifying Cognition.* New York, NY: Oxford University Press; 2002.

Gabbard GO. *Psychodynamic Psychiatry in Clinical Practice.* 3rd ed. Washington, DC: American Psychiatric Press; 2000.

Gabbard GO. Psychodynamic approaches to personality disorders. *Focus J Lifelong Learn Psychiatry.* 2005;3(3):363.

Gesell A. *Mental Growth in the Preschool Child.* New York: Macmillan; 1925.

Green WH. *Child and Adolescent Clinical Psychopharmacology.* 2nd ed. Baltimore, MD: Williams & Wilkins; 1995.

Goodwin FK, Ebert MH, Bunney WE. Mental effects of reserpine in man: a review. In: Shader RI, ed. *Psychiatric Complications of Medical Drugs.* New York, NY: Raven; 1972:75-101.

Hales R, Yudofsky S. *The American Psychiatric Publishing Testbook of Clinical Psychiatry.* Washington, DC: American Psychiatric Association; 2002.

Hansen L, Salmon D, Galasko D, et al. The Lewy body variant of Alzheimer's disease: a clinical and pathologic entity. *J Neurol.* 1990;40(1):1.

Hebert LE, Scherr PA, Bienias JL, Evans DA. Alzheimer disease in the US population: prevalence estimates using the 200 census. *Arch Neurol.* 2003;60(8):1119.

Hietala J, Koivisto H, Anttila P, et al. Comparison of the combined marker GGT-CDT and the conventional laboratory markers of alcohol abuse in heavy drinkers, moderate drinkers and abstainers. *Alcohol Alcohol Suppl.* 2006;41(5):528.

IsHak WW, Mikhail A, Amiri SR, et al. Sexual dysfunction. *Focus J Lifelong Learn.* 2005;3(4):520.

Jacobsen LK, Rapaport JL. Research update: childhood-onset schizophrenia: implications of clinical and neurobiological research. *J Clin Psycho Psychiatry.* 1998;39:101.

Jacoby R, Oppenheimer C, eds. *Psychiatry in the Elderly.* New York, NY: Oxford University Press; 1997.

Jenike MA. Psychiatric illnesses in the elderly: a review. *J Geriatr Psychiatry Neurol.* 1996;9:65.

Jensvold MF, Halbreich U, Hamilton J, eds. *Psychopharmacology and Women: Sex, Gender and Hormones.* Washington, DC: American Psychiatric Press; 1996.

Jeste DV, Caligiuri MP. Tardive dyskinesia. *Schizophr Bull.* 1993;19(2):305.

Kanner L. Autistic disturbances of affective contact. *Nerv Child.* 1943;2:217.

Kaplan HI, Saddock BJ. *Synopsis of Psychiatry.* 6th ed. Baltimore, MD: William & Wilkins; 1991.

Kaplan HI, Saddock BJ. *Kapland and Sadok's Pocket Handbook of Psychiatric Drug Treatment.* 3rd ed. Baltimore, MD: Williams & Wilkins; 2001.

Kaplan HI, Saddock BJ. *Kaplan and Sadok's Synopsis of Psychiatry.* 9th ed. Baltimore, MD: William & Wilkins; 2002.

Kaplan HI, Saddock BJ. *Kaplan and Sakok's Comprehensive Textbook of Psychiatry.* 8th ed. Baltimore, MD: Lippincott Williams & Wilkins; 2004.

Kaufman DM. *Clinical Neurology for Psychiatrists.* 5th ed. Philadelphia, PA: WB Saunders; 2001.

Kessler RC, Berglaund P, Demler O, et al. The epidemiology of major depressive disorder: results from the National Comorbidity Survey Replication (NCS-R). *JAMA.* 2003;289:3095.

Lewis M, ed. *Child and Adolescent Psychiatry: A Comprehensive Textbook.* 3rd ed. Baltimore, MD: Williams & Wilkins; 2002.

Liebson E, White RF, Albert ML. Cognitive inconsistencies in abnormal illness behavior and neurological disease. *J Nerv Ment Dis.* 1996;184(2):122.

Marsh L. Psychosis in Parkinson's disease. *Prim Psychiatry.* 2005;12(7):56.

Maxmen JS, Ward NG. *Essential Psychopathology and Its Treatment.* 2nd ed. New York, NY: WW Norton; 1995.

McDonald WM, Nemeroff CB. The diagnosis and treatment of mania in the elderly. *Bull Menninger Clin.* 1996;60:174.

McIntyre RS, Konarski JZ. Obesity and psychiatric disorders: frequently encountered clinical questions. *Focus J Lifelong Learn.* 2005;3(4):511.

Mokdad AH, Bowman BA, Ford ES, et al. Increased prevalence of obesity and diabetes in the United States. *JAMA.* 2001;286:1195.

Morgan MY, Colman JC, Sherlock S. The use of a combination of peripheral markers for diagnosing alcoholism and monitoring for continued abuse. *Alcohol Alcohol Suppl.* 1981;16:167.

Murray CJL, Lopez AD. Global mortality, disability, and the contribution of risk factors: Global Burden of Disease Study. *Lancet.* 1997;349:1436.

Murray CJL, Lopez AD. Alternative projections of mortality and disability by cause 1990-2020: Global Burden of Disease Study. *Lancet.* 1997;349:1498.

Neinstein LS. *Adolescent Health Care: A Practical Guide.* 2nd ed. Baltimore, MD: Urban & Schwarzenberg; 1991.

Nemeroff CB, DeVane CL, Pollock BG. Newer antidepressants and the cytochrome P450 system. *Am J Psychiatry.* 1996;153(3):311.

Nierenberg AA, Eidelman P, Wu Y, et al. Depression: an update for the clinician. *Focus J Lifelong Learn Psychiatry.* 2005;3(1):3.

Oldham JM. Personality disorders. *Focus J Lifelong Learn Psychiatry.* 2005;3(3):372.

Pennington BF. *Diagnosing Learning Disorders: A Neuropsychological Framework.* New York, NY: Guilford Press; 1991.

Pollock BG. Recent developments in drug metabolism of relevance to psychiatrists. *Harv Rev Psychiatry.* 1994;2:204.

Porsolt RD, Bertin A, Jalfre M. Behavioral despair in mice: a primary screening test for antidepressants. *Ach Int Parmacodyn Ther.* 1977;229(2):327.

Richelson E. Pharmacokinetic drug interactions of new antidepressants: a review of the effects on the metabolism of other drugs. *Mayo Clin Proc.* 1997;72:835.

Rifai MA, Rosenstein DL. Hepatitis C and psychiatry. *Focus J Lifelong Learn Psychiatry.* 2005;3(2):194.

Rizvi SL, Linehan MM. Dialectical behavior therapy for personality disorders. *Focus J Lifelong Learn Psychiatry.* 2005;3(3):489.

Rosenberg DA. Web of deceit: a literature review of Munchausen syndrome by proxy. *Child Abuse Negl.* 1987;11:547.

Rosenstein DL, Nelson JC, Jacobs SC. Seizures associated with antidepressants: a review. *J Clin Psychiatry.* 1993;54(8):289.

Rourke BP, Fuerst DR. *Learning Disabilities and Pyschosocial Functioning: A Neuropsychological Perspective.* New York, NY: Guilford Press; 1991.

Roy-Byrne PP, Hommer D. Benzodiazepine withdrawal: overview and implications for the treatment of anxiety. *Am J Med.* 1988;84(6):1041.

Russ E, Shedler J, Bradley R, Westen D. Redefining the construct of narcissistic personality disorder: diagnostic criteria and subtypes. *Am J Psychiatry.* 2008;165;1473.

Russell AT. Childhood-onset schizophrenia. In: Gabbard GO, ed. *Treatments of Psychiatric Disorders.* Vol 1. 2nd ed. Washington, DC: American Psychiatric Press; 1995.

Rutter M, Taylor E, Herson L, eds. *Child and Adolescent Psychiatry: Modern Approaches.* 2nd ed. Oxford, UK: Blackwell Scientific Publications; 1994.

Rutter M, Tizard J, Whitmore K (eds). *Education, Health, and Behavior.* London: Longmans; 1970.

Rutter ML, Yale W, Graham PJ. Enuresis and behavioral deviance: some epidemiological considerations, In: Kolvin I, MacKeith R, Meadow SR (eds). *Bladder Control and Enuresis.* London: Spastics International Medical Publications, in association with Heineman; 1973;137. (*Clinics in Developmental Medicine, Nos. 48,49*)

Sadavoy J, Lazarus LW, Jarvik LF, Grossberg GT, eds. *Comprehensive Review of Geriatric Psychiatry-II.* 2nd ed. Washington, DC: American Psychiatric Press; 1996.

Salloway S, Malloy P, Cummings J. *Neuropsychiatry of the Limbic and Subcortical Disorders.* Washington, DC: American Psychiatric Press; 1997.

Scates AC, Doraiswamy PM. Focus on citalopram. *Formulary.* 1998;33:725.

Schatzberg AF. Recent studies of the biology and treatment of depression. *Focus J Lifelong Learn Psychiatry.* 2005;3(1):14.

Schatzberg AF, Nemeroff CB, eds. *The American Psychiatric Press Textbook of Psychopharmacology.* 3rd ed. Washington, DC: American Psychiatric Press, 2003.

Schulman JK, Muskin PR, Shapiro PA. Psychiatry and cardiovascular disease. *Focus J Lifelong Learn Psychiatry.* 2005;3(2);208.

Schulz SC, Findling RL, Wise A, Friedman L, Kenny J. Child and adolescent schizophrenia. *Psychiatr Clin North Am.* 1998;21:43.

Semenchuk MR, Labiner DM. Gabapentin and lamotrigine: prescribing guidelines for psychiatry. *J Pract Psychiatry Behav Health.* 1998;334.

Semrud-Clikeman M, Hynd GW. Right hemispheric dysfunction in nonverbal learning disabilities: social, academic, and adaptive functioning in adults and children. *Psychol Bull.* 1990;107(2):196.

Shapiro PA, Lesperance F, Frasure-Smith N, et al. An open-label preliminary trial of sertraline for treatment of major depression after acute myocardial infarction (the SADHAT Trial). Sertraline Anti-depressant Heart Attack Trial. *Am Heart J.* 1999;137: 1100.

Shelton CI. Long-term management of major depressive disorder: are differences among antidepressant treatments meaningful? *J Clin Psychiatry.* 2004;65(17):29-33.

Shirayama Y, Chen ACH, Nakagawa S, Russell DS, Duman RS. Brain-derived neurotrophic factor produces antidepressant effects in behavioral models of depression. *J Neurosci.* 2002;22:3251.

Sigman GS. Eating disorders in children and adolescents. *Pediat Clin N Am.* 2003;50(5):11139.

Slavney PR, Teitelnaum ML. Patients with medically unexplained symptoms: DSM-III diagnoses and demographic characteristics. *Gen Hosp Psychiatry.* 1985;7(1):21.

Smith FA, Querques J, Levenson JL, Stern TA. Psychiatric assessment and consultation. In: Levenson JL, ed. *The American Psychiatric Publishing Textbook of Psychosomatic Medicine.* Washington, DC: American Psychiatric Publishing; 2005:3-14.

Spiegel D, Dhadwal N, Gill F. 'I'm sober, doctor, really': best biomarkers for underreported alcohol use. *Curr Psychiatry.* 2008;7(9):15.

Stahl SM. *Essential Psychopharmacology: The Prescriber's Guide.* Cambridge, UK: Cambridge University Press; 2004.

Striegel-Moore RH, Cachelin FM, Dohm FA, Pike KM, Wiffley DE, Fairburn CG. Comparison of binge eating disorder and bulimia nervosa in a community sample. *Int J Eat Disord.* 2001;29:15.

Tasman A, Kay J, Lieberman JA. *Psychiatry.* 2nd ed. Philadelphia, PA: WB Saunders; 2003.

Toth EL, Baggaley A. Coexistence of Munchausen's syndrome and multiple personality disorder: detailed report of a case and theoretical discussion. *Psychiatry.* 1991;54(2):176.

Victor M, Ropper AH. *Principles of Neurology.* 7th ed. New York, NY: McGraw-Hill; 2001.

Vieweg WV, Adler RA, Fernandez A. Weight control and antipsychotics:how to tip the scales away from diabetes and heart disease. *Curr Psychiatry.* 2002;1(8):10.

Volavka J. *Neurobiology of Violence.* 2nd ed. Washington, DC: American Psychiatric Press; 2002.

Volkmar FR. Childhood and adolescent psychosis: a review of the past 10 years. *J Am Acad Child Adolesc Psychiatry.* 1996;35:843.

Wise MD, Rundell JR, eds. *The American Psychiatric Press Textbook of Consultation-Liaison Psychiatry: Psychiatry in the Medically Ill.* 2nd ed. Washington, DC: American Psychiatric Press; 2002.

Wong Bernice, ed. *Learning About Learning Disabilities.* 3rd ed. San Diego, CA: Academic Press; 2004.

Xu H, Richardson JS, Li X. Dose –related effects of chronic antidepressants on neuroprotective proteins BDNF, Bcl-2 and Cu/Zn-SOD in rat hippocampus. *Neuropsychopharmacology.* 2003;28:53.

Yager J, Devlin M, Halmi K, et al. Eating disorders. *Focus J Lifelong Learn.* 2005;3(4):503.

Yonkers KA, Winner KL, Stowe Z, et al. Management of bipolar disorder during pregnancy and the postpartum period. *Am J Psychiatry.* 2004;161:608.

Zhang X, Gainetdinov RR, Beaulieu JM, et al. Loss-of-function mutation in tryptophan hydroxylase-2 identified in unipolar depression. *Neuron.* 2005;45(1):11–16.

Zucker KL, Bradley SJ. Gender Identity and psychosexual disorders. In: Weiner JM, Dulcan MK, eds. *The American Psychiatric Publishing Textbook of Child and adolescent Psychiatry.* 3rd ed. Washington, DC: American Psychiatric Publishing; 2004:813.